LYME BORRELIOSIS IN EUROPE AND NORTH AMERICA

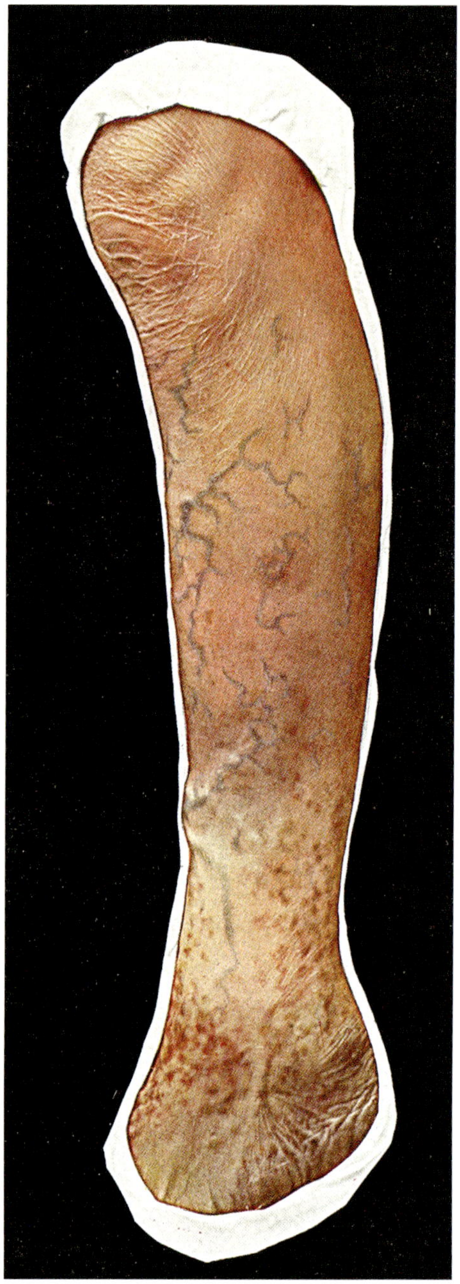

Atrophia cutis idiopathica. *Source: Atlas der hautkrankheiten Volume II*, Prof. Dr. E. Jacobi, 6th edition, 1918, original publishers: Urban and Schwarzenberg (now Elsevier). Courtesy of Prof. Robert R. Müllegger.

LYME BORRELIOSIS IN EUROPE AND NORTH AMERICA

Epidemiology and Clinical Practice

EDITED BY
Sunil K. Sood

WILEY-BLACKWELL
A JOHN WILEY & SONS, INC., PUBLICATION

Published by John Wiley & Sons, Inc., Hoboken, New Jersey

Published simultaneously in Canada

Wiley-Blackwell is an imprint of John Wiley & Sons, formed by the merger of Wiley's global Scientific, Technical, and Medical business with Blackwell Publishing.

Library of Congress Cataloging-in-Publication Data:

Lyme borreliosis in Europe and North America : epidemiology and clinical practice / [edited by] Sunil Kumar Sood.
p. ; cm
Includes bibliographical references and index.
ISBN 978-0-470-64752-3 (cloth)
1. Lyme disease–Europe. 2. Lyme disease–North America. I. Sood, Sunil Kumar
[DNLM: 1. Lyme Disease–diagnosis–Europe. 2. Lyme Disease–diagnosis–North America.
3. Lyme Disease–epidemiology–Europe. 4. Lyme Disease–epidemiology–North America.
5. Lyme Disease–therapy–Europe. 6. Lyme Disease–therapy–North America. WC 406]
RA644. L94L96 2011
362.196′9246—dc22

2010028569

Printed in Singapore

oBook ISBN: 978-0-470-93396-1
ePDF ISBN: 978-0-470-93395-4

10 9 8 7 6 5 4 3 2 1

CONTENTS

PREFACE

Today Lyme borreliosis is diagnosed and treated in the early stages of the illness in the vast majority of patients, yet this has not diminished its public health importance. It continues to be an emerging infectious disease, with the expanding range of tick vectors a key factor in its increased incidence. Although probably a disease of antiquity, many of the features of Lyme borreliosis were discovered in Europe beginning 128 years ago, and the discovery of Lyme arthritis in the mid-1970s set off an accelerated phase of investigation that resulted in confirmation of the infectious etiology. Extensive clinical and laboratory research has yielded significant advances in understanding the pathogenesis, diagnosis, and treatment of *Borrelia burgdorferi* infection, and in elucidation of the pathogen–host–vector interactions. Moreover our understanding of other tick-borne diseases has been enhanced by the application of research tools developed to study Lyme borreliosis.

This book is designed to be a clinically oriented guide that presents the state-of-the-art knowledge base in a historical and basic science perspective. It also strives to expand the clinician's overall awareness of tick-borne zoonotic infections. Contributing to this book are scientists with mastery in studying the pathogen, and experts who have vast clinical experience in treating it have compiled evidence-based information on the diagnosis and management of Lyme borreliosis. Specialists, primary care practitioners, and scientists alike will herein find practical and current information on this interesting vector-borne infection. For an authoritative treatise on other tick-borne diseases the reader is referred to *Tick-Borne Diseases of Humans* by Jesse Goodman, David Dennis, and Daniel Sonenshine (2005, ASM Press), and for details on the biology and epidemiology of Lyme borreliosis to *Lyme Borreliosis: Biology, Epidemiology and Control* by Jeremy Gray, Olaf Kahl, Robert Lane, and Gerold Stanek (2002, CAB International) and *Borrelia: Molecular Biology, Host Interaction and Pathogenesis* by D. Scott Samuels and Justin Radolf (2010, Caister Academic Press.)

Lyme borreliosis exhibits some differences on the North American and Eurasian continents. A unique feature of this book is its equal emphasis on the disease as it occurs on each continent. Some other books on Lyme borreliosis relegate the heterogeneous and extensive European clinical experience to a single chapter on European Lyme disease. This book does not employ the conventional division by chapter of biology, systemwise manifestations, European, pediatric, and chronic Lyme disease. Instead, each chapter attempts to present a balanced perspective and a complete description of its subject by combining the European and North American experiences.

It is unfortunate that an unwarranted mystique has become attached to this infectious disease. We have learned that Lyme borreliosis is amenable to cure with antibiotics at any stage of detection. Although the infection manifests in a limited number of clinical forms, it has somehow acquired the mantle of an ill-understood malady with "protean" manifestations. The entire spectrum of Lyme borreliosis is discussed in this book. Following a review of epidemiology of the disease, the causative spirochete genospecies, and tick vectors in the first two chapters, the next six chapters review pathogenesis, diagnosis, and treatment of Lyme borreliosis. The subsequent chapters detail the role of serologic, culture, and molecular diagnostic methods. An important feature of the book is a separate chapter on prognosis that is an evidence-based review of outcome studies. This chapter also includes practical advice to physicians to help them manage the challenging clinical scenario of a chronic illness ascribed to Lyme disease. A guide to prevention strategies, especially the management of a tick bite, is detailed in the final chapter.

The editor and authors hope that this first edition will be a comprehensive reference for clinicians and scientists who are working diligently to treat and control Lyme borreliosis, and will serve as a source of the information they need to dispel the misconceptions and myths built around this infectious disease.

Bay Shore, NY SUNIL K. SOOD

ACKNOWLEDGMENTS

I am indebted to Betty C. Hobbs, who introduced me to bacteria; to Lorry Rubin who gave me wise counsel to study Lyme disease; to Robert Daum and my Tulane ID mentors; to Jinnie Kim who helped conceive the project; to Jyoti for her patience and for not letting me lose mine; and to Arpana, Vandana, and Rishi for their editorial assistance and counsel.

I dedicate the book to all my residents and fellows, who will read it cover-to-cover.

S. K. S.

CONTRIBUTORS

Maria E. Aguero-Rosenfeld, New York University School of Medicine, New York, NY, USA

Leif Dotevall, Department of Communicable Disease Control, Vastra Gotaland, Sweden

Frank Dressler, Kinderklinik, Medizinische Hochschule Hannover, Hannover, Germany

Fadi A. Haddad, Sharp Grossmont Hospital, La Mesa, CA and Scripps Mercy Hospital, San Diego, CA, USA

John J. Halperin, Overlook Hospital and Mount Sinai School of Medicine, Summit, NJ, USA

Pierre-François Humair, Via Aprica 26, 6900 Lugano, Switzerland

Hans-Iko Huppertz, Klinikum Bremen-Mitte and University of Göttingen, Bremen, Germany

Norman T. Ilowite, Children's Hospital at Montefiore, Albert Einstein College of Medicine, Bronx, NY, USA

Patricia I. Irigoyen, Children's Hospital at Montefiore, Albert Einstein College of Medicine, Bronx, NY, USA

Barbara J. B. Johnson, Division of Vector-Borne Diseases, National Center for Zoonotic, Vector-Borne and Enteric Diseases, CDC, Fort Collins, CO, USA

Peter J. Krause, Yale University School of Public Health and Yale School of Medicine, New Haven, CT, USA

Paul M. Lantos, Duke University School of Medicine, Durham, NC, USA

Robert R. Müllegger, State Hospital Wiener Neustadt, Wiener Neustadt, Austria

Susan O'Connell, Health Protection Agency and Southampton University Hospitals Trust, Southampton, UK

Joseph Piesman, Division of Vector-Borne Diseases, National Center for Zoonotic, Vector-Borne and Enteric Diseases, CDC, Fort Collins, CO, USA

Mark B. Salzman, Kaiser Permanente, West Los Angeles Medical Center, Los Angeles, CA, USA

Eugene D. Shapiro, Yale University School of Medicine and Yale Graduate School of Arts and Sciences, New Haven, CT, USA

Vijay K. Sikand, Tufts University School of Medicine, Boston, MA, and Lawrence and Memorial Hospital, New London, CT, USA

Sunil K. Sood, Steven & Alexandra Cohen Children's Medical Center of New York, New Hyde Park, NY and Southside Hospital, Bay Shore, NY, USA

Guiqing Wang, New York Medical College, Valhalla, NY, USA

Klaus Weber, Eichgrabenstr. 17, 82340 Feldafing, Germany

Bettina Wilske, Harthauser Strasse 8b, 81545 Munich, Germany

Gary P. Wormser, New York Medical College, Valhalla, NY, USA

1

THE EMERGENCE AND EPIDEMIOLOGY OF LYME BORRELIOSIS IN EUROPE AND NORTH AMERICA

Sunil K. Sood, Susan O'Connell, and Klaus Weber

Lyme borreliosis, also known as Lyme disease, is an infectious disease caused by the spirochete *Borrelia burgdorferi.* Several genospecies are included within *B. burgdorferi* sensu lato ("in a broad sense"). In North America all the well-characterized isolates of *Borrelia* obtained from patients with Lyme borreliosis are *B. burgdorferi* sensu stricto ("in a strict sense"). At least two other genospecies not present in the United States, *B. afzelii* and *B. garinii*, are additional proven agents of Lyme borreliosis in Europe, causing more than 70% of European-acquired infections (Wang et al., 1999). Probably owing to differences in tissue tropism, there are variations in the spectrum of clinical manifestations of the disease between genospecies, resulting also in some differences in clinical presentation between the continents. There are also some differences in serologic immune responses, which has implications for diagnostic testing (Chapter 10) and for vaccine development.

There is evidence, based on multilocus sequence typing of bacterial housekeeping genes, that *B. burgdorferi* existed in North America thousands of years before its discovery, and that it originated in Europe (Qiu et al., 2008, Hoen et al., 2009, Margos et al., 2009, Margos et al., 2008). The organism probably was carried across the Atlantic Ocean to the northeast by migratory birds, and then spread westward (Comstedt et al., 2006; Ginsberg et al., 2005).

Lyme Borreliosis in Europe and North America: Epidemiology and Clinical Practice, First Edition.
Edited by Sunil K. Sood

HISTORICAL OVERVIEW

Lyme disease appeared in contemporary medical textbooks in the early 1980s, but most manifestations of the infection were known in Europe in the latter part of the nineteenth century and the early twentieth century. Undoubtedly the modern North American description spearheaded efforts to identify the etiology, leading to identification of the causative spirochete in 1983. It also led, in stages, to retroactive correlations of the "old" European manifestations. The story of that ground-breaking description has by now been told repeatedly, often with much flourish, and an engaging account directed at a broad audience was published recently (Edlow, 2004). For more detailed accounts of the discoveries pertaining to this spirochetal syndrome in Europe, see the well-researched chapters by Klaus Weber and by Willy Burgdorfer, in Weber's *Aspects of Lyme Borreliosis* (Weber and Burgdorfer, 1993). Brief historical perspectives on various manifestations of the disease are presented in individual chapters in this book. A brief recounting of the chronology and seminal events that gave us the complete clinical picture is presented here.

Acrodermatitis Chronica Atrophicans

In 1883 the German physician Buchwald presented the case of a 36-year-old man with a "diffuse idiopathic skin atrophy" of 16 years duration (Buchwald, 1883). This is now recognized as the first description of acrodermatitis chronica atrophicans (ACA), a late manifestation of Lyme borreliosis. Herxheimer and Hartmann introduced the term "acrodermatitis chronica atrophicans" in 1902, with a review of about 12 cases published in the interim, and 12 of their own cases. (Herxheimer and Hartmann, 1902) A few years later 202 patients with "atrophy cutis" were reviewed; two-thirds of those likely had ACA (Weber and Pfister, 1993). Patients with arthralgia, bone atrophy, arthropathy, and synovial thickening were described during the next few decades (Weber and Burgdorfer, 1993). Other dermatologists in Germany noted that the "pallida reaction" (*Treponema pallidum*) was positive in several ACA patients' serum.

An infectious etiology was proposed in 1946 by Svarts, who described improvement of ACA on penicillin (Svarts, 1946). At the University of Munich, between 1954 and 1955, dermatologist Hans Götz transplanted affected skin from an ACA patient into himself and three other physician volunteers (Gotz, 1954; 1955). He documented ACA-like chronic inflammation that lasted up to 312 days that resolved with penicillin but speculated that a "large virus" was the cause.

In 1949 Thyresson reported on the partial or complete success of penicillin therapy in 40 of 57 patients with ACA (Thyresson, 1949). Finally, Asbrink confirmed the common spirochetal etiology of acrodermatitis chronica atrophicans and erythema migrans in 1984 after spirochetes were isolated on culture from an ACA lesion (Asbrink et al., 1984). In the United States ACA had been seen as far back as 1895, although it appears to have occurred mostly in immigrants from Europe (Sweitzer and Laymon, 1935).

Erythema (Chronicum) Migrans

An "erythema migrans" rash occurring after a tick bite was first mentioned at a meeting of the Swedish Dermatological Society by Swedish physician Arvid Afzelius in 1909 as a ring-like expanding lesion with central clearing (Afzelius, 1910). It was described in more detail, as "erythema chronicum migrans" (ECM), by the Austrian dermatologist Lipschütz and by Riehl in 1913 (Lipschütz, 1913). The relationship between tick bite and erythema migrans was further specified by Afzelius in 1921 (Afzelius, 1921). Lipschütz in 1923 had astutely suggested that the tick intestinal tract and salivary glands be studied microscopically to look for bacteria as the cause of ECM, but this had to wait until Burgdorfer's discovery, 59 years later, in the United States (Lipschütz, 1923). In fact the Swedish dermatologist Sven Hellerström is credited with the first formal proposal of a tick-borne spirochetal etiology of ECM in 1930 (Scrimenti and Scrimenti, 1993; Hellerstrom, 1930). Meanwhile, in a report entitled *Spirochetes in Aetiologically Obscure Diseases* (1948), the dermatologist Carl Lennhoff performed mercury chloride staining of biopsies in a variety of skin diseases, including erythema migrans. In retrospect, his visualization of spirochetes in so many different disorders was deemed nonspecific (Burgdorfer, 1993).

Better evidence of an infectious cause came from the success in clearing ECM with penicillin. (Hellerstrom, 1951; Hollstrom, 1951) The experiments of Binder et al. in 1955 in Würzburg yielded the first persuasive evidence of the infectious etiology of ECM (Binder et al., 1955). They reproduced ECM in three volunteers by transplanting skin from the edge of a patient with the typical rash, and re-transmitting it between volunteers. The incubation period was one to three weeks, and penicillin treatment successfully cleared the rash in each case.

The first recorded case of ECM in North America was diagnosed in 1969, by Rudolph Scrimenti, a physician in Wisconsin. He published the histopathology, consisting of lymphocytic and plasma cell periadenexal infiltrate, and treated the patient successfully with penicillin, based on his knowledge of the European disease and the description by Hellerström (Scrimenti, 1970; Scrimenti and Scrimenti, 1993). His patient also had symptoms of radiculitis, headache, and fever, and he associated the extremely large ring-like rash with the bite of what Scrimenti generically called a wood tick. Then in 1975 Mast and Burrows described a cluster of four cases in southeastern Connecticut (Mast and Burrows, 1976). (An earlier case series, published in 1962, described erythema migrans in American servicemen, but they had become infected while stationed in the Air Force base in Wiesbaden, Germany; Flanagan, 1962).

Weber summarized the knowledge obtained by 1986, stating that the term "erythema migrans" (used by Afzelius originally) should be the generally used designation because it is "shorter, self-explanatory, and older" and is more accurate, and the rash is not prolonged more than a few weeks in most cases (Weber, 1986). Erythema migrans (EM) has become the generally accepted term.

Borrelial Lymphocytoma

In 1911 the Swiss pathologist Burckhardt described a patient with a solitary cutaneous pseudolymphoma, which could have been the first documented example of a borrelial lymphocytoma (Burckhardt, 1911). However, "pseudolymphomas" described by Spiegler and Fendt in 1894 and 1900 could also have been borrelial lymphocytoma (see Chapter 7). The designation "lymphocytoma" was first used by Kaufmann-Wolf in 1921 and Biberstein in 1923 (Kaufmann-Wolf, 1921; Biberstein, 1923). These terms included both borrelial and nonborrelial types of benign hyperplasias of the skin. When it became clear through clinical observations and positive serological tests that a certain kind of benign cutaneous hyperplasia was of borrelial origin, the designation borrelial lymphocytoma was introduced for this cutaneous sign of Lyme borreliosis (Weber et al., 1985). Another term, "lymphadenosis benigna cutis," had been coined by Bäfverstedt from Sweden in 1943, when he presented a large series of patients with benign cutaneous hyperplasia associated in a few cases with erythema migrans (Bäfverstedt, 1943).

Paschoud in 1954 may have made the initial association of borrelial lymphocytoma with neuroborreliosis in describing a large plaque that followed a tick bite in a patient with meningoradiculitis (Paschoud, 1954). He also performed a transmission experiment in Lausanne wherein the recipients developed borrelial lymphocytoma in about six weeks (Paschoud, 1957).

Neuroborreliosis

In 1922, the French physicians, Charles Garin and A. Bujadoux reported on a case of facial palsy and meningoradiculoneuritis after a tick bite (Garin and Bujadoux, 1922). The Swedish dermatologist Hellerström read a paper to the Southern Medical Association in Cincinnati in 1929, describing meningitis associated with ECM Afzelius in European patients (Hellerstrom, 1930, 1951). In 1941 in Munich, the German neurologist Alfred Bannwarth presented three groups of patients who had either intensely painful meningoradiculoneuritis, facial palsy (four of six were children), or "chronic lymphocytic meningitis with cerebral symptoms" (Bannwarth, 1941). All had a lymphocytic pleocytosis, albeit much less prominent in the first group. Headache, vomiting, and neck stiffness were prominent only in the third group. It is interesting that papilledema, abducens paralysis, and prolonged CNS inflammation were noted in one patient each in the last group, complications that have been described recently in Lyme neuroborreliosis, notably in children (Dayan et al., 2004; Rothermel et al., 2001). Thus Bannwarth provided a description of the natural course of what we now call early neurological manifestations of Lyme borreliosis, or neuroborreliosis. In 1949 and 1962, Georg Schaltenbrand made an important postulation regarding the association of CNS manifestations and tick bites, and recorded improvement after treatment with corticosteroids and tetracycline (Schaltenbrand, 1949; 1962). Hellerström's patient treated with penicillin in 1951 had ECM and meningitis.

Note that the following additional designations have been used in Europe: "paralysie par les tiques" (Garin and Bujadoux, 1922), "meningitis after erythema migrans and tick bite" (Hellerström 1930), "chronische lymphozytäre meningitis" (Bannwarth, 1941), "meningomyeloradiculitis after tick bite with erythema" (Bammer and Schenk, 1965), "peripheral neuropathy in ACA" (Hopf, 1966), "meningopolyneuritis Garin-Bujadoux-Bannwarth" (Horstrup and Ackermann, 1973), "erythema chronicum migrans meningitis" (Weber, 1974), "Bannwarth's syndrome" (Weber and Burgdorfer, 1993), "progressive borrelien-enzephalomyelitis" (Ackermann et al., 1985), "cerebral vasculitis" (Weber and Burgdorfer, 1993), "neuroborreliosis" (Stiernstedt et al., 1988), "chronic peripheral neuropathy" (Kristoferitsch, 1993), and "Lyme neuroborreliosis" (Dotevall et al., 1988; Pfister et al., 1991). These terms span the spectrum of the neurological manifestations of Lyme borreliosis.

Setting the Stage for the Unified Etiology of Diverse Clinical Presentations

In Würzburg, Germany, W. Hauser concluded that the three cutaneous manifestations were related to each other and to the distribution of *I. ricinus ticks* (Hauser, 1965). Hopf described

92 patients that established the relationship between ACA and a chronic neuropathy, as well as a few cases of concomitant arthritis, facial palsy, and other neurologic symptoms that he thought were coincidental (Hopf, 1966).

In 1976 Weber systematically ruled out other possible causes in a case of meningitis that followed erythema migrans and responded to intravenous penicillin. He proposed a bacterial species, unlikely to be *Borrelia*, as a possible etiologic agent, given the knowledge that relapsing fever borreliae were transmitted by soft (argasid) and not hard (ixodid) ticks (Weber, 1974). Thus the connection between cutaneous and neurological manifestations was recognized in Europe, but the knowledge remained mainly restricted to the fields of dermatology and neurology.

Lyme Arthritis

In 1975 phone calls by members of the public to the Connecticut Health Department and the CDC led to a retrospective investigation into a remarkable cluster of new arthritis cases. Two very perceptive mothers, Polly Murray and Judith Mensch, were concerned that the majority of cases were children diagnosed as juvenile rheumatoid arthritis (JRA), often in the same family, dating at least back to 1972 (Steere et al., 1986). Their insistence on an investigation was heeded by David Snydman at the health department, who invited Allen Steere, a rheumatology fellow at Yale University, Stephen Malawista, the Chief of Rheumatology, and their colleagues to jointly conduct an epidemiologic investigation. Snydman began by plotting all the reported cases on a map of the towns of Lyme and Old Lyme (Edlow, 2004). All patients with arthritis were examined and a distinct geographic and seasonal (summer–fall) pattern was noted, which was inconsistent with JRA and instead pointed to an infectious etiology.

Their findings were published in stages, leading up to the complete picture of this emerging infection that closely clustered in and around the towns of Lyme, Old Lyme, and East Haddam in southeastern Connecticut. Of 39 children and 12 adults, 13 had a history of an expanding red rash that resembled European ECM descriptions. As arthritis had never been formally linked to ECM, Steere and co-investigators considered the arthritis to be a novel disease, and named it after the town of Lyme, where the first case was thought to have occurred (Steere et al., 1977). (The term "Lyme arthritis" first appeared in the literature in letters to JAMA in 1976 when the physicians referred to the ongoing investigation at Yale, before the seminal 1977 report was published; Mast and Burrows, 1976; Hazard et al., 1976). Epidemiologic evidence suggested an arthropod vector, and the investigators suspected transmission of a viral agent. Extensive viral testing yielded no putative agent. Through their continued observations on old and new patients, they were able to tie in the skin lesion with migratory joint pains, monoarticular or oligoarticular arthritis, neurologic abnormalities, myocardial conduction abnormalities, nonspecific systemic symptoms, and nonspecific serum inflammatory markers in 32 patients with onset in 1976, whom they followed prospectively (Steere et al., 1977). They specifically proposed the ixodid tick *I. scapularis* as the vector because some patients with ECM and Lyme arthritis reported tick bites (one identified as *I. scapularis*), and tick survey results were consistent with a dramatically raised risk of acquiring Lyme disease in communities on one bank of the river (Steere et al., 1978).

Further data on the incidence of cases and the distribution of *Ixodes* ticks expanded our understanding of the epidemiology of Lyme borreliosis, with recognition of distinct foci along the northeastern coast, in Wisconsin, and on the west coast in California and Oregon

(Steere and Malawista, 1979). Other locations on the continent, notably Minnesota and Ontario, were added as endemic areas for the "tick-borne dermatitis-encephalitis-arthritis syndrome" that was now firmly established in medical nomenclature as Lyme disease (Schrock, 1982, 1981; Steere and Malawista, 1979). Based on the prior European experience and anecdotal American experience, Steere and colleagues conducted an open-label randomized trial of three antibiotics for ECM. They demonstrated shortened duration of rashes as well as a decreased rate of later stage manifestations compared to untreated controls (Steere et al., 1980).

Discovery of the Spirochetal Etiology of Lyme Borreliosis

In 1981 Willy Burgdorfer of the NIH Rocky Mountain Laboratories in Montana, who was collaborating with Jorge Benach at Stony Brook, was dissecting *Ixodes* ticks collected on Shelter Island, New York, off the east end of Long Island, partly in pursuit of an additional vector of *R. rickettsii*, when he made a discovery. Burgdorfer himself called it serendipitous, although his prior expertise in tick microscopy and knowledge of historical observations undoubtedly fostered his discovery (Burgdorfer, 1993a,b).

As a graduate student in Switzerland, Burgdorfer had dissected thousands of *Ornithodoros* ticks, looking for infection with *B. duttoni*, the spirochetal agent of relapsing fever in Africa. He had moved to the Montana laboratory in 1951. In 1978, a few months after speaking with Steere about methods to identify pathogens in ticks, he spent a sabbatical in Switzerland, where he discovered certain deer parasite microfilariae in *I. ricinus*, the European sheep tick. The hemolymph from Benach's Shelter Island ticks was negative for rickettsiae, but he noticed large microfilariae-like organisms. In order to determine how the microfilariae in ticks had entered the hemolymph, he dissected the midgut, but they were negative. Instead, he noted faintly stained spirochete-like structures. They were better visualized on Giemsa stains and on wet preparations by dark field microscopy.

Burgdorfer recalled the European literature and Hellerström's presentation on ECM to the Southern Medical Association in Cincinnati, and decided to follow his hunch. The spirochetes reacted positively with sera from Lyme disease patients in indirect immunofluorescence tests. Burgdorfer stained some slides that he had brought back from the Swiss Plateau and found morphologically and antigenically similar organisms in smears from *Ixodes ricinus* ticks, and subsequently in the guts of a few *Ixodes pacificus* from the western United States (Burgdorfer, 1984; Burgdorfer et al., 1985). Alan Barbour, his colleague at the Rocky Mountain Laboratories, successfully cultured the spirochete in modified Kelly's medium in November 1981 (Burgdorfer et al., 1982). One clone, the original "Shelter Island isolate," was given the designation B31 and continues to be a standard lab research strain (ATCC 35210; Barbour, 1984). The investigators were able to reproduce erythema migrans lesions in rabbits by allowing infected *I. dammini* to feed on them. The lesions were mostly at distant sites from the tick attachment site, indicating a bacteremic spread.

In twin papers published in 1983, Steere et al. and Benach et al. established the bacterial cause of human Lyme disease with their isolation of the "*I. dammini* spirochete" from the blood, ECM skin lesions, or CSF of five patients from Connecticut and Long Island (Steere et al., 1983; Benach et al., 1983). The organism was also linked to European ECM in a paper published the same month, following studies on live ticks from Europe supplied to Burgdorfer by André Aeschlimann, his Swiss collaborator from his 1978 sabbatical (Burgdorfer et al., 1983). With these studies the etiology of Lyme disease was established beyond doubt, and in 1984 the borrelial species was named for Willy Burgdorfer (Johnson

RC, 1984). Culture evidence of *B. burgdorferi* sensu lato in ACA from Asbrink followed in 1984 and from Hovmark in borrelial lymphocytoma in 1986 (Asbrink et al., 1984; Hovmark et al., 1986). The unified etiology and clinical picture of Lyme borreliosis on either side of the Atlantic were finally established.

Because the global distribution of this disease was now recognized, the First International Symposium on Lyme disease was organized at Yale University where scientists and physicians from Europe and North America shared their experience (Schmid, 1984). In that symposium, and at a dermatology meeting in Germany, one of the authors (KW) and coworkers announced their finding of elevated antibody titers against *B. burgdorferi* in 100% of ACA and borrelial lymphocytoma patients and in some patients with erythema migrans. Steere's group as well as other European investigators reported similar findings in their patients with erythema migrans or Lyme arthritis. This was followed by similar reports in patients with meningoradiculoneuritis. Today Lyme borreliosis is regarded as the most important human tick-borne illness in the Northern Hemisphere, and experts in numerous disciplines continue to elucidate the biology of an organism that has probably been with us for millennia (Marshall et al., 1994; Dennis, 2002).

Meticulous observations—at times using human inoculation experiments that would be unthinkable today—allowed investigators over a 100-year period to describe and begin to treat this spirochetal infection, without the benefit of modern microbiologic tools. This fascinating, multifaceted, and bicontinental story is valuable to all students and practitioners of science, most important because it proves the Pasteurian principle of how chance favors the prepared mind.

EPIDEMIOLOGY OF LYME BORRELIOSIS IN NORTH AMERICA

Lyme borreliosis in North America occurs in the temperate climate zone. Although the North American vectors, black-legged ticks of the genus *Ixodes*, are widely distributed, only a few regions are considered endemic for Lyme disease. Lyme borreliosis has been called a disease of place (Brown et al., 2005). The incidence of reported cases ranges from 0 in several states to 111.2/100,000 in Delaware (CDC, 2011). The highest incidence states, all in the northeastern and northern midwestern regions, had an average annual rate of 29.2 cases per 100,000 population in the three-year period 2003 to 2005 and for 1992 to 2006 accounting for more than 90% of cases on the continent (Bacon et al., 2008). From 2005 to 2009, incidence areas leveled off or declined in several high incidence states, but rose sharply in Delaware and in New England (CDC, 2011). During 2003 to 2005, 64,382 Lyme disease cases were reported to the CDC, for an average of over 20,000 cases/year, and this number was unchanged for 2006 (Figure 1.1). A doubling of the reported cases from 1992 to 2006 is ascribed to multiple reasons: enhanced surveillance, true increase in infections, increased diagnosis, misdiagnosis, and reporting errors (Bacon et al., 2008). In 2009, there were 29,959 confirmed and 8509 probable cases, for an incidence of 13.4 confirmed cases per 100,000 population. Underreporting to the extent of 10 to 12-fold has been shown in some studies. One estimate of the actual number is 60 to 100,000 per year, which would result in overall national case rates of about 20–30/100,000 (Steere, 2006; CDC, 2007).

Further the prevalence is focal within most endemic regions, correlating with local ecologic factors (see below). Even within townships and counties, the prevalence can vary

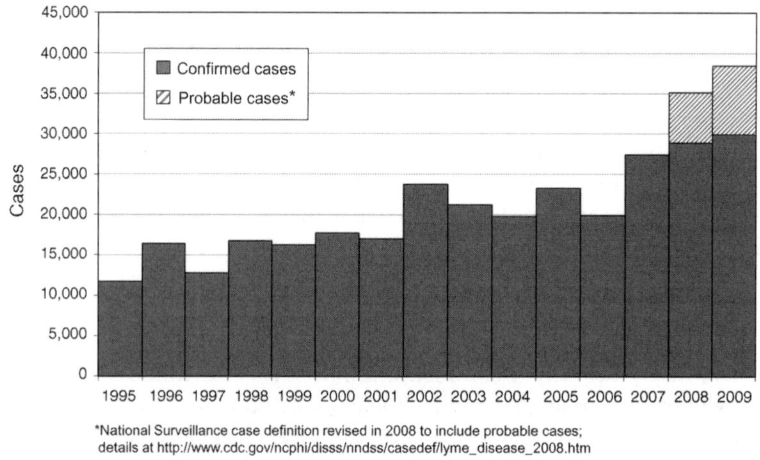

Figure 1.1 Reported cases of Lyme disease by year, United States, 1991–2009. Source: CDC. http://www.cdc.gov/ncidod/dvbid/lyme/ld_upclimblymedis.htm.

greatly. In fact 90% of cases in 1999 occurred in 109 counties, out of 3143 counties in the United States (CDC, 2001). During 2002 to 2006 the annual rate per 100,000 ranged from 219 to 962 in the 10 highest rate counties (Bacon et al., 2008). A dot plot map of reported cases is generated by the CDC (Figure 1.2). It is useful to look at this map when considering

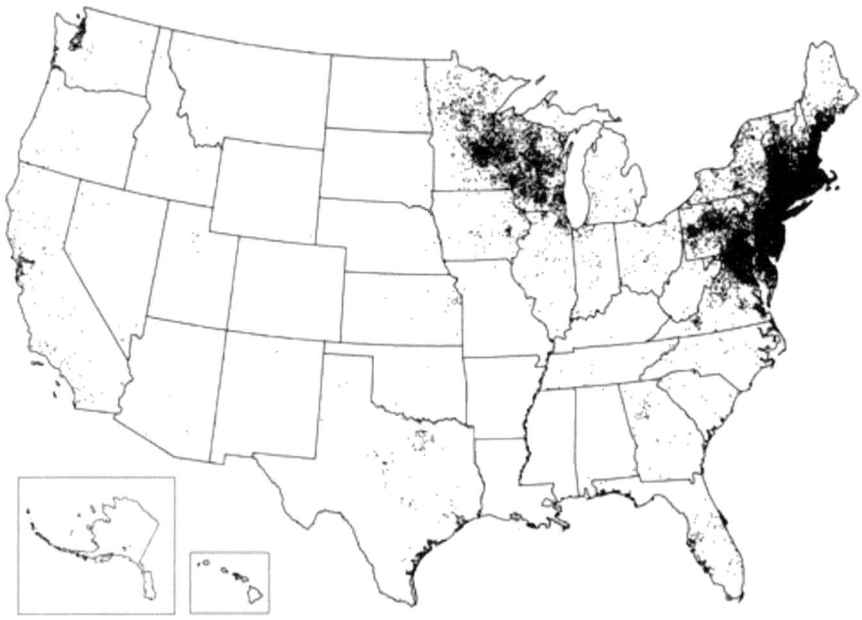

Figure 1.2 Reported cases of Lyme disease, United States, 2009. Source: CDC. http://www.cdc.gov/ncidod/dvbid/lyme/ld_Incidence.htm.

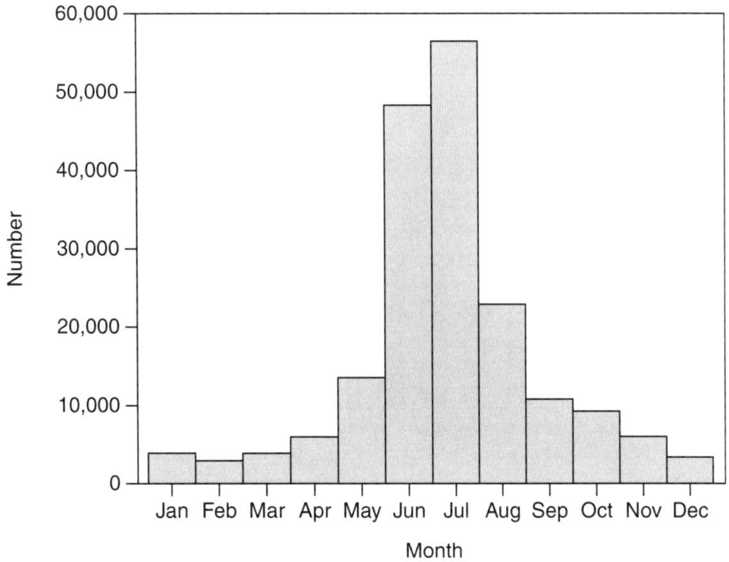

Figure 1.3 Reported cases of Lyme disease by month of illness onset United States, 1992–2006. Source: Bacon et al., 2008.

the diagnosis of Lyme borreliosis, as the epidemiologic setting is key to predictive values of both symptoms and laboratory tests (CDC, 2007). In addition to this overview map, physicians should consult a county-by-county map (see Figure 10.4, Chapter 10). The infection is uncommon in Canadian provinces, and very rare instances in Mexico have been reported in the literature (see below).

Human Factors

During 1992 to 2006 about 70% of cases occurred from June to August, consistent with the months during which nymph and adult *Ixodes* ticks are actively seeking hosts, and people are exposed more often because of recreational and occupational activities (Bacon et al., 2008) (Figure 1.3). A bimodal age distribution of Lyme borreliosis has been established in United States surveillance (Figure 1.4). The first peak (5–9 years) can be explained by outdoor activity habits of the post–toddler-years age group. The second peak starts after the fifth decade of life. The intervening trough probably reflects the relative preoccupation with study and employment in the third and fourth decades. There is a slight male predominance (53%), and an unexplained disproportionate increase in the males aged 5 to 19 years occurred from 1992 to 2006 (Bacon et al., 2008).

Tick Vectors and Environmental Aspects

The maintenance of *B. burgdorferi* in nature in North America is sustained by the multi-host life-cycle of *I. scapularis* (Figure 1.5). The reason that Lyme borreliosis is highly endemic in the northeastern and north-central regions is that high populations of white-tailed deer and rodents, particularly white-footed mice and chipmunks, sustain

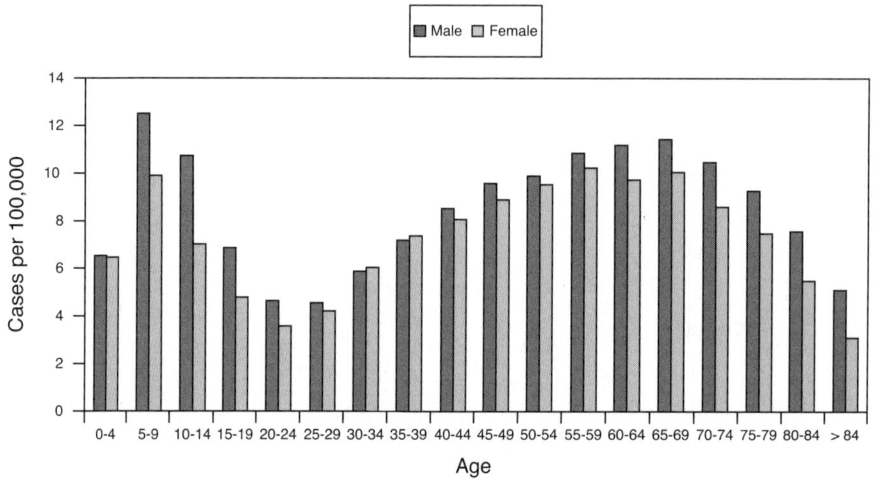

Figure 1.4 Average annual incidence of reported cases of Lyme disease by age group and sex, United States, 1992–2004. Source: CDC. http://cdc.gov/ncidod/dvbid/lyme/ld_MeanAnnualIncidence.htm.

transmission of the spirochete in nature, resulting in a higher infection rate in the deer tick variety of *Ixodes* (LoGiudice et al., 2003) (see Chapter 2). The rodents harbor the spirochete, serving as a ready reservoir that allows tick infection, while deer appear to serve primarily as a mating ground. In contrast, the most important host for *I. pacificus* ticks in the western United States and British Columbia is the western fence lizard (*Sceloporus occidentalis*), which is not a competent reservoir of *B. burgdorferi*

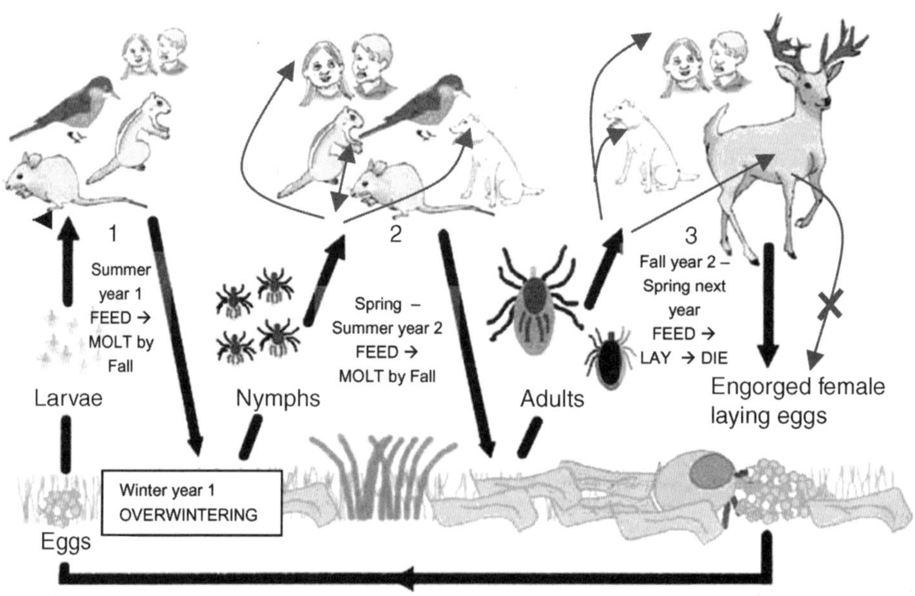

Figure 1.5 Life cycle of the blacklegged tick or "deer" tick, *Ixodes scapularis*. 1, 2, 3 = Feeding on new host. During feeding, infection is transmitted as shown by direction of red arrow. X = transmission blocked. Source: Modified from Kirby Stafford. (*See insert for color representation*).

(Brown et al., 2005). Its blood is borreliacidal, so the role of lizards is termed zooprophylactic, that is lowering the efficiency of transmission to other hosts (Lane and Quistad, 1998). The enzootic cycle of infection is maintained because *I. pacificus* can also feed on western grey squirrels (*Sciurus griseus)* which were recently identified as competent reservoir hosts for *B. burgdorferi.* It is also mainatained by interactions with secondary hosts such as woodrats, and another tick, *I. spinipalpis* (Eisen, 2004). The zooprophylactic effect of lizards may also be a factor in explaining the lack of endemic Lyme borreliosis in the southern United States.

In the northeast and north-central endemic regions the distribution of cases mirrors the presence of *Ixodes* ticks, competent reservoir rodents, and white-tailed deer in the same environment. The two major ecological factors that make for a prime habitat for *Ixodes* are high humidity and frequenting by small rodents and deer. Wooded areas or brush near water (coastal or inland, especially along rivers and estuaries), as well as unmaintained areas around gardens and domestic properties, especially where there is a lot of leaf litter, harbor such conditions. Rodents can carry ticks into areas from which deer can be kept out, giving rise to risk to small children and pets even if they do not play in woods or brush, the so-called peridomestic or periresidential risk (Dennis, 1998). Seropositivity rates among dogs have in fact been used to predict the distribution of *B. burgdorferi* (Lindenmayer et al., 1991). In the Pacific coast endemic areas the ecological components are oak and bay tree woodlands where *I. pacificus* ticks feed mainly on lizards (Lane and Loye, 1991).

It is important to understand the distinction between endemicity of Lyme disease and presence of enzootic *B. burgdorferi.* The latter refers to established maintenance of the spirochete in animal reservoirs but does not equate with spread to humans, as environmental conditions may not be conducive to tick-borne transmission to people. For example, it is likely that borreliae do not survive long enough in the mid-gut of *Ixodes* ticks in the warmer southern climate of the United States to threaten transmission at the ticks' subsequent feeds. So, although *B. burgdorferi* is enzootic contiguous to Lyme borreliosis endemic areas (chiefly along the Atlantic coast south to Florida, and in areas of Minnesota, Illinois, and northern Michigan), cases of human Lyme borreliosis occur only sporadically in these enzootic areas. Given the frequent reporting of cases from "nonendemic" states and counties, it is important for clinicians to carefully consider whether suitable ecologic and zoonotic factors are present locally when considering the diagnosis in a patient with compatible symptoms and signs. Of course, presence of the right conditions can presage the emergence of human cases in an area.

A classic illustration of such a diagnostic dilemma is seen in the well-documented cases of tick-bite associated erythematous rash illnesses in Missouri that were initially labeled erythema migrans (Masters and Donnell, 1995). Investigative evidence to date indicates that erythema migrans-like rash illnesses in the southern United States are not caused by *B. burgdorferi* (Wormser et al., 2005; Philipp et al., 2006). It is postulated that an organism provisionally named *B. lonestari* may be transmitted by *Amblyomma americanum*, the lone-star tick, which is highly prevalent across the southern United States (Varela et al., 2004). PCR evidence of *B. lonestari* or a closely related bacterium has been demonstrated in a single case of erythema migrans-like rash lesion in a patient who was probably exposed in Maryland and in an *A. americanum* tick that was found to be attached at the center of the rash (Dennis, 2005). It is also conceivable that one or more other, as yet undiscovered, tick- or insect-borne pathogens are the etiology of erythema migrans-like rashes.

US Clinical Case Definitions

The CDC developed and has recently revised the case definition for national reporting of Lyme disease under the National Notifiable Diseases Surveillance System (CDC, 2008, 2009). It is unequivocally stated that this definition is for surveillance and is not intended for use in clinical diagnosis. The definition encompasses erythema migrans, and three late manifestations—musculoskeletal system, nervous system, and cardiovascular system Lyme disease. Laboratory evidence (a positive culture, positive two-tier testing interpreted using established criteria, or positive IgG immunoblot interpreted using established criteria) is an essential criterion for the case definition, with the exception of erythema migrans after a known exposure. Cases reported with laboratory evidence alone are considered *Suspected.* Approximately two-thirds of cases reported have erythema migrans, a third have arthritis, about 12% have neurologic symptoms, and fewer than 1% have second- or third-degree atrioventricular block. During 1992 to 2006 of the reported cases 13% had more than one clinical manifestation (Bacon et al., 2008). This spectrum of clinical manifestations based on passive reporting differs from that found in a prospective study of newly diagnosed Lyme disease in children in Connecticut (Gerber et al., 1996). Only 6% presented with arthritis. Cases of arthritis are more likely to be reported because serologic confirmation is available, whereas there is an underreporting of erythema migrans due to a failure of physicians to report an established and treatable disease.

Lyme Borreliosis—An Emerging Infection

Lyme borreliosis remains an emerging disease, designated by the Institute of Medicine as one of the most rapidly emerging in the United States. There is a small body of evidence for its gradual geographic spread. After its initial identification in one county in Connecticut, cases were identified in all counties by 1985 (Petersen et al., 1989). Increases in incidence and of cumulative prevalence of human cases have been documented in longitudinal studies on Fire Island, NY, and Great Island, MA (Handrahan et al., 1984; Steere et al., 1986). In three high-incidence states there was a documented increase in the number of counties reporting Lyme disease between 1992 and 2006 (Bacon et al., 2008). Several factors are at play in the emergence of Lyme borreliosis in North America. The distribution of the tick vector *Ixodes scapularis* advanced inland up major river valleys from the coast in Maine and New York State, resulting in more counties being counted as endemic in these states as well (Rand et al., 2007; White et al., 1991). It has been proposed that the propensity of *B. burgdorferi* to be transmitted among several mammalian species has allowed Lyme borreliosis to spread rapidly in the northeast (Hanincova et al., 2006). Focal outbreaks can rapidly emerge, chiefly attributable to proliferation of deer in the local area (Lastavica et al., 1989; Steere et al., 1986). Deer are important feeding hosts for the adult (reproductive) stage of *I. scapularis.* In fact the emergence and increase of Lyme borreliosis in the United States is primarily due to ecological conditions that have allowed increases in deer populations as colonial farmlands gave way to forested areas during the past few decades (Steere, 1994). Presently the US northeast, despite having some of the largest metropolitan areas in the country, is forested for about 60% of its area, with approximately 80% forest cover in New England and Maine (Mac et al., 1998). The outward expansion of suburban developments into wooded areas, and the trend toward building new homes in rural settings in parts of the north and northeast are also major factors in the increased number of human cases (Dennis, 2002).

It appears more than coincidental that the main endemic areas on three continents are situated along the terminal moraine of glaciers that retreated after the last ice age, since emergence of new forests in these locations was conducive to increases in white-tailed deer populations (Steere et al., 2004; Mac et al., 1998).

It is important that primary care clinicians continue to report new cases to local health authorities so that accurate statistics can be maintained. These can be used to plan environmental measures and future immunization strategies.

Canada

Lyme borreliosis is rare in Canada (Anon., 1991, 2006). Both tick vectors of *B. burgdorferi* are present in the country (*I. scapularis* in eastern and central Canada *and I. pacificus* in British Columbia). Range expansions for *I. scapularis* have been observed in parts of southern Manitoba, eastern Ontario, and Nova Scotia in recent years. Ongoing surveillance efforts include preparation of risk maps for potential expansion of the range of *I. scapularis* in eastern and central Canada. Current and projected climate change models have been used to make predictions because data on rising mean temperatures in northern climes are biologically consistent with increases in vector populations (Ogden et al., 2006. 2008a,b). However, data are relatively sparse, and systematic sampling and ecological risk modeling will be key to developing more accurate predictive risk maps. Most reported cases are from Ontario, but reporting from Quebec, the other large eastern province, is considered incomplete. The infection rate of *I. pacificus* ticks in British Columbia is very low, and only two human cases of Lyme borreliosis were reported from British Columbia in 2006. A National Lyme Disease Meeting was held in March 2006 under the auspices of the Public Health Agency of Canada (Anon, 2006). Data sources included the Canadian Institute for Health Information, a hospital morbidity database, Statistics Canada's Morbidity and Mortality Database, and cases reported by the provinces to the Public Health Agency's Notifiable Disease Reporting System (NDRS). Of the 345 cases reported to the NDRS between 1994 and 2004, 193 (56%) were related to travel outside Canada. As in the United States the age distribution is bimodal (data from 1992–2002) with peaks in children 5 to 15 years and adults 50 to 60 years.

Mexico

Borrelial lymphocytoma and erythema migrans were reported from Mexico in four patients who had never traveled outside the country (Gordillo-Perez et al., 2007). In two patients with clinical features of borrelial lymphocytoma, the histopathological findings, although not pathognomonic, were consistent with those seen in European borrelial lymphocytoma. Sera from both lymphocytoma patients and from one erythema migrans patients were positive for antibodies to *B. burgdorferi* by immunoblot, and skin biopsies from all four patients were positive by PCR for *B. burgdorferi* DNA, using primers for the *B. burgdorferi* sensu lato flagellin (*fla*) gene. All lesions disappeared after antibiotic treatment. A report of seropositivity (only 9 of almost 3000 samples tested) is much less convincing (Gordillo et al., 1999). Sera were from individuals from all states of Mexico, without any indication that a history of tick exposure or of illness compatible with Lyme borreliosis was elicited. Only three bands were required for a positive by immunoblot, which is not standard in the United States. Nevertheless, and despite the lack of culture evidence of *B. burgdorferi* to date (Johnson, 2008), it is possible that rare cases of human *B. burgdorferi* infections occur in Mexico.

Congenital Lyme Disease: Lack of Evidence from Epidemiological Studies

Case reports of suspected congenital infection with *B. burgdorferi*, all in the 1980s, were based upon "morphologically compatible" spirochetes on histology at autopsy, including brain and cardiac tissue, without accompanying evidence of inflammation (Weber et al., 1988; Schlesinger et al., 1985). Specific immunohistochemical stains for *B. burgdorferi* were not used in these cases, and microscopic visualization and silver staining are prone to false-positives. Large epidemiologic investigations, one of them a study of 2000 pregnancies, have yielded no association between the mothers' prenatal or in-pregnancy exposure and fetal death, prematurity, or congenital malformations (Strobino et al., 1993; Gerber and Zalneraitis, 1994; Strobino et al., 1999). The authors of a recent comprehensive literature review concluded that despite evidence that *B. burgdorferi* can cross the placenta, a teratogenic effect or congenital Lyme borreliosis in infants has not been found. There is a theoretical potential for fetal loss, based on animal studies, but recommendations for the treatment of Lyme borreliosis or of tick bites in pregnancy are not modified, with the exception of avoidance of tetracyclines (Elliott et al., 2001).

EPIDEMIOLOGY OF LYME BORRELIOSIS IN EUROPE

In Europe, as in the United States, Lyme borreliosis is the most common arthropod-borne infection of human beings (Anon, 2004). European Lyme borreliosis is similar in many respects to American-acquired infection, but there are some significant variations in clinical presentations and epidemiology, related to the greater diversity of borrelial genospecies found in Europe and to environmental factors (Stanek and Strle, 2003; Stanek et al., 2011, in press).

Tick Vectors and Environmental Aspects

The main European vectors of *Borrelia burgdorferi* are *Ixodes ricinus* and *Ixodes persulcatus. Ixodes ricinus,* the sheep tick or castor-bean tick, is widely distributed throughout Europe, extending south from Scandinavia to Mediterranean countries, and from the western edge of the continent to Russia. In Russia and the Baltic republics the eastern range of *I. ricinus* overlaps with that of *I. persulcatus,* the taiga tick, which is widely distributed throughout temperate Asia to the Far East (Gern and Humair, 2002).

The vector ticks occur in areas of deciduous woodlands and mixed forests throughout Europe. They require high humidity levels and are protected from desiccation in leaf litter. They can also be found in heathlands and pasturelands of regions that have mild, damp climates, such as the British Isles, but arid areas of southern Europe are not suitable habitats (Gray et al., 1998). Altitude is also a limiting factor for tick survival, with fewer ticks found above 1000 meters, although several recent studies have shown that their ranges are gradually extending into higher altitudes and higher latitudes, which may be related to climate change (Daniel et al., 2005; Lindgren and Jaenson, 2006; Gern et al., 2008).

The potential for human Lyme borreliosis acquisition is more focal, as it depends on interactions of numerous factors, including the presence of ticks, borrelial reservoir-competent hosts, and human activities within the tick habitats, particularly at times of peak tick feeding activity in spring, early summer, and autumn. An optimal habitat for Lyme borreliosis acquisition is mixed deciduous woodland with a rich variety of the small mammals and birds that are potential borrelial reservoir hosts, and larger mammals—particularly deer—which are feeding hosts for adult ticks and thus help maintain tick populations at their reproductive stage (Gray et al., 1998). Expansions of deer populations and ranges have contributed significantly to increased tick abundance in many parts of Europe. There is greater variety of borrelial reservoir hosts in Europe than in North America, with many species of small- and medium-sized mammals and birds involved as reservoir hosts, depending on the *B. burgdorferi* genospecies (Gern and Humair, 2002; EUCALB, 2011) (Figure 1.6).

Changes in land utilization, including forestry practice, influence the suitability of habitats for Lyme borreliosis endemicity. In many parts of Europe reinstatement of

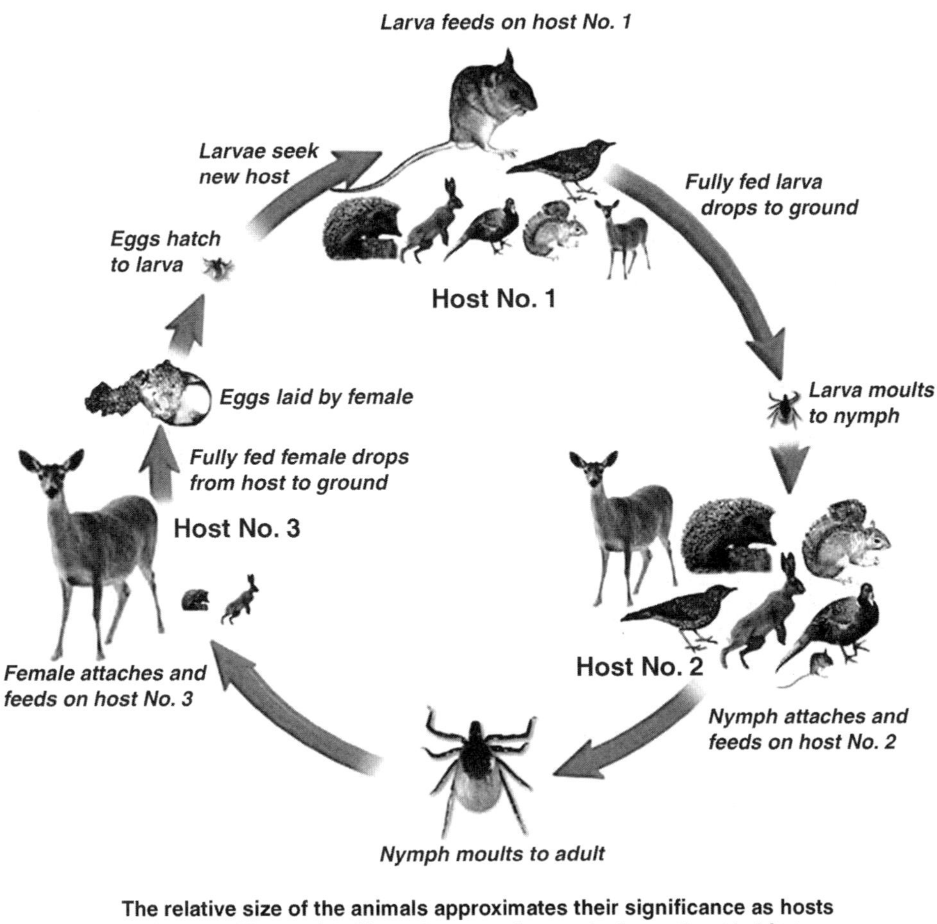

Figure 1.6 Life cycle of *Ixodes* in Europe, to illustrate diversity of hosts. Source: Jeremy Gray, University of Dublin.

deciduous and mixed woodland in areas previously used as pine forest monoculture is likely to increase tick population densities (Anon, 2004). Many other changes in agricultural practices, land management, and residential housing can also increase or decrease tick populations, borrelial reservoir hosts, and human access, thus affecting Lyme borreliosis risk (Linard et al., 2007). Local risk assessments can be helpful in indicating need for disease awareness and for reinforcing the importance of primary prevention measures, particularly tick awareness and the early removal of attached ticks (Linard et al., 2007; EUCALB, 2011).

Borrelial Genospecies

Several pathogenic genospecies of *Borrelia burgdorferi* are present in Europe, and there are some differences in their geographic distribution. There are also variations in clinical presentations associated with the different genospecies, which are related to organotropisms and other factors. The major pathogenic genospecies are *B. garinii* and the closely related *B. bavariensis* (formerly *B. garinii* serotype 4), *B. afzelii* and *B. burgdorferi* sensu stricto. *Borrelia garinii* and *B. afzelii* are widely distributed in Europe and Eurasia. *Borrelia burgdorferi* sensu stricto has been found more focally, and can cause disease presentations similar to those seen in North America. It does not appear to be present in *I. persulcatus* ticks.

All four major pathogenic genospecies can cause erythema migrans and meningitis. *Borrelia garinii* is particularly neurotropic and is strongly associated with radiculopathic and encephalomyelitic presentations (Rupprecht et al., 2008). *Borrelia afzelii* can also cause neurological complications but is less frequently identified in CSF than *B. garinii.* It can cause the late skin manifestation, acrodermatitis chronica atrophicans (ACA), and patients with this condition may also have vasculitic peripheral neuropathy (Wang et al., 1999; Kristoferitsch, 1993). Borrelial lymphocytoma, an uncommon early skin manifestation, is caused predominantly by *B. afzelii* (Maraspin et al., 2002). Lyme arthritis is associated with all three genospecies, but mainly with *B. burgdorferi* sensu stricto and *B. garinii* (Lunemann et al., 2001). There have been a few case reports associating other genospecies, including *B. spielmanii, B. valaisiana,* and *B. lusitaniae,* with significant clinical manifestations, mainly erythema migrans. The most convincing evidence so far for pathogenicity in these genospecies has come from the isolation of *B spielmanii* from a few patients with erythema migrans (Fingerle et al., 2008).

There are relatively high prevalences of *B. valaisiana* in tick populations in some of the most westerly countries of Europe, including Ireland and the United Kingdom (Kirstein et al., 1997). The significant presence in tick populations of this essentially nonpathogenic organism may be a contributing factor to the lower prevalence of clinically significant reported disease in these countries than in regions where pathogenic genospecies are predominant. Similarly *B. lusitaniae* is the most prevalent genospecies identified in ticks in Portugal, a very low disease-prevalence country, where fewer that 40 serologically confirmed cases of Lyme borreliosis were reported annually between 2000 and 2004 (0.4/100,000), following the introduction of mandatory reporting in 1999 (Lopes de Carvalho and Nuncio, 2006).

There are also intraspecies variations that may correlate with some variations in disease presentations and severity, and also with reservoir host competency. For example, most *B. garinii* serotypes are associated with avian reservoirs, particularly ground-feeding birds

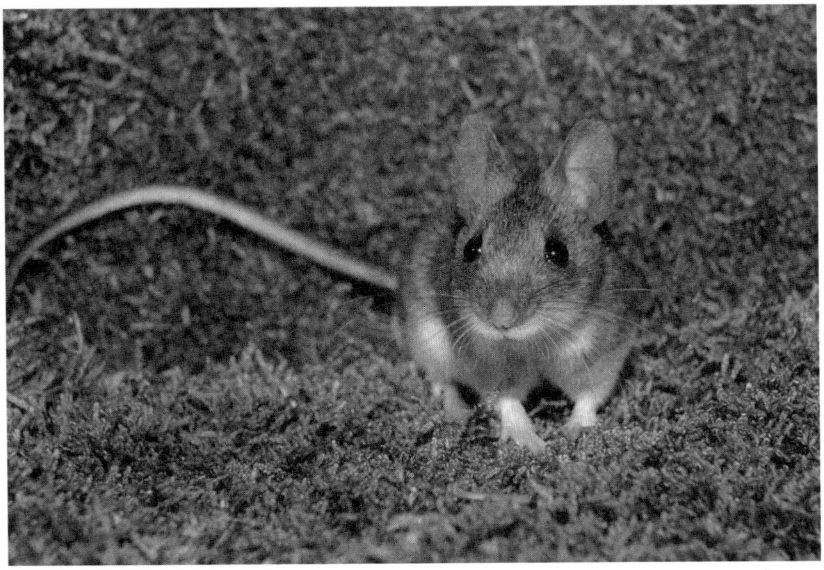

Figure 1.7 Yellow–necked field mouse (*Apodemus flavicollis*). Source: Jiri Bohdal.

such as blackbirds and pheasants, but *B. bavariensis* (formerly *B. garinii* serotype 4) is maintained in nature by *Apodemus* mice (Huegli et al., 2002) (Figure 1.7).

Human Factors

Risk of Lyme borreliosis can result from people's residential, occupational, or recreational activities, and in some cases it can be difficult to assign infection acquisition definitively to a single risk category. Many people living in Lyme disease endemic areas also take part in outdoor leisure activities there, away from their immediate home environments. Some are also employed in jobs such as forestry work or deer management that place them at significantly higher risk of tick bites than other local residents. In many high prevalence areas throughout Europe, traditional woodland activities such as wild berry-picking and mushroom gathering remain very popular, and for some people, especially in eastern countries, they may be important sources of food and income. Other activities such as professional or recreational deer-hunting also increase risk of infection acquisition. Housing developments in previously rural Lyme disease-endemic areas also expose new populations to risk of infection

A population-based prospective study of nearly 5000 people in southeastern Bavaria in 1996 and 1997 showed an incidence of Lyme disease of 7.1/1000 patient observation years (33 cases), and asymptomatic infection occurring in 7.6/1000 patient observation years (35 seroconversions, Reimer et al., 2002). Tick bites were reported by 1072 participants. The overall seroprevalence at the start of the study was 11%, which rose with increasing age and outdoor activity or employment. Residential risk is significant, especially for people who have gardens backing on to woodlands, but residential risk alone seems less marked in Europe than in the United States (Linard et al., 2007; Fitzner et al., 2002).

Recreational risk both at home and abroad seems to be very significant, and has risen in the past 15 years, correlating with the rising popularity of outdoor activities and holidays such as hiking, mountain-biking, and wildlife observation. There have been major developments in activity holiday travel to many regions within the expanded European Union and neighboring countries that have areas of high endemicity for Lyme borreliosis. The most popular times for outdoor recreation and vacations coincide with peak periods for tick feeding activities.

Epidemiological data, reviewed below, indicate that in most European countries there is a bimodal age effect for disease acquisition, with peaks occurring in the 5 to 15 and 40 to 60 age groups. Peak periods for the diagnosis of erythema migrans are late spring and summer, following the peak tick feeding periods. Acute neuroborreliosis cases peak 1 to 2 months later but may be diagnosed at any time through the year.

The age at which a person acquires infection may have some bearing on the clinical features of disseminated disease. The most common complication of Lyme borreliosis reported in children is facial palsy. Painful radiculopathy is more commonly diagnosed in older adults and is rare in children. Acrodermatitis chronica atrophicans is principally seen in older people and is reported more frequently in women than in men (Stanek and Strle, 2003).

European Clinical Case Definitions

European clinical case definitions, initially published in 1996 and updated in 2010, were developed as part of the EUCALB (European Union Concerted Action on Lyme Borreliosis) initiative http://meduni09.edis.at/eucalb/cms/index.php?lang=en (Stanek et al., 2010). They encompass the more common clinical presentations occurring in Europe, and have been helpful both in clinical practice and toward the standardization of epidemiological data (Stanek et al., 2010). Guidelines for the diagnosis and treatment of neuroborreliosis in Europe were published by the European Federation of Neurological Societies in 2010 (Mygland et al., 2009). Several other evidence-based diagnostic and treatment guidelines are also available from national authorities or specialist groups in Europe (HPA, 2011).

European Epidemiological Data

There is no standardized or centralized method of collecting epidemiological data on Lyme borreliosis in Europe (Hubálek, 2009), and there are currently no plans to add Lyme borreliosis to the listed diseases covered the coordinated disease surveillance by the European Community (Smith and Takkinen, 2006). The European Centre for Disease Control has commissioned an epidemiologic situation analysis, reporting in 2011 (http://www.ecdc.europa.eu/en/Pages/home.aspx). Epidemiological evidence is obtained piecemeal from numerous sources, including national or regional mandatory notification schemes in a few countries, surveillance schemes in some endemic regions, primary care surveys, seroprevalence studies, and reporting systems based on laboratory-confirmed cases. Some examples are given below and in Table 1.1.

Overall national figures have only limited value, especially in the larger, more industrialized countries where most of the population is urban dwelling, as they do not indicate regional and subregional variations in risk, which can be very marked. Regional and local

TABLE 1.1 Reported incidence of Lyme borreliosis/100,000 population in selected European countries

Country (Approx pop 10^6)	2001	2005	2008	Other Data	Comments
Portugal (10) *(MN)*	0.03	0.04	ND		See text and Lopes de Carvalho and Nuncio (2006)
Spain (40)	ND	ND	ND	9.8 in La Rioja (Lindgren and Jaenson, 2006)	Focal areas mainly in northern Spain
Ireland (3.8)	ND	ND	ND	1997 seroprevalence: park rangers: 3.4%; gen pop: 0.6% (Robertson et al., 1998)	Focal areas include Connemara, West Cork and Kerry
England and Wales (53.3) *(LC)*	0.5	1.1	1.72 (LD)	17% of confirmed cases acquired abroad	Estimated 15 in one focal area in 2007 (HPA, 2011)
Scotland (5.1) *(MN)*	0.6	1.7	5.5 (LD)	285 cases in 2008 (LD)	High prevalences in parts of highlands (HPA, 2011)
France (60)	ND	ND	ND	1999–2000: 9.4 national PC survey (Letrilliart et al., 2005) 2001–2003: 180–232 Alsace (prospective) (InVS, 2008)	Information on other endemic areas also available from InVS
Belgium (10.3)	9.7	16	ND	<3.65 – >31.78 in municipalities (Linard et al., 2007)	Additional data available in Linard et al. (2007)
Netherlands (16)	74 (est)	103 (est)	ND	43 (est) in 1995(De Mik et al., 1997); 103 (est) in 2005 (Hofhuis et al., 2006)	PC estimates for EM
Germany (82)	ND	ND	ND	60,000 cases/year estimated in 2002 (Mehnart and Krause, 2005)	See text and Reimer et al. (2002), Fitzner et al. (2002), Smith and Takkinen, (2006), Rath et al. (1996), Huppertz et al. (1999)
Switzerland (7.2)	ND	ND	ND	30.4 (Lindgren and Jaenson, 2006)	95 in Neuchatel canton 1996–1997 (Nahimana et al., 2000)

(continued)

TABLE 1.1 (*Continued*)

Country (Approx pop 10^6)	2001	2005	2008	Other Data	Comments
Italy (57.5)	0.02	ND	ND		
Denmark (5.3) (*MN of NB*)	ND	1.7-	1.1	1994–2004: 471 NB cases (EpiNorth, 2010)	82 NB cases in 2004 (Christiansen and Molbak, 2005)
Norway (4.5) *(MN of late stage disease)*	2.7	6.2	7.2	Marked increase in NB cases in 2004; reasons unclear (Nygard et al., 2005)	Prevalent in southern and central coastal counties (Nygard et al., 2005)
Sweden (8.8)	ND	ND	ND	1992–3: 69 in southern Sweden (Berglund et al., 1995) 1997–1998: 464 EM in PC (Bennet et al., 2006)	Prospective study 1992–1993 (Berglund et al., 1995). Retrospective case search 1997–2003 (Bennet et al., 2006)
Finland (5.2) *(LC)*	13	24	24.1	1999 est. 200 in southern archipelago (Junttila et al., 1999)	Seroprevalence in Aland islands adults 19.7% in 1996 (Carlsson et al., 1998)
Lithuania (3.7) *(LC)*	33	34	106.6		
Latvia (2.4) *(LC + C)*	16	21	31.8		
Estonia (1.4) *(LC)*	25	21	133.3		Highest risk around Finnish Gulf coast
Poland (38.6) *(MN)*	6.4	12	21.6	> 11.55 nationally in 2005 (Stefanoff et al., 2006)	100 focally in northeastern region (Flisiak and Prokopowicz, 1999)
Czech Republic (10.3) *(MN)*	35	36	—		
Slovakia (5.4)	13	16	—	2001 seroprevalence: gen pop: 5.4%; risk pop.: 16.8% (Stefancikova et al., 2001)	
Hungary (9.9)	13	12	—		

Austria (8.1)	ND	135 (est)	—	1997 seroprevalence: gen pop: 7.7% (Santino et al., 1997)	National data from physician estimate
Slovenia (2) *(MN)*	163	206	—		See text
Croatia (4.7)	ND	ND	—	3317 cases reported 1987–2003 (Mulic et al., 2006)	Northwest has highest incidence
Greece (10.6)	ND	ND	—	0.27% seroprevalence in naval recruits (Stamouli et al., 2000)	
Romania (22.4)	ND	ND	—	1999 seroprevalence: gen pop: 4–8%; risk pop. 9.3–31.7% (Hristea et al., 2001)	
Bulgaria (7.9)	4.5	13	—		

Note: Data for 2001 and 2005 from Eurosurveillance (Smith and Takkinen, 2006), for 2008 from EpiNorth (EpiNorth, 2010) and local reports; additional data from other sources.
Approx pop 10^6: approximate population in millions (Source: *Times Atlas of the World Mini Edition*, 2003, Times Books, Ltd.)

Abreviations

Est: estimated
Gen pop: general population
LC: laboratory-confirmed cases
LC + C: laboratory confirmed cases and clinical cases
LD: local data
MN: mandatory notification
NB: neuroborreliosis
ND: no data given in reference.
PC: primary care
Risk pop: risk population (forestry workers, etc.)

data analysis is important for the appropriate targeting of public health and clinical interventions.

About 85,000 cases are reported annually in Europe, but this is a considerable underestimate, both because of inconsistent case reporting mechanisms and underrecognition of disease manifestations, particularly erythema migrans (Lindgren and Jaenson, 2006). In 2002 it was estimated that at least 60,000 cases are likely to occur annually in Germany alone, giving an approximate incidence rate of 75/100,000 in that country (Mehnert and Krause, 2005).

Mandatory Reporting Schemes

Erythema migrans and other manifestations of the disease are mandatorily reportable nationally in Slovenia. Data for 2005 indicated an incidence rate of 206/100,000 (Smith and Takkinen, 2006). Despite the high degree of local awareness of Lyme borreliosis, it is recognized that notifications there are incomplete, especially with regard to erythema migrans (Strle, 1999). Slovenian data related to disseminated and late complications are likely to be more accurate because most patients with these presentations are managed within a few research-orientated medical institutions.

Neuroborreliosis has been notifiable in Denmark since 1994. Case notifications ranged from 41 in 2002 to 104 in 2006; the annual average is 83 (1.5/100,000) (Christiansen and Molbak, 2005). Cases of disseminated and late borreliosis have been notifiable in Norway since 1995 (Nygard et al., 2005). Annual incidence of neuroborreliosis varied from 75 to 200 cases in the 10 years 1995 to 2004 (average 3/100,000). There was a marked increase of nearly 100 cases between 2003 and 2004. As neurological complications are the most significant manifestations of disseminated and late Lyme borreliosis in Europe, data on neuroborreliosis obtained from the Slovenian, Danish, and Norwegian notification schemes give useful information on epidemiological trends in widely geographically separated areas of Europe.

Regional Clinical Surveillance and Prospective Studies

In some other countries case surveillance is regionally focused on areas of known high endemicity, such as Alsace and Limousin in France and in six eastern states of Germany (Mehnert and Krause, 2005, 2008; InVS, 2010). A French national primary care–based prospective study estimated an overall national incidence rate of 9.4/100,000 (Letrilliart et al., 2005), whereas data from the Alsace study suggested a regional rate of 180-232/100,000, which varied from 30 to 511/100,000 between individual cantons in the region. Erythema migrans was the only manifestation of disease in 90% of the cases; a further 5% had evidence of neuroborreliosis. Similar detailed and useful study reports are available for several other regions of France from L'Institut Veille Sanitaire (http://www.invs.sante.fr/surveillance/lyme/index.htm).

The extended notification scheme in the six eastern German states (Berlin, Brandenburg, Mecklenburg-Vorpommern, Sachsen, Sachsen-Anholt, and Thuringen) reported 3019 cases (17.8/100,000) in 2002 and 3968 (23.3/100,000) in 2003 (Mehnert and Krause, 2005). Most cases were erythema migrans (89.3% and 86.7%), with neuroborreliosis accounting for less than 4% of cases in either year. Two states, Brandenburg and Sachsen, accounted for 81% of the case reports. The incidence in Brandenburg was 74/100,000 in

2003, and it ranged from 10 to 237/100,000 in districts within the state. A prevalence study of forestry workers in Brandenburg performed in 1992 had shown a seroprevalence of 8% (Rath et al., 1996). Another German prospective study, which was performed in the Wurzburg region in 1996 following an extensive awareness campaign, reported an incidence rate of 111/100,000 (313 cases). Erythema migrans was the only manifestation in 89% of cases (Huppertz et al., 1999).

A primary care–based prospective study was performed in southern Sweden in 1992 to 1993 (Berglund et al., 1995). The overall annual incidence was 69/100,000 (1471 cases) and ranged focally from 26 to 160/100,000. Erythema migrans was the presenting feature in 77%; 16% had neuroborreliosis and 7% had arthritis. A later primary care–based retrospective study in southeastern Sweden estimated a mean annual incidence rate for erythema migrans of 464/100,000 between 1997 and 2003 (Bennet et al., 2006).

In addition to their epidemiological value, prospective community-based studies can provide longer term benefits to study populations, as they raise awareness of the condition, its clinical features, management, and prevention within primary and secondary care health care providers and the general community.

Laboratory-Based Surveillance

The great majority of specialized diagnostic tests for Lyme borreliosis in England and Wales are performed in a single laboratory, enabling development of an enhanced surveillance system based on detailed clinical and epidemiological information from laboratory-confirmed cases. Annual incidence of laboratory-confirmed cases rose from 268 (0.5/100,000) in 2001 to 973 (1.79/100,000) in 2009 (HPA, 2011). Erythema migrans cases are certainly underreported. Neuroborreliosis is the most common complication (10–20% of reported cases annually). Between 15% and 20% of infections annually were acquired abroad, mainly through recreational activities in mainland Europe or the United States. Most patients acquiring infection abroad are UK residents, but migrants from other European countries, including Poland, Hungary, and the Baltic republics, have featured significantly in this subgroup in recent years, following changes in employment opportunities in the enlarged European Union. About 70% of indigenously acquired cases occurred in southern counties and were associated mainly with recreational or residential risks. In the southwest, which includes several well-known endemic areas, the overall annual rate for 2007 was 4.7/100,000 and was estimated at 15/100,000 in one focal area. Few occupationally acquired symptomatic infections are identified annually. A small prevalence study of forestry workers showed an overall seroprevalence of 25% by two-tier testing, which increased with tick exposure risk and duration of employment, but no study participant had current disease and only 10% had Lyme disease–related symptoms in the past (Guy et al., 1989). A national study of agricultural workers showed a seroprevalence of only 0.2% (Thomas et al., 1999).

Some other countries also use laboratory-based surveillance, mainly as an adjunct to clinically-based studies or notification schemes (Mehnert and Krause, 2005). Variability in test requesting patterns and diagnostic methods limit the validity of direct comparisons of laboratory-based surveillance findings between countries. Nevertheless, some useful demographic, geographic, and seasonality data may be obtained, and referring clinicians and patients are approached for additional clinical and tick exposure risk information in some schemes.

Summary

Some general conclusions can be drawn from the available data, despite the difficulties posed by lack of a standardized European reporting system. It is also possible to assess trends from year to year in countries or regions that have stable reporting systems, be they based on mandatory notification, regional clinical reporting, or laboratory surveillance. Data on neuroborreliosis incidence could be particularly valuable as a sentinel for monitoring trends and for informing public health activities, as neurological manifestations are the most common and potentially most serious complications of European-acquired Lyme disease, and are likely to have a high degree of diagnostic specificity.

Lyme borreliosis is by far the most common vector-borne infection in Europe, with a widespread distribution, correlating overall with the distribution of *Ixodes ricinus* and *Ixodes persulcatus* ticks. Disease incidence increases from the west to the east of the continent, and decreases from south to north in Scandinavia and from north to south in Italy, Spain, Portugal, and Greece. The highest prevalence regions are included in the area extending eastward from a longitude of about 5° east and southward between latitudes 62° and 42° north, but there focal areas of high prevalence elsewhere. It is interesting that the early descriptions of various clinical presentations of Lyme borreliosis originated from physicians working in the areas of Europe where recent ecological, epidemiological, and clinical studies have indicated high infection prevalence.

Reported incidence has increased very significantly throughout Europe in recent years for several reasons. Public health efforts and media attention have led to far greater awareness of the disease, leading to diagnoses of cases that might otherwise have been unrecognized. There has also been a significant genuine increase in incidence, related to expansion in density and range of tick populations and increased recreational and residential human activities in tick habitats.

Asymptomatic or minimally symptomatic infections are common in many endemic areas. Seroprevalence in high-risk occupational groups is significant in many parts of Europe, and increases with age and years of exposure risk, but incidence of occupationally acquired clinical disease seems to be low.

Borrelia burgdorferi, A VERSATILE ZOONOTIC BACTERIUM

Borrelia burgdorferi is a eubacterial species (phylum Spirochaetes) that uses a variety of small mammals as its reservoir, and thus is a vector-borne, accidental, zoonotic infection of humans. A review of the voluminous literature on the biology of the organism is beyond the scope of this book. The reader is referred to the books *Lyme Borreliosis: Biology, Epidemiology and Control* and *Borrelia: Molecular Biology, Host Interaction and Pathogenesis* (Gray et al., 2002; Samuels and Radolf, 2010). Among many others, scientists at the Rocky Mountain laboratories of the NIH in Hamilton, Montana, continue to build on the knowledge spawned by isolation of the organism at their institute in 1981. The following brief summary is based in part on a current review by members of this group (Tilly et al., 2008).

Published genomes of the three major *Borrelia burgdorferi* genospecies reveal that all have a linear chromosome and several linear or circular plasmids (Fraser et al., 1997; Casjens, 2000; Casjens et al., 2000). The linear structure of the chromosome and plasmids is unusual in bacteria, which raises the question of whether it confers an evolutionary advantage for *Borrelia* species. It is clear that in several species certain plasmid-encoded genes are essential for infectivity or persistence in different hosts. In contrast with other disease-causing eubacteria, it has been difficult to define specific virulence factors in this species, leading to the concept of *B. burgdorferi* as an obligate parasite rather than a primary pathogen of mammals. A relatively small genome also distinguishes this spirochete from most free-living bacteria. *Borrelia burgdorferi* lacks many metabolic synthesis pathways and presumably derives essential nutrients and cofactors from the host. This also necessitates the use of highly enriched media for culture in the laboratory, most often containing rabbit serum (see Chapter 9).

Surface lipoproteins are perhaps the best fit for virulence factors in *B. burgdorferi*, as antibody responses to these are predictably present in disease. Certain lipoproteins, notably outer surface protein A (OspA), have a role in protecting against re-infection. The bacterium regulates the differential expression of these outer-surface proteins to cycle between its mammalian and tick hosts because it must adapt to different temperature and pH conditions in each host's internal environment. For example OspA is expressed while in the gut of the unfed tick, but OspC expression is detectable only after the tick has attached to a vertebrate host. Later during the course of mammalian infection the spirochete expresses other putative virulence factors, including antigenic variants from the variable major protein-like sequence expression locus (VlsE), which may help it evade the host immune system. Transcription of genes for differential lipoprotein expression such as OspC has been shown to be regulated by the rpoS and rpoN encoded alternative sigma factors, which modulate gene expression in response to certain environmental stresses. Studies done on plasmid retention and clonal variation of *B. burgdorferi* strain B31 passaged in mice showed that loss of two linear plasmids in particular, lp25 and lp28-1, abrogates the ability of the organism to invade multiple tissue sites. This indicates an essential role in virulence for their best-characterized gene products, nicotinamidase and VlsE proteins (Purser and Norris, 2000).

Several animal models have yielded valuable information on the pathogenesis of *B. burgdorferi* infection from either needle-injection or tick bite infection studies (Philipp and Johnson, 1994). Erythema migrans, bacteremia, and meningitis has been investigated in the rabbit model. Mice have been used to study facets of the immune response, protection from OspA vaccine, persistence of infection, carditis, and arthritis (Steere et al., 2005). Hamsters were an early model to study disseminated infection and arthritis. Dogs develop arthritis and CNS infection and have yielded data on response to antibiotic treatment. The rhesus macaque has been valuable in studying the course of neurologic infection, treatment studies, and development of diagnostic assays.

Mammalian toll-like receptor 2 [TLR2] is key to innate immune recognition of *B. burgdorferi* lipoprotein antigens components by phagocytic and antigen-presenting cells, which serve to limit the load of invading spirochetes. *Borrelia burgdorferi* genospecies also vary in their susceptibility to complement-mediated killing. Whereas *B. garinii* is highly susceptible, *B. afzelii* and *B. burgdorferi* ss express surface proteins, notably Erp proteins (Stevenson et al., 2002). These proteins confer resistance to complement-mediated killing by binding with host "H factors" that coat the bacterial surface. An argument has been made that complement factors play a role in the global ecology of Lyme borreliosis, being a key determinant of host specificity for particular genospecies (Kurtenbach et al., 1998, 2006). Neutralizing antibodies also mediate mammalian immunity, whereas transfer of T cells in a mouse model does not confer protection against

Borrelia. Neither the innate or adaptive immune responses alone are always sufficient to clear *Borrelia* infection. The concept of bacterial persistence in tissue sanctuaries, postulated to occur even after treated infection, has been cause for extensive investigation, but it is debatable whether interaction with extracellular matrix protects the bacteria from neutralizing antibodies (Cabello et al., 2007; Coburn et al., 2005). Recent findings contradict the concept that decorin and fibronectin binding proteins have a significant role in interaction with host extracellular matrix (Shi et al., 2006; Tilly et al., 2008). In tissue culture, spirochetes have been visualized inside a variety of cell types, but intracellular persistence of organisms has not been demonstrable in infected tissue from Lyme borreliosis patients or in animal models (Duray, 1987; Barthold et al., 1993; Steere et al., 2005).

The study of animal and human pathogenesis of *B. burgdorferi* infections is a burgeoning and vibrant area of research that spans genomics, immunology, molecular microbiology, entomology, veterinary biology, and field biology. *Borrelia* and tick researchers share and develop their research at a variety of scientific forums worldwide, and they have not only contributed greatly to better understanding of human infection but have also advanced the field of tick-borne diseases. Moreover elucidating the fundamental processes employed by the organism to infect and survive in such varied hosts has implications for other disease processes. Just one example is how the study of Lyme arthritis can provide clues to possible infectious triggers of other forms of arthritis.

The chapters that follow explain the biologic basis for the current approaches to diagnosis and management of Lyme borreliosis.

REFERENCES

Ackermann R, Gollmer E, Rehse-Kupper B: Progressive *Borrelia* encephalomyelitis. Chronic manifestation of erythema chronicum migrans disease of the nervous system. *Dtsch Med Wochenschr* 110:1039–1042; 1985.

Afzelius A: Verhandlungen der Dermatologischen Gesellschaft zu Stockholm, 28 Oct 1909. *Arch Dermatol Syph* 101:404; 1910.

Afzelius A: Erythema chronicum migrans. *Acta Derm Venereol* 2:120–125; 1921.

Anon: Lyme disease in Canada. *CMAJ* 144:177; 1991.

Anon: *The Vectorborne Human Diseases of Europe: Their Distribution and Burden on Public Health*. World Health Organization Regional Office for Europe; 2004.

Anon: National Lyme Disease Meeting March 8–9, 2006. Public Health Agency of Canada; 2006.

Asbrink E, Hovmark A, Hederstedt B: The spirochetal etiology of acrodermatitis chronica atrophicans Herxheimer. *Acta Derm Venereol* 64:506–512; 1984.

Bacon RM, Kugeler KJ, Mead PS: Surveillance for Lyme disease. United States, 1992–2006. *MMWR Surveill Summ* 57:1–9; 2008.

Bäfverstedt B: Uber Lymphadenosis benigna cutis. *Acta derm Venereol (Stockh)* 24:1–202; 1943.

Bammer H, Schenk K: Meningo–Myelo. Radiculitis after a tick bite with erythema. *Dtsch Z Nervenheilkd* 187:25–34; 1965.

Bannwarth A: Chronische lymphocytäre Meningitis, entzündliche Polyneuritis und "Rheumatismus." *Arch Psychiatr Nervenkr* 113:284–376; 1941.

Barbour AG: Isolation and cultivation of Lyme disease spirochetes. *Yale J Biol Med* 57:521–525; 1984.

Barthold SW, De Souza MS, Janotka JL, Smith AL, Persing DH: Chronic Lyme borreliosis in the laboratory mouse. *Am J Pathol* 143:959–971; 1993.

Benach JL, Bosler EM, Hanrahan JP, Coleman JL, Habicht GS, Bast TF, Cameron DJ, Ziegler JL, Barbour AG, Burgdorfer W, Edelman R, Kaslow RA: Spirochetes isolated from the blood of two patients with Lyme disease. *N Engl J Med* 308:740–742; 1983.

Bennet L, Halling A, Berglund J: Increased incidence of Lyme borreliosis in southern Sweden following mild winters and during warm, humid summers. *Eur J Clin Microbiol Infect Dis* 25:426–432; 2006.

Berglund J, Eitrem R, Ornstein K, Lindberg A, Ringer A, Elmrud H, Carlsson M, Runehagen A, Svanborg C, Norrby R: An epidemiologic study of Lyme disease in southern Sweden. *N Engl J Med* 333:1319–1327; 1995.

Biberstein H: Lymphozytome. *Zentralbl Hautkr* 6:70–71; 1923.

Binder E, Doepfmer R, Hornstein O: Experimental transmission of chronic erythema migrans from man to man. *Hautarzt* 6:494–496; 1955.

Brown RN, Lane RS, Dennis DT: Geographic distributions of tick-borne diseases and their vectors. *In* Goodman JL, Dennis DT, Sonenshine DE (eds): *Tick-Borne Diseases of Humans*. Washington, DC, American Society for Microbiology; 2005.

Buchwald A: Ein Fall von diffuser idiopathischer Haut-Artophie. *Arch Derm Syphilol* 10:553–556; 1883.

Burckhardt JL: Zur Frage der Follikel und Keimzentrenbildung in der haut. *Frankf Z Pathol* 6:352–359; 1911.

Burgdorfer W: Discovery of the Lyme disease spirochete and its relation to tick vectors. *Yale J Biol Med* 57:515–520; 1984.

Burgdorfer W: The historical road to the discovery of *Borrelia burgdorferi*. *In* Weber K, Burgdorfer WE (eds): *Aspects of Lyme Borreliosis*. Berlin, Springer; 1993a.

Burgdorfer W: How the discovery of *Borrelia burgdorferi* came about. *Clin Dermatol*, 11:335–338; 1993b.

Burgdorfer W, Barbour AG, Hayes SF, Benach JL, Grunwaldt E, Davis JP: Lyme disease. A tick-borne spirochetosis? *Science* 216:1317–1319; 1982.

Burgdorfer W, Barbour AG, Hayes SF, Peter O, Aeschlimann A: Erythema chronicum migrans. A tickborne spirochetosis. *Acta Trop* 40:79–83; 1983.

Burgdorfer W, Lane RS, Barbour AG, Gresbrink RA, Anderson JR: The western black-legged tick, *Ixodes pacificus*. A vector of *Borrelia burgdorferi*. *Am J Trop Med Hyg* 34:925–930; 1985.

Cabello FC, Godfrey HP, Newman SA: Hidden in plain sight. *Borrelia burgdorferi* and the extracellular matrix. *Trends Microbiol* 15:350–354; 2007.

Carlsson SA, Grandlund H, Nyman D, Wahlberg P: IgG seroprevalence of Lyme borreliosis in the population of the Aland Islands in Finland. *Scand J Infect Dis*, 30:501–503;1998.

Casjens S: *Borrelia* genomes in the year 2000. *J Mol Microbiol Biotechnol* 2:401–410; 2000.

Casjens S, Palmer N, van Vugt R, Huang WM, Stevenson B, Rosa P, Lathigra R, Sutton G, Peterson J, Dodson RJ, Haft D, Hickey E, Gwinn M, White O, Fraser CM: A bacterial genome in flux. The twelve linear and nine circular extrachromosomal DNAs in an infectious isolate of the Lyme disease spirochete *Borrelia burgdorferi*. *Mol Microbiol* 35:490–516; 2000.

CDC: Lyme disease. United States, 1980. *MMWR Morb Mortal Wkly Rep* 30:489–482, 497; 1981.

CDC: Lyme disease. United States, 1999. *MMWR Morb Mortal Wkly Rep* 50:181–185; 2001.

CDC: Lyme disease. United States, 2003–2005. *MMWR Morb Mortal Wkly Rep* 56:573–576; 2007.

CDC: Lyme disease (*Borrelia burgdorferi*) 2008 case definition; 2008.

CDC: Notice to readers: final 2008 reports of nationally notifiable infectious diseases. *MMWR Morb Mortal Wkly Rep* 58:856–869; 2009.

CDC: http://www.cdc.gov/ncidod/dvbid/lyme/ld_statistics.htm [Accessed January 26, 2011].

Christiansen AH, Molbak K: Neuroborreliosis 1994–2004. Statens Serum Institut; 2005.

Coburn J, Fischer JR, Leong JM: Solving a sticky problem. New genetic approaches to host cell adhesion by the Lyme disease spirochete. *Mol Microbiol* 57:1182–1195; 2005.

Comstedt P, Bergstrom S, Olsen B, Garpmo U, Marjavaara L, Mejlon H, Barbour AG, Bunikis J: Migratory passerine birds as reservoirs of Lyme borreliosis in Europe. *Emerg Infect Dis* 12:1087–1095; 2006.

Daniel M, Kriz B, Danielova V, Materna J, Rudenko N, Holubova J, Schwarzova L, Golovchenko M: Occurrence of ticks infected by tickborne encephalitis virus and *Borrelia* genospecies in mountains of the Czech Republic. *Euro Surveill* 10:E0503311; 2005.

Dayan NE, Rubin LG, Di John D, Sood SK: Hypoglycorrhachia in Lyme meningitis. *Pediatr Infect Dis J* 23:370–371; 2004.

De Mik EL, van Pelt W, Doctors-van Leeuwen BD, van der Veen A, Schellekens JF, Borgdorff MW: The geographical distribution of tick bites and erythema migrans in general practice in the Netherlands. *Int J Epidemiol* 26:451–457; 1997.

Dennis DT: Epidemiology, ecology, and prevention of Lyme disease. *In* Rahn DW, Evans J (eds): *Lyme Disease*. Philadelphia, American College of Physicians; 1998.

Dennis DT: Epidemiology of Lyme borreliosis. *In* Gray J, Kahl O, Lane RS, Stanek G (eds): *Lyme Borreliosis. Biology, Epidemiology and Control.* New York, CAB International; 2002.

Dennis DT: Rash decisions: Lyme disease, or not? *Clin Infect Dis* 41:966–968; 2005.

Dotevall L, Alestig K, Hanner P, Norkrans G, Hagberg L: The use of doxycycline in nervous system *Borrelia burgdorferi* infection. *Scand J Infect Dis Suppl* 53:74–79; 1988.

Duray PH: The surgical pathology of human Lyme disease. An enlarging picture. *Am J Surg Pathol*, 11 Suppl 1, 47–60; 1987.

Edlow JA: *Bull's Eye. Unraveling the Medical Mystery of Lyme Disease.* New Haven, Yale University Press; 2004.

Eisen L: The roles of birds, lizards, and rodents as hosts for the western black-legged tick *Ixodes pacificus*. *J Vector Ecol* 29:295–308; 2004.

Elliott DJ, Eppes SC, Klein JD: Teratogen update. Lyme disease. *Teratology* 64:276–281; 2001.

EpiNorth. http://www.epinorth.org/eway/default.aspx?pid=230&trg=MainArea_5260&MainArea_5260=5279:0:15,2937:1:0:0:::0:0 [Accessed May 8, 2010].

European Union Concerted Action on Lyme Borreliosis (EUCALB). *Prevention and Control.* http://meduni09.edis.at/eucalb/cms/index.php?lang=en [Accessed Jan. 22, 2011].

Fingerle V, Schulte-Spechtel UC, Ruzic –Sabljic E, Leonhard S, Hofmann H, Weber K, Pfister K, Strle F, Wilske B: Epidemiological aspects and molecular characterization of *Borrelia burgdorferi* s.l. from southern Germany with special respect to the new species *Borrelia spielmanii* sp. nov. *Int J Med Microbiol* 298:279–290; 2008.

Fitzner J, Ammon A, Baumann I, Talaska T, Schonberg A, Stobel K, Fingerle V, Wilske B, Petersen L: Risk factors in Lyme borreliosis. A German case-control study. *Int J Med Microbiol* 291(suppl 33): 220; 2002.

Flanagan BP: Erythema chronicum migrans Afzelius in Americans. *Arch Dermatol*, 86,410–411; 1962.

Flisiak R, Prokopowicz D: [Clinical picture of Lyme boreliosis]. *Wiad Parazytol* 45:143–149; 1999.

Fraser CM, Casjens S, Huang WM, Sutton GG, Clayton R, Lathigra R, White O, Ketchum KA, Dodson R, Hickey EK, Gwinn M, Dougherty B, Tomb JF, Fleischmann RD, Richardson D, Peterson J, Kerlavage AR, Quackenbush J, Salzberg S, Hanson M, van Vugt R, Palmer N, Adams MD, Gocayne J, Weidman J, Utterback T, Watthey L, McDonald L, Artiach P, Bowman C, Garland S, Fuji C, Cotton

MD, Horst K, Roberts K, Hatch B, Smith HO, Venter JC: Genomic sequence of a Lyme disease spirochaete, *Borrelia burgdorferi*. *Nature* 390:580–586; 1997.

Garin C, Bujadoux A: Paralysie par les tiques. *J Med Lyon* 71:765–767; 1922.

Gerber MA, Zalneraitis EL: Childhood neurologic disorders and Lyme disease during pregnancy. *Pediatr Neurol* 11:41–43; 1994.

Gerber MA, Shapiro ED, Burke GS, Parcells VJ, Bell GL: Lyme disease in children in southeastern Connecticut. Pediatric Lyme Disease Study Group. *N Engl J Med*, 335:1270–1274; 1996.

Gern L, Humair PF: Ecology of *Borrelia burgdorferi* sensu lato in Europe. *In* Gray J, Kahl O, Lane RS, Stanek G (eds): *Lyme Borreliosis: Biology, Epidemiology and Control*. Wallingford, Oxon, UK, CABI Publishing; 2002.

Gern L, Moran Cadenas F, Burri C: Influence of some climatic factors on *Ixodes ricinus* ticks studied along altitudinal gradients in two geographic regions in Switzerland. *Int J Med Microbiol;* 298 (Suppl 1): 55–59; 2008.

Ginsberg HS, Buckley PA, Balmforth MG, Zhioua E, Mitra S, Buckley FG: Reservoir competence of native North American birds for the lyme disease spirochete, *Borrelia burgdorferi*. *J Med Entomol* 42:445–449; 2005.

Gordillo G, Torres J, Solorzano F, Cedillo-Rivera R, Tapia-Conyer R, Munoz O: Serologic evidences suggesting the presence of *Borrelia burgdorferi* infection in Mexico. *Arch Med Res* 30:64–68; 1999.

Gordillo-Perez G, Torres J, Solorzano-Santos F, De Martino S, Lipsker D, Velazquez E, Ramon G, Onofre M, Jaulhac B: *Borrelia burgdorferi* infection and cutaneous Lyme disease, Mexico. *Emerg Infect Dis* 13:1556–1558; 2007.

Gotz H: [Acrodermatitis chronica atrophicans Hexheimer as an infectious disease.]. *Hautarzt* 5:491–504; 1954.

Gotz H: Die Acrodermatitis chronica atrophicans Herxheimer als Infektionskrankheit. *Hautarzt* 6:249–252; 1955.

Gray JS, Kahl O, Robertson JN, Daniel M, Estrada-Pena A, Gettinby G, Jaenson TG, Jensen P, Jongejan F, Korenberg E, Kurtenbach K, Zeman P: Lyme borreliosis habitat assessment. *Zentralbl Bakteriol* 287:211–228; 1998.

Gray J, Kahl O, Lane RS, Stanek G: *Lyme Borreliosis: Biology, Epidemiology and Control*. New York, CAB International; 2002.

Guy EC, Bateman DE, Martyn CN, Heckels JE, Lawton NF: Lyme disease. Prevalence and clinical importance of *Borrelia burgdorferi* specific IgG in forestry workers. *Lancet* 1:484–486; 1989.

Hanincova K, Kurtenbach K, Diuk-Wasser M, Brei B, Fish D: Epidemic spread of Lyme borreliosis. Northeastern United States. *Emerg Infect Dis* 12:604–611; 2006.

Handrahan JP, Benach JL, Coleman JL, Bosler EM, Morse DL, Cameron DJ, Edelman R, Kaslow RA: Incidence and cumulative frequency of endemic Lyme disease in a community. *J Infect Dis* 150:489–496; 1984.

Hauser W: Wahrscheinliche Infektionskrankheiten der Haut. *Handbuch Haut-und Geschlechtskrankheiten*. Berlin, Springer; 1965.

Hazard GW, Leland K, Mathewson HO: Erythema chronicum migrans and "Lyme arthritis." *JAMA* 236:2392; 1976.

Health Protection Agency (HPA): http://www.hpa.org.uk/Topics/InfectiousDiseases/InfectionsAZ/LymeDisease/ [Accessed Jan. 22, 2011].

Hellerström S: Erythema chronicum migrans Afzelii. *Acta Derm Venereol (Stockh)* 2:315; 1930.

Hellerström S: Erythema chronicum migrans Afzelius with meningitis. *Acta Derm Venereol* 31:227–234; 1951.

Herxheimer K, Hartmann K: [Uber acrodermatitis chronica atrophicans]. *Arch Dermatol Syph* 61:57–76; 1902.

Hoen AG, Margos G, Bent SJ, Diuk-Wasser MA, Barbour A, Kurtenbach K, Fish D: Phylogeography of *Borrelia burgdorferi* in the eastern United States reflects multiple independent Lyme disease emergence events. *Proc Natl Acad Sci USA* 106:15013–15008; 2009.

Hofhuis A, van der Giessen JW, Borgsteede FH, Wielinga PR, Notermans DW, van Pelt W: Lyme borreliosis in the Netherlands. Strong increase in GP consultations and hospital admissions in past 10 years. *Euro Surveill* 11:E0606222; 2006.

Hollstrom E: Successful treatment of erythema migrans Afzelius. *Acta Derm Venereol* 31:235–243; 1951.

Hopf HC: [Acrodermatitis chronica atrophicans (Herxheimer) and the nervous system. Analysis of clinical, physiologic, histologic and electromyographic findings]. *Monogr Gesamtgeb Neurol Psychiatr* 114:1–130; 1966.

Horstrup P, Ackermann R: [Tick born meningopolyneuritis (Garin-Bujadoux, Bannwarth) (author's transl)]. *Fortschr Neurol Psychiatr Grenzgeb* 41:583–606; 1973.

Hovmark A, Asbrink E, Olsson I: The spirochetal etiology of lymphadenosis benigna cutis solitaria. *Acta Derm Venereol* 66:479–484; 1986.

Hristea A, Hristescu S, Ciufecu C, Vasile A: Seroprevalence of *Borrelia burgdorferi* in Romania. *Eur J Epidemiol* 17:891–896; 2001.

Hubálek Z: Epidemiology of Lyme borreliosis. *Curr Probl Dermatol* 37:31–50; 2009.

Huegli D, Hu CM, Humair PF, Wilske B, Gern L: Apodemus species mice are reservoir hosts of *Borrelia garinii* OspA serotype 4 in Switzerland. *J Clin Microbiol* 40:4735–4737; 2002.

Huppertz HI, Bohme M, Standaert SM, Karch H, Plotkin SA: Incidence of Lyme borreliosis in the Wurzburg region of Germany. *Eur J Clin Microbiol Infect Dis* 18:697–703; 1999.

Institut de veille sanitaire (INVS): *La maladie de Lyme: Donnees de reseau du surveillance de la maladie en Alsace Mars 2001–Fev 2003* (2008). http://www.nvs.sante.fr/publications/2005/lyme_alsace/index.html [Accessed May 8, 2010].

Institut de veille sanitaire (INVS): *Surveillance de la maladie de Lyme - Réseau Alsace, 2001–2003.* http://www.invs.sante.fr/surveillance/lyme/reseau_alsace.htm [Accessed Jan. 22, 2011].

Johnson BJB: Personal Communication; 2008.

Johnson RC, Schmid GP, Hyde FW, Steigerwalt AG, Brenner DJ: *Borrelia burgdorferi* sp. nov. Etiologic agent of Lyme disease. *International Journal of Systematic Bacteriology* 34, 496–497; 1984.

Junttila J, Peltomaa M, Soini H, Marjamaki M, Viljanen MK: Prevalence of *Borrelia burgdorferi* in *Ixodes ricinus* ticks in urban recreational areas of Helsinki. *J Clin Microbiol* 37:1361–1365; 1999.

Kaufmann-Wolf M: [Uber guartige lymphocytare Neubildungen der Scrotalhaut des Kindes]. *Arch fur Dermatol Syph (Berlin)* 130:425–435; 1921.

Kirstein F, Rijpkema S, Molkenboer M, Gray JS: Local variations in the distribution and prevalence of *Borrelia burgdorferi* sensu lato genomospecies in *Ixodes ricinus* ticks. *Appl Environ Microbiol* 63:1102–1106; 1997.

Kristoferitsch W: Neurologic manifestations in Lyme borreliosis. *Clin Dermatol* 11:393–400; 1993.

Kurtenbach K, Sewell HS, Ogden NH, Randolph SE, Nuttall PA: Serum complement sensitivity as a key factor in Lyme disease ecology. *Infect Immun* 66:1248–1251; 1998.

Kurtenbach K, Hanincova K, Tsao JI, Margos G, Fish D, Ogden NH: Fundamental processes in the evolutionary ecology of Lyme borreliosis. *Nat Rev Microbiol* 4:660–669; 2006.

Lane RS, Loye JE: Lyme disease in California. Interrelationship of ixodid ticks (Acari), rodents, and *Borrelia burgdorferi*. *J Med Entomol* 28:719–725; 1991.

Lane RS, Quistad GB: Borreliacidal factor in the blood of the western fence lizard (*Sceloporus occidentalis*). *J Parasitol* 84:29–34; 1998.

Lastavica CC, Wilson ML, Berardi VP, Spielman A, Deblinger RD: Rapid emergence of a focal epidemic of Lyme disease in coastal Massachusetts. *N Engl J Med* 320:133–137; 1989.

Letrilliart L, Ragon B, Hanslik T, Flahault A: Lyme disease in France. A primary care-based prospective study. *Epidemiol Infect* 133:935–942; 2005.

Linard C, Lamarque P, Heyman P, Ducoffre G, Luyasu V, Tersago K, Vanwambeke SO, Lambin EF: Determinants of the geographic distribution of Puumala virus and Lyme borreliosis infections in Belgium. *Int J Health Geogr* 6:15; 2007.

Lindenmayer JM, Marshall D, Onderdonk AB: Dogs as sentinels for Lyme disease in Massachusetts. *Am J Public Health* 81:1448–1455; *1991*.

Lindgren E, Jaenson TGT: Lyme borreliosis in Europe. Influences of climate and climate change, epidemiology, ecology and adaptation measures. Geneva, World Health Organization Regional Office for Europe; 2006.

Lipschütz B: Über eine seltene Erythemform (Erythema chronicum migrans). *Archiv fur Dermatologic und Syphilis* 118:349–356; 1913.

Lipschütz B: Weiterer Beitrag zur Kenntnis des "Erythema chronicum migrans." *Arch Dermatol Syph* 143:365–374; 1923.

Logiudice K, Ostfeld RS, Schmidt KA, Keesing F: The ecology of infectious disease. Effects of host diversity and community composition on Lyme disease risk. *Proc Natl Acad Sci USA* 100:567–571; 2003.

Lopes de Carvalho I, Nuncio MS: Laboratory diagnosis of Lyme borreliosis at the Portuguese National Institute of Health (1990–2004). *Euro Surveill* 11:257–260; 2006.

Lunemann JD, Zarmas S, Priem S, Franz J, Zschenderlein R, Aberer E, Klein R, Schouls L, Burmester GR, Krause A: Rapid typing of *Borrelia burgdorferi* sensu lato species in specimens from patients with different manifestations of Lyme borreliosis. *J Clin Microbiol* 39:1130–1133; 2001.

Mac MJ, Opler PA, Puckett Haecker CE, Doran PD: Northeast: Forest changes. *In* U.S. Geological Survey (ed): *Status and Trends of the Nation's Biological Resources*. Vol. 2. Reston, VA, U.S. Department of the Interior; 1998.

Maraspin V, Cimperman J, Lotric-Furlan S, Ruzic-Sabljic E, Jurca T, Picken RN, Strle F: Solitary borrelial lymphocytoma in adult patients. *Wien Klin Wochenschr* 114:515–523; 2002.

Margos G, Gatewood AG, Aanensen DM, Hanincova K, Terekhova D, Vollmer SA, Cornet M, Piesman J, Donaghy M, Bormane A, Hurn MA, Feil EJ, Fish D, Casjens S, Wormser GP, Schwartz I, Kurtenbach K: MLST of housekeeping genes captures geographic population structure and suggests a European origin of *Borrelia burgdorferi*. *Proc Natl Acad Sci USA* 105:8730–8735; 2008.

Margos G, Vollmer SA, Cornet M, Garnier M, Fingerle V, Wilske B, Bormane A, Vitorino L, Collares-Pereira M, Drancourt M, Kurtenbach K: A new *Borrelia* species defined by multilocus sequence analysis of housekeeping genes. *Appl Environ Microbiol* 75:5410–5416; 2009.

Marshall W F III, Telford S R III, Rys PN, Rutledge BJ, Mathiesen D, Malawista SE, Spielman A, Persing DH: Detection of *Borrelia burgdorferi* DNA in museum specimens of Peromyscus leucopus. *J Infect Dis* 170:1027–1032; 1994.

Mast WE, Burrows WM: Erythema chronicum migrans and "Lyme arthritis." *JAMA* 236:2392; 1976a.

Mast WE, Burrows WM Jr: Erythema chronicum migrans in the United States. *JAMA* 236:859–860; 1976b.

Masters EJ, Donnell HD: Lyme and/or Lyme-like disease in Missouri. *Mo Med* 92:346–353; 1995.

Mehnert WH, Krause G: Surveillance of Lyme borreliosis in Germany, 2002 and 2003. *Euro Surveill* 10:83–85; 2005.

Mulic R, Antonijevic S, Klismanic Z, Ropac D, Lucev O: Epidemiological characteristics and clinical manifestations of Lyme borreliosis in Croatia. *Mil Med* 171:1105–1109; 2006.

Mygland A, Ljostad U, Fingerle V, Rupprecht T, Schmutzhard E, Steiner I: European Federation of Neurological Societies. EFNS guidelines on the diagnosis and management of European Lyme neuroborreliosis. *Eur J Neurol* 17:8–16; 2010.

Nahimana I, Gern L, Peter O, Praz G., Moosmann Y, Francioli P: [Epidemiology of Lyme borreliosis in French-speaking Switzerland]. *Schweiz Med Wochenschr* 130:1456–1461; 2000.

Nygard K, Brantsaeter AB, Mehl R: Disseminated and chronic Lyme borreliosis in Norway, 1995–2004. *Euro Surveill* 10:235–238; 2005.

Ogden NH, Marouf A, Barker IK, Bigras-Poulin M, Lindsay LR, Morshed MG, O'Callaghan CJ, Ramay F, Waltner-Toews D, Charron DF: Climate change and the potential for range expansion of the Lyme disease vector *Ixodes scapularis* in Canada. *Int J Parasitol* 36:63–70; 2006.

Ogden NH, Lindsay LR, Hanincova K, Barker IK, Bigras-Poulin M, Charron DF, Heagy A, Francis CM, O'Callaghan CJ, Schwartz I, Thompson RA: Role of migratory birds in introduction and range expansion of *Ixodes scapularis* ticks and of *Borrelia burgdorferi* and *Anaplasma phagocytophilum* in Canada. *Appl Environ Microbiol* 74:1780–1790; 2008a.

Ogden NH, Lindsay LR, Morshed M, Sockett PN, Artsob H: The rising challenge of Lyme borreliosis in Canada. *Can Commun Dis Rep* 34:1–19; 2008b.

Paschoud JM: [Lymphocytoma after tick bite]. *Dermatologica* 108:435–437; 1954.

Paschoud JM: [*Lymphadenosis benigna cutis* as a communicable infectious disease; new viewpoints on its course, histology and therapy]. *Hautarzt* 8:197–211; 1957.

Petersen LR, Sweeney AH, Checko PJ, Magnarelli LA, Mshar PA, Gunn RA, Hadler JL: Epidemiological and clinical features of 1,149 persons with Lyme disease identified by laboratory-based surveillance in Connecticut. *Yale J Biol Med* 62:253–262; 1989.

Pfister HW, Preac-Mursic V, Wilske B, Schielke E, Sorgel F, Einhaupl KM: Randomized comparison of ceftriaxone and cefotaxime in Lyme neuroborreliosis. *J Infect Dis* 163:311–318; 1991.

Philipp MT, Johnson BJ: Animal models of Lyme disease: pathogenesis and immunoprophylaxis. *Trends Microbiol* 2:431–437; 1994.

Philipp MT, Masters E, Wormser GP, Hogrefe W, Martin D: Serologic evaluation of patients from Missouri with erythema migrans-like skin lesions with the C6 Lyme test. *Clin Vaccine Immunol* 13:1170–1171; 2006.

Piesman J, Gern L: Lyme borreliosis in Europe and North America. *In* Bowman AS, Nuttall, PA (eds): *Ticks: Biology, Disease, and Control.* Cambridge University Press, Cambridge, UK, 2008, pp. 220–252.

Purser JE, Norris SJ: Correlation between plasmid content and infectivity in *Borrelia burgdorferi. Proc Natl Acad Sci USA* 97:13865–13870; 2000.

Qiu WG, Bruno JF, McCaig WD, Xu Y, Livey I, Schriefer ME, Luft BJ: Wide distribution of a high-virulence *Borrelia burgdorferi* clone in Europe and North America. *Emerg Infect Dis* 14:1097–1104; 2008.

Rand PW, Lacombe EH, Dearborn R, Cahill B, Elias S, Lubelczyk CB, Beckett GA, Smith RP Jr: Passive surveillance in Maine, an area emergent for tick-borne diseases. *J Med Entomol* 44:1118–1129; 2007.

Rath PM, Ibershoff B, Mohnhaupt A, Albig J, Eljaschewitsch B, Jurgens D, Horbach I, Fehrenbach FJ: Seroprevalence of Lyme borreliosis in forestry workers from Brandenburg, Germany. *Eur J Clin Microbiol Infect Dis* 15:372–377; 1996.

Reimer B, Erbas B, Lobbichler K, Truckenbrodt R, Gartner-Kothe U, Kapeller N, Hansen M, Fingerle V, Wilske B, von Sonnenberg F: Seroprevalence of Borrelia infection in occupational tick-exposed people in Bavaria (Germany). *Int J Med Microbiol* 291(suppl 33): 215; 2002.

Robertson JN, Gray JS, Macdonald S, Johnson H: Seroprevalence of *Borrelia burgdorferi* sensu lato infection in blood donors and park rangers in relation to local habitat. *Zentralbl Bakteriol* 288:293–301; 1998.

Rothermel H, Hedges T.R. III, Steere AC: Optic neuropathy in children with Lyme disease. *Pediatrics* 108:477–481; 2001.

Rupprecht TA, Koedel U, Fingerle V, Pfister HW: The pathogenesis of Lyme neuroborreliosis. From infection to inflammation. *Mol Med* 14:205–212; 2008.

Samuels DS, Radolf JD (eds): *Borrelia. Molecular Biology, Host Interaction and Pathogenesis.* Norfolk, UK, Caister Academic Press; 2010.

Santino I, Dastoli F, Sessa R, Del Piano M: Geographical incidence of infection with *Borrelia burgdorferi* in Europe. *Panminerva Med* 39:208–214; 1997.

Schaltenbrand G: Chronische aseptische Meningitis. *Nervenarzt* 20:433–442; 1949.

Schaltenbrand G: Radikulomyelomeningitis nach Zeckenbiss. *Munch Med Wochenschr* 104:829–834; 1962.

Schlesinger PA, Duray PH, Burke BA, Steere AC, Stillman MT: Maternal-fetal transmission of the Lyme disease spirochete, *Borrelia burgdorferi*. *Ann Intern Med* 103:67–68; 1985.

Schmid GP: The global distribution of Lyme disease. *Yale J Biol Med* 57:617–618; 1984.

Schrock CG: Lyme disease: additional evidence of widespread distribution. Recognition of a tick-borne dermatitis-encephalitis-arthritis syndrome in an area of known ixodes tick distribution. *Am J Med* 72:700–706; 1982.

Scrimenti RJ: Erythema chronicum migrans. *Arch Dermatol* 102:104–105; 1970.

Scrimenti RJ, Scrimenti M: Lyme disease redux: the legacy of Sven Hellerstrom. *Wis Med J* 92:20–21; 1993.

Shi Y, Xu Q, Seemanapalli SV, McShan K, Liang FT: The dbpBA locus of *Borrelia burgdorferi* is not essential for infection of mice. *Infect Immun* 74:6509–6512; 2006.

Smith R, Takkinen J: Lyme borreliosis. Europe-wide coordinated surveillance and action needed? *Euro Surveill* 11:E0606221: 2006.

Stamouli M, Totos G, Braun HB, Michel G, Gizaris V: Very low seroprevalence of Lyme borreliosis in young Greek males. *Eur J Epidemiol* 16:495–496; 2000.

Stanek G, Strle F: Lyme borreliosis. *Lancet* 362:1639–1647; 2003.

Stanek G, Fingerle V, Hunfeld KP, Jaulhac B, Kaiser R, Krause A, Kristoferitsch W, O'Connell S, Ornstein K, Strle F, Gray J: Lyme borreliosis. Clinical case definitions for diagnosis and management in Europe. *Clin Microbiol Infect;* 17:69–79; 2011.

Stanek G, Wormser GP, Gray J, Strle F: Lyme borreliosis. *Lancet* 2011 (in press).

Steere AC: Lyme disease. A growing threat to urban populations. *Proc Natl Acad Sci USA* 91:2378–2383; 1994.

Steere AC: Lyme borreliosis in 2005, 30 years after initial observations in Lyme Connecticut. *Wien Klin Wochenschr* 118:625–633; 2006.

Steere AC, Malawista SE, Hardin JA, Ruddy S, Askenase W, Andiman WA: Erythema chronicum migrans and Lyme arthritis. The enlarging clinical spectrum. *Ann Intern Med* 86:685–698; 1977a.

Steere AC, Malawista SE, Snydman DR, Shope RE, Andiman WA, Ross MR, Steele FM: Lyme arthritis. An epidemic of oligoarticular arthritis in children and adults in three Connecticut communities. *Arthritis Rheum* 20:7–17; 1977b.

Steere AC, Broderick TF, Malawista SE: Erythema chronicum migrans and Lyme arthritis. Epidemiologic evidence for a tick vector. *Am J Epidemiol* 108:312–321; 1978.

Steere AC, Malawista SE: Cases of Lyme disease in the United States. Locations correlated with distribution of *Ixodes dammini*. *Ann Intern Med* 91:730–733; 1979.

Steere AC, Malawista SE, Newman JH, Spieler PN, Bartenhagen NH: Antibiotic therapy in Lyme disease. *Ann Intern Med* 93:1–8; 1980.

Steere AC, Grodzicki RL, Kornblatt AN, Craft JE, Barbour AG, Burgdorfer W, Schmid GP, Johnson E, Malawista SE: The spirochetal etiology of Lyme disease. *N Engl J Med* 308:733–740; 1983.

Steere AC, Snydman D, Murray P, Mensch J, Main AJ Jr, Wallis RC, Shope RE, Malawista SE: Historical perspective of Lyme disease. *Zentralbl Bakteriol Mikrobiol Hyg [A]* 263:3–6; 1986a.

Steere AC, Taylor E, Wilson ML, Levine JF, Spielman A: Longitudinal assessment of the clinical and epidemiological features of Lyme disease in a defined population. *J Infect Dis* 154:295–300; 1986b.

Steere AC, Coburn J, Glickstein L: The emergence of Lyme disease. *J Clin Invest* 113:1093–1101; 2004.

Steere AC, Coburn J, Glickstein L: Lyme borreliosis. *In* Goodman JL, Dennis DT, Sonenshine DE (eds): *Tick-Borne Diseases of Humans*. Washington, DC, American Society for Microbiology; 2005.

Stefancikova A, Pet'ko B, Rozicka I, Salyova N, Ohlasova D: Epidemiological survey of human borreliosis diagnosed in eastern Slovakia. *Ann Agric Environ Med* 8:171–1715; 2001.

Stefanoff P, Rosinska M, Zielinski A: [Epidemiology of tick-borne diseases in Poland]. *Przegl Epidemiol*, 60(suppl 1):151–159; 2006.

Stevenson B, El-Hage N, Hines MA, Miller JC, Babb K: Differential binding of host complement inhibitor factor H by *Borrelia burgdorferi* Erp surface proteins. A possible mechanism underlying the expansive host range of Lyme disease spirochetes. *Infect Immun* 70:491–497; 2002.

Stiernstedt G, Gustafsson R, Karlsson M, Svenungsson B, Skoldenberg B: Clinical manifestations and diagnosis of neuroborreliosis. *Ann NY Acad Sci* 539:46–55; 1988.

Strle F: Lyme borreliosis in Slovenia. *Zentralbl Bakteriol* 289:643–652; 1999.

Strobino BA, Williams CL, Abid S, Chalson R, Spierling P: Lyme disease and pregnancy outcome. A prospective study of two thousand prenatal patients. *Am J Obstet Gynecol* 169:367–374; 1993.

Strobino B, Abid S, Gewitz M: Maternal Lyme disease and congenital heart disease. A case-control study in an endemic area. *Am J Obstet Gynecol* 180:711–716; 1999.

Svarts N: Penicillinbehandling vid dermatitis atrophicans Herxheimer. *Nord Med* 32:2783; 1946.

Sweitzer SE, Laymon CW: *Acrodermatitis Chronica Atrophicans*. *Arch Derm Syphilol*, 31:196–211; 1935.

Thomas DR, Salmon RL, Coleman TJ, Morgan-Capner P, Sillis M, Caul EO, Morgan KL, Paiba GA, Bennett M, Ribeiro D, Lloyd G, Kench SM, Meadows D, Softley P, Chalmers RM: Occupational exposure to animals and risk of zoonotic illness in a cohort of farmers, farmworkers, and their families in England. *J Agricultural Safety Health* 5:373–382; 1999.

Thyresson N: The penicillin treatment of acrodermatitis atrophicans chronica (Herxheimer). *Acta Derm Venereol* 29:572–621; 1949.

Tilly K, Rosa PA, Stewart PE: Biology of infection with *Borrelia burgdorferi*. *Infect Dis Clin North Am* 22:217–234; 2008.

Varela AS, Luttrell MP, Howerth EW, Moore VA, Davidson WR, Stallknecht DE, Little SE: First culture isolation of *Borrelia* lonestari, putative agent of southern tick-associated rash illness. *J Clin Microbiol* 42:1163–1169; 2004.

Wang G, van Dam AP, Schwartz I, Dankert J: Molecular typing of *Borrelia burgdorferi* sensu lato. Taxonomic, epidemiological, and clinical implications. *Clin Microbiol Rev* 12:633–653; 1999.

Weber K: [Erythema chronicum migrans meningitis—a bacterial infectious disease? (author's transl))]. *MMW Munch Med Wochenschr* 116:1993–1998; 1974.

Weber K: Remarks on the infectious disease caused by *Borrelia burgdorferi*. *Zentralbl Bakteriol Mikrobiol Hyg [A]* 263:206–208; 1986.

Weber K, Bratzke HJ, Neubert U, Wilske B, Duray PH: *Borrelia burgdorferi* in a newborn despite oral penicillin for Lyme borreliosis during pregnancy. *Pediatr Infect Dis J* 7:286–289; 1988.

Weber K, Burgdorfer W: *Aspects of Lyme Borreliosis*. Berlin, Springer; 1993.

Weber K, Pfister HW: History of Lyme borreliosis in Europe. *In* Weber K, Burgdorfer WE (eds): *Aspects of Lyme Borreliosis*. Berlin, Springer; 1993.

Weber K, Schierz G, Wilske B, Preac-Mursic V: [Lymphocytoma—a borreliosis?] *Z Hautkr* 60:1585–1598; 1985.

White DJ, Chang HG, Benach JL, Bosler EM, Meldrum SC, Means RG, Debbie JG, Birkhead GS, Morse DL: The geographic spread and temporal increase of the Lyme disease epidemic. *JAMA* 266:1230–1236; 1991.

Wormser GP, Masters E, Liveris D, Nowakowski J, Nadelman RB, Holmgren D, Bittker S, Cooper D, Wang G, Schwartz I: Microbiologic evaluation of patients from Missouri with erythema migrans. *Clin Infect Dis* 40:423–428; 2005.

2

THE SPIROCHETES AND VECTOR TICKS OF LYME BORRELIOSIS IN NATURE

Joseph Piesman and Pierre-François Humair

The ticks that transmit Lyme disease spirochetes are a group of closely related species in the genus *Ixodes*: *I. scapularis* and *I. pacificus* in North America, *I. ricinus* in Europe, and *I. persulcatus* in Eurasia (Table 2.1). Although all four of these tick species have unique aspects to their biology and ecology, they share important traits that result in their remarkable public health impact. They are widely distributed over large areas of the Northern Hemisphere, where rainfall is high and deciduous forests predominate (Figure 2.1). The six-legged larval ticks generally acquire infection with the Lyme disease spirochete by feeding on a rodent or a bird, molt to the nymphal stage, and transmit infection to another animal host or human as eight-legged nymphs. The nymphs are quite small (<2 mm), and are often able to transmit spirochetes to their victim while escaping detection. Nymphs are the principal vector stage where *I. scapularis, I. pacificus,* and *I. ricinus* are the primary vectors (Piesman, 1989). Adults generally feed on a larger host, like deer. In some areas of Eurasia where *I. persulcatus* is the primary vector, transmission by adult ticks may be common (Korenberg et al., 2002). All three active life stages quest on forest vegetation or in the edge habitat called ecotone (Maupin et al., 1991) where they are likely to come into contact with humans. Thus they serve as excellent vectors of zoonotic disease agents, transmitting pathogens from animals to humans. In different parts of the world they transmit the etiologic agents that cause Lyme disease, human granulocyctic anaplasmosis (previously known as HGE), human babesiosis, as well as tick-borne encephalitis.

Lyme Borreliosis in Europe and North America: Epidemiology and Clinical Practice, First Edition. Edited by Sunil K. Sood

TABLE 2.1 Principal vector ticks and spirochetes associated with Lyme borreliosis

Ticks Species	Distribution	Genotype of *B. burgdorferi*
Ixodes scapularis	Eastern North America	*B. burgdorferi* sensu stricto
Ixodes pacificus	Western North America	*B. burgdorferi* sensu stricto
Ixodes ricinus	Western and central Europe[a]	*B. garinii, B. afzelii, B. burgdorferi* sensu stricto
Ixodes persulcatus	Central Europe and Asia	*B. garinii, B. afzelii*

[a]*B. spielmanii, B. lusitaniae,* and *B. valaisiana* occasionally isolated from humans; *B. garinii* serotype 4 aka *B. bavariensis.*

The blacklegged tick or "deer tick," *Ixodes scapularis*, is the principal vector of Lyme disease spirochetes in North America. Although populations of this tick might have once covered the entire eastern half of North America, land use practices around the end of the nineteenth century had a dramatic impact on its distribution. As forests were cleared for agricultural purposes, and deer aggressively hunted to near extinction in much of the eastern United States (Spielman, 1988), the distribution of *I. scapularis* probably shrunk to a few refugia where deer were still found. After World War II much of this land converted from agriculture to suburban housing with secondary growth of the forest; this resulted in a huge upsurge in white-tailed deer. The white-tailed deer population was estimated to be as high as 17 million animals in 1997 (McCabe and McCabe, 1997), and is undoubtedly higher today. Slowly but surely, *I. scapularis* has regained much of its former range (Dennis et al., 1998) and come into increasing contact with people. This has helped fuel the Lyme disease epidemic in North America over the last 30 years. The role of climate change and the future of Lyme disease expansion in North America have received considerable recent attention (Ogden et al., 2008b).

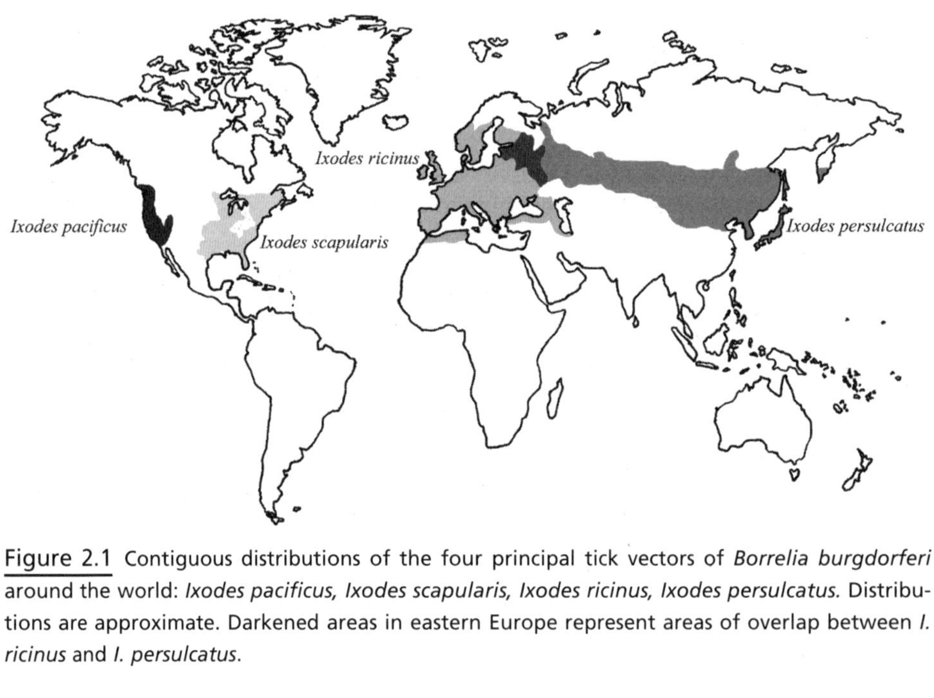

Figure 2.1 Contiguous distributions of the four principal tick vectors of *Borrelia burgdorferi* around the world: *Ixodes pacificus, Ixodes scapularis, Ixodes ricinus, Ixodes persulcatus.* Distributions are approximate. Darkened areas in eastern Europe represent areas of overlap between *I. ricinus* and *I. persulcatus.*

The castor-bean tick or "sheep tick," *I. ricinus*, is the primary vector of Lyme disease spirochetes in Europe. Although clinical manifestations of the disease were described at the end of the nineteenth century in Europe, it took a century to bring out the involvement of *I. ricinus* (Burgdorfer et al., 1983). This tick is found in a variety of habitats in Europe, from urban parks in Berlin to remote island locations in the Baltic Sea. In Europe exposure to *I. ricinus* may be more common in recreational settings than in residential areas.

The taiga tick (so named for the coniferous forests that dominate northern latitudes particularly in Siberia), *I. persulcatus,* is the primary vector of Lyme disease spirochetes in eastern Europe and Asia. The current chapter will focus on the biological and ecological characteristics of *I. scapularis* and *I. ricinus* that make these two tick species such efficient vectors of Lyme disease spirochetes in North America and Europe.

DIVERSITY OF SPIROCHETES

North America

In North America several genospecies of *Borrelia burgdorferi* sensu lato (s.l.). have been described in *Ixodes* ticks. Clearly, the predominant spirochete found in *I. scapularis* populations throughout its range is *B. burgdorferi* sensu stricto (s.s.) (Qiu et al., 2002). Approximately 25% of nymphal *I. scapularis* and 50% of adults are infected with *B. burgdorferi* s.s. in areas of the northeastern United States where the cycle is most efficient. Another genospecies, *B. bissettii*, was first reported from a single *I. scapularis* tick from New York State (Anderson et al., 1988). Subsequently isolates of *B. bissettii* from *I. scapularis* have been extremely rare, whereas isolates of this genospecies from the non–person-biting tick *I. spinipalpis* in the western United States have been frequent (Postic et al., 1998; Norris et al., 1999). A third genospecies of *B. burgdorferi* s.l. present in North American *Ixodes*, *B. andersonii* (Marconi et al., 1995), appears to be limited to infecting cottontail rabbits and the associated rabbit tick *I. dentatus*. Recently *B. californiensis* was described infecting kangaroo rats in the western United States (Postic et al., 2007), and *B. carolinensis* was described from rodents in South Carolina (Rudenko et al., 2009). A spirochete that more closely resembles relapsing fever spirochetes than *B. burgdorferi* s.l. has been described in *I. scapularis* (Scoles et al., 2001). This spirochete has been found to be closely related to an isolate made from *I. persulcatus* in Japan; indeed all the "hard tick relapsing fever" isolates found in *Ixodes* are closely related and have been termed *B. miyamotoi* s.l. (Bunikis et al., 2004). Another hard tick relapsing fever spirochete, *B. lonestari*, has been isolated from the lone star tick, *Amblyomma americanum* (Varela et al., 2004). Although a diversity of *Borrelia* have been isolated from ticks in North America, it is important to stress that all well-characterized human isolates of *Borrelia* from Lyme disease patients in North America have proved to be *B. burgdorferi* s.s. to date (Liveris et al., 1999; Terekhova et al., 2006).

Europe

In Europe seven genospecies of *B. burgdorferi* s.l. have been described within the *I. ricinus* tick vector: *B. burgdorferi* s.s., *B. afzelii, B. garinii* (various serotypes have been described for *B. garinii* [Wilske et al., 1993], and serotype 4 has been named *B. bavariensis* [Margos et al., 2009]), *B. valaisiana, B. spielmanii*, and *B. lusitaniae*. The first three genospecies are clearly pathogenic to humans, since they have been repeatedly isolated or detected in patients, and tend to cause distinct clinical manifestations (van Dam et al., 1993). *Borrelia valaisiana* and *B. lusitaniae* were thought to be nonpathogenic, but evidence suggests they may also be human pathogens (Diza et al., 2004; Collares-Pereira et al., 2004). *Borrelia spielmanii* has been isolated from human skin on several occasions (Richter et al., 2006; Fingerle et al., 2008). In eastern Europe where *I. persulcatus* is present, only *B. garinii* and *B. afzelii* have been observed in the taiga tick (Korenberg et al., 2002).

The infection prevalence of *B. burgdorferi* s.l. in populations of questing *I. ricinus* ticks vary throughout Europe, ranging generally from 0% to 50% (Hubalek and Halouzka, 1998), but this range can be exceptionally exceeded as, for example, in Portugal where 75% of *I. ricinus* adults were found infected (De Michelis et al., 2000). Overall, *I. ricinus* nymphs (range 0–42.9%, average 10.8%) and adults (range 2.9–46.7%, average 17.4%) are much more infected than larvae (range 0–10.8%, average 1.9%) (Hubalek and Halouzka, 1998). In eastern Europe where *I. ricinus* and *I. persulcatus* are sympatric, the infection prevalence is noticeably lower in *I. ricinus* than in *I. persulcatus* (Korenberg et al., 2002). A novel *Borrelia* related to relapsing fever spirochetes (usually known for efficient transovarial transmission) has been observed in *I. ricinus* ticks (Fraenkel et al., 2002). Larval *I. ricinus* reported to be infected with *B. burgdorferi* may actually be infected with this hard tick relapsing fever spirochete (= *B. miyamotoi* s.l.).

Borrelia burgdorferi s.l. has been reported from many European countries, and their geographic distribution hypothetically follows the distribution of the main tick vector, *I. ricinus* (Figure 2.1). The geographic distribution of diverse *B. burgdorferi* s.l. genospecies in western Europe shows regional variations. However, *B. garinii* and *B. afzelii* are the most prevalent and the most widely distributed genospecies in *I. ricinus*, whereas *B. burgdorferi* s.s., *B. valaisiana,* and *B. lusitaniae* are less frequent. Diverse genospecies—but not necessarily all—are generally present in the same endemic area. Mixed infections with two or more genospecies are generally rare but have been documented across western Europe in *I. ricinus* (Gern and Humair 2002).

Borrelia bissettii, usually distributed in North America, has been observed in cultures of human tissue in Slovenia (Picken et al., 1996), but the isolation of *B. bissettii* has not yet been reported either in tick vectors or in reservoir hosts, and remains to be confirmed in nature on the European continent. Another genospecies (isolate A14S) was initially cultured from a skin biopsy of a patient in the Netherlands (Wang et al., 1999). This novel *Borrelia* has been named *Borrelia spielmanii* (Richter et al., 2006); *B. spielmanii* has been found in *I. ricinus* ticks in Germany and France and in garden dormice reservoirs in France (Richter et al., 2004).

TICK ECOLOGY

North America

Ixodes scapularis is a tick species that is closely tied to forests and leaf litter. This is due in part to the fact that leaf litter provides a moist microclimate where the ticks can survive between host feedings. These ticks need high moisture content (>95% relative humidity) or they will rapidly desiccate. The key role of leaf litter was demonstrated in New Jersey: when leaf litter was removed from the forest floor, *I. scapularis* populations were reduced by 73% to 100% (Schulze et al., 1995). Although the most abundant populations of *I. scapularis* are generally found in deciduous forest with deep leaf litter, mixed evergreen-deciduous forest can also contain high populations of ticks, as can coastal habitats dominated by shrubs and bushes. In suburban properties containing woodlots, landscape ecology studies demonstrated that the abundance of ticks displayed the following pattern: woods > ecotone > ornamental plantings > mowed lawn (Maupin et al., 1991). Mowed lawns, however, can contain modest populations of *I. scapularis* in areas that are not exposed to direct sunlight.

Many abiotic factors have been suggested as possible limitations on the distribution of *I. scapularis*, including rainfall, a greenness–wetness index, maximum and minimum temperatures, the number of degree days during the summer months, soil types and drainage, as well as altitude (Brownstein et al., 2003; Guerra et al., 2002; Rand et al., 2004a). The need is urgent for a predictive model, one that incorporates all the important factors that affect the distribution of *I. scapularis* and predicts what areas are most likely to be invaded by *I. scapularis* in the near future (Diuk-Wasser et al., 2006).

Europe

Two major vectors of *B. burgdorferi* s.l. are present in Europe: *I. ricinus* and *I. persulcatus*. *I. ricinus* is almost distributed all over Europe as westward as Portugal and as eastward as Russia, and as southward as Italy and as northward as Scandinavia (Figure 2.1). The *I. ricinus* distribution even goes over European boundaries, since this tick species is present in North Africa. *I. persulcatus*, on the contrary, has a limited occurrence in eastern Europe (Russia, Estonia, Latvia) (Figure 2.1) compared to its huge distribution in Asia, mainly throughout Asian Russia as far as Sakhalin Island, as well as Japan, China, and Korea. In parts of eastern Europe *I. ricinus* and *I. persulcatus* are sympatric species, since their respective distributions do overlap (Figure 2.1).

As for any organism, the habitats of *I. ricinus* are defined by abiotic and biotic factors. The two most important abiotic factors are humidity and temperature. *Ixodes ricinus* is sensitive to desiccation and requires a high level of relative humidity over 80% (Kahl and Knulle, 1988). This tick is able to maintain a stable water balance for a long period of time, as long as the hygrometric requirement is satisfied. *Ixodes ricinus* lives in the low vegetation strata and the leaf litter of deciduous woodlands and mixed forests. In these sheltered humid microhabitats, *I. ricinus* finds suitable life conditions all year round either on the low vegetation during questing activity or in the leaf litter during diapause, a form of quiescence (molt, oogenesis, overwintering). The density of *I. ricinus* and the prevalence of infected ticks both decrease with altitude (Jouda et al., 2004). *Ixodes ricinus* was rare above 1200 m (Aeschlimann, 1972) but becomes more frequent with climate change. The presence of suitable hosts for each tick stage in the habitat is obviously an essential biotic factor. *Ixodes ricinus* is also prevalent in open habitats like cattle and sheep pastures as, for example, in the British Isles where cool and wet climates occur (Gray, 1991).

The life cycle of *I. ricinus* usually takes three years to complete (range 2–6 years), each stage taking one year to develop to the next instar (Gray, 1991). The questing activity of *I. ricinus* ticks generally occurs from March to October in most of their geographic distribution, but local climatic conditions can modulate the onset and the end of tick activity. The questing activity of *I. ricinus* is particularly important in spring and early summer. This time of the year is at higher risk for humans visiting tick habitats. The tick activity decreases during warm summer months and increases again in autumn. The annual tick activity is longer at lower altitudes and shows much more variation over the years than at higher altitudes (Jouda et al., 2004).

Two other tick species, *I. hexagonus* and *I. uriae*, have been described as vectors of *B. burgdorferi* s.l. in Europe (Gern et al., 1997; Olsen et al., 1993). These two species have an endophilic or nidicolous behavior, squatting in the nests of their hosts. *I. hexagonus* mainly parasitizes mustelidae, hedgehogs, and foxes, whereas *I. uriae* feeds on seabirds. Both species have only a very limited contribution in terms of Lyme borreliosis transmission to humans. The risk with *I. hexagonus* is more obvious, since this tick species may be present in urban parks and gardens due to the presence of suitable hosts (cats, dogs, hedgehogs) (Gern et al., 1997). The risk with *I. uriae* would be limited to ornithologists in contact with seabirds and seabird colonies.

HOSTS

North America

Immature *I. scapularis* (larvae and nymphs) take a blood meal from a very different range of hosts compared to the adult females (adult males generally do not take a blood meal). Females will not feed on small vertebrates like rodents, lizards, or birds. Female *I. scapularis* can be found on a variety of medium or large mammals (raccoons, skunks, foxes, wild pigs, cats, dogs, etc.), but their primary hosts are white-tailed deer (*Odocoileus virginianus*) (Piesman et al., 1979). The central role of deer in supporting populations of *I. scapularis* has been dramatically illustrated by the eradication of deer from an isolated island off the coast of Maine, followed by the virtual disappearance of ticks over several years (Rand et al., 2004b). Curiously, although deer are central to the support of the tick population, they are absolutely refractory to infection with *B. burgdorferi* s.l. Although the reason for this refractory status of deer remained a mystery for an extended period of time, an elegant series of experiments demonstrated that the host complement present in deer blood lyses *B. burgdorferi* almost instantaneously (Kurtenbach et al., 1998). Thus deer do not serve as reservoirs of *B. burgdorferi* infection.

Larval and nymphal *I. scapularis* feed on a wide range of small vertebrates, including rodents, shrews, lizards, and birds. In the northeastern United States where infection rates with *B. burgdorferi* s.s. are extremely high in *I. scapularis*, the primary hosts for immature *I. scapularis* are white-footed mice (*Peromyscus leucopus*) and the eastern chipmunk (*Tamias striatus*). Both white-footed mice and eastern chipmunks are extremely efficient reservoirs of *B. burgdorferi* s.s. (Hanincova et al., 2006) as are shrews (Brisson et al., 2008). Rodent complement does not lyse these spirochetes, and the majority of larval *I. scapularis* that feed on these hosts become infected with spirochetes and molt to infected nymphs. The nymphal stage of *I. scapularis* is the primary vector of *B. burgdorferi* s.s. to humans (Piesman, 1989). In general, larval *I. scapularis* feed on rodents in late summer (August–September), molt to nymphs that overwinter, and feed the next spring–summer (May–July). This perpetuates an efficient enzootic cycle of Lyme disease spirochetes in parts of the northeastern and midwestern United States, and isolated locations in parts of southern Ontario (Canada).

The diversity of small vertebrates changes on the Atlantic coast of North America along a north–south cline. In more northern latitudes, rodents predominate, serving as efficient reservoirs of *B. burgdorferi* s.s. In the south, rodent populations are much less significant, and reptiles are the predominant small vertebrates moving along the forest floor and serving as hosts for immature *I. scapularis*. Like deer, lizard complement is quite lytic for *B. burgdorferi* s.s. (Kuo et al., 2000; Ullmann et al., 2003). Thus infection with *B. burgdorferi* s.s. is extremely rare in the lizard-fed nymphal *I. scapularis* in the southern United States. In addition nymphal *I. scapularis* rarely feed on people in the southeast United States, whereas thousands of nymphal *I. scapularis* are removed from people each year in the northeastern United States. Although southern populations of *I. scapularis* are fully competent to transmit *B. burgdorferi* s.s., the zooprophylactic effect of lizards and varying nymphal questing patterns dramatically reduces the prospect for humans acquiring infection with *B. burgdorferi* s.s. south of the Maryland border. Population genetics studies of *I. scapularis* along this north–south cline may yield answers regarding the variant behaviors of this important vector species, thus leading to a better understanding of their public health impact (Oliver et al., 1993; Telford, 1998). Ground-feeding birds are often infested with immature *I. scapularis* and can serve as reservoir hosts for *B. burgdorferi* s.s., but infestation levels on birds are generally lower than on rodents or lizards. Birds may be especially important in moving spirochete-infected *I. scapularis* to new locations (Ogden et al., 2008a). They also may reintroduce ticks to areas where tick eradication has been attempted.

Europe

Ixodes ricinus feeds on a large spectrum of vertebrates, including small-, medium-, large-sized mammals, birds, and reptiles. As in North America, hosts in Europe are important because they ensure the maintenance of populations of ticks and the maintenance of populations of *B. burgdorferi* s.l. The presence and abundance of suitable hosts for *I. ricinus* adults such as deer is a key factor for the maintenance of a tick population in a determined habitat, and this has a direct impact on the tick density in an endemic area of Lyme borreliosis (Gray et al., 1992). Also the maintenance of *Borrelia* species related to Lyme borreliosis is ensured by the existence of reservoir hosts in endemic areas. In this context, hosts for both subadult tick stages (larvae and nymphs) are of major importance. The ecology of Lyme borreliosis shows a more complex picture in Europe than in North America, mainly because of the diversity of *Borrelia* genospecies. Several vertebrate species have been identified as efficient reservoirs for *B. burgdorferi* s.l., and included are small- and medium-sized mammal species as well as bird species (Gern and Humair 2002; Gern et al., 1998; Humair, 2002). The identification of reservoirs has been undertaken in many European countries, and efforts have mainly focused on small rodents that can be easily captured, handled, and maintained in captivity. Among terrestrial mammals, the most important reservoir species are undoubtedly *Apodemus flavicollis*, *A. sylvaticus*, *A. agrarius*, and *Clethrionomys glareolus*. The contribution of these rodent species in the maintenance of *B. burgdorferi* s.l. in nature is important for many reasons. They usually show an important host density in wooded areas, their infestation by larval ticks is high, and their infectivity to feeding ticks is high as well. In addition they can sustain *Borrelia* infection during overwintering months and even as long as a rodent lifetime. Larger rodents like squirrels (*Sciurus vulgaris*, *S. carolinensis*), and dormice (*Myoxus glis*, *Eliomys quercinus*) are also involved as reservoirs of *Borrelia*. Insectivores such as shrews (*Sorex*,

Neomys) and hedgehogs (*Erinaceus europaeus*) contribute to the maintenance of *B. burgdorferi* s.l. Among lagomorphs, hares (*Lepus europaeus*, *L. timidus*) appear to more efficiently transmit *Borrelia* to ticks than rabbits (*Oryctolagus cuniculus*) do. But what is valid for one endemic area may be different in another. In urban or suburban habitats, rats (*Rattus rattus*, *R. norvegicus*) as well as hedgehogs can be more efficient reservoirs than any other rodent species previously mentioned.

Birds have been investigated less extensively than mammals and have been the subject of some controversy (Humair, 2002). However, passerine birds like blackbirds (*Turdus merula*) and game birds like pheasants (*Phasianus colchicus*) were clearly demonstrated as reservoirs (Humair et al., 1998; Kurtenbach et al., 1998a). Other ground-frequenting species are suspected to have a role in the natural maintenance. This mainly includes passerines of the Turdidae family such as thrushes (*Turdus* sp.) and robins (*Erithacus rubecula*) but also some species belonging to Paridae, Sylvidae, and Fringillidae. The involvement of seabirds have also been demonstrated in a closed enzootic cycle involving only colony-nesting seabirds and the seabird tick, *I. uriae* (Olsen et al., 1993). Such a cycle is not restricted to the European continent but has been observed in diverse isolated locations in the bi-circumpolar distribution of *I. uriae* (Olsen et al., 1995).

The most interesting point about the ecology of Lyme borreliosis in Europe is the specific host associations of *B. burgdorferi* s.l. In continental Europe, *B. afzelii* is associated with small rodents (mainly *Apodemus* mice and *Clethrionomys* voles) (Humair et al., 1995, 1999; Hanincova et al., 2003), and *B. burgdorferi* s.s. is associated with squirrels (Humair and Gern, 1998). *Borrelia garinii* is associated with birds (Humair et al., 1998; Hanincova et al., 2003) with the exception of *B. garinii* serotype 4 (*B. bavariensis*), which is related to *Apodemus* mice (Huegli et al., 2002). *Borrelia valaisiana* is specifically maintained by birds (Humair et al., 1998; Hanincova et al., 2003). *B. spielmanii* was shown to be maintained by the garden dormice (*E. quercinus*) (Richter et al., 2004). The reservoir hosts of *B. lusitaniae* have been identified to be lizards (Richter and Matuschka, 2006). In the United Kingdom, in endemic areas where *B. afzelii* is absent, *B. burgdorferi* s.s. is associated with small rodents (Kurtenbach et al., 1998b), but with much less efficiency. In summary, *B. burgdorferi* s.l. genospecies are maintained in Europe by differential transmission cycles. The host complement system is clearly involved in this phenomenon of host specificity.(Kurtenbach et al., 1998c)

Large mammals like deer (*Capreolus capreolus*, *Cervus elaphus*, *Dama dama*) and moose (*Alces alces*) are clearly not reservoirs of *B. burgdorferi* s.l., although they have a crucial role in the reproduction of the tick. Additionally the red fox (*Vulpes vulpes*) seems to have a limited role.

PERSONAL PROTECTION AND CONTROL

North America

The first line of defense against contracting Lyme disease is personal protection. Knowing where the ticks are and avoiding tick habitat (forest leaf litter and ecotone) when the ticks are most active (May–July for nymphal *I. scapularis*) is key. When the high risk habitat must be entered, long pants (tucked into socks) and long sleeve shirts seem like a prudent precaution, but formal scientific evidence that this strategy actually reduces the risk of Lyme disease is lacking. Treatment of skin or clothing with the tick repellent DEET, and treatment of clothing only with permethrin (as per label instructions) presents an additional barrier to tick feeding. Numerous studies using animal models for transmission have shown that nymphal *I. scapularis* must feed for >48 hours before the risk of *B. burgdorferi* s.s. transmission starts to rapidly increase (des Vignes et al., 2001). In two studies of *I. scapularis* bites in humans there was a significant increase in risk of acquiring *B. burgdorferi* infection if the tick was attached more than 72 hours, as measured objectively by a scutal index method (see Chapter 12). This may be due in part to the downregulation during tick feeding of outer surface protein A (OspA), which binds to tick midgut epithelium and keeps spirochetes trapped in the midgut until after feeding commences; it may also be due in part to the upregulation of outer surface protein C (OspC). OspC may facilitate migration to the tick salivary glands and/or may be required for infection of the vertebrate host (Schwan and Piesman, 2002). OspC also binds to a tick salivary gland protein, salp15, that may protect it from the host immune response (Ramamoorthi et al., 2005; Dai et al., 2009). Whatever the mechanism, daily tick checks by residents of hyperendemic regions should lead to the removal of many attached nymphal *I. scapularis* before the two days they require to effectively transmit spirochetal infection to the tick-bite victim. The reason that adult female *I. scapularis* do not transmit spirochetal infection efficiently in North America, despite the fact that approximately half of them are infected with *B. burgdorferi* s.s. in some areas, is that their large size relative to the nymph often allows for their prompt detection and removal (Falco et al., 1996).

Tick control remains an essential part of the strategy to prevent Lyme disease. A single area-wide acaricide application timed to kill nymphal *I. scapularis* just as their feeding activity begins (end of May, early June), can effectively eliminate 70% to 100% of tick populations. Acaricides commonly used include carbaryl, cyfluthrin, deltamethrin, fulvalinate, and permethrin. Although these chemicals can be extremely effective, the majority of residents living in hyperendemic regions perceive them as being toxic to nontarget organisms as well as humans and will not consider their use. This has led to the search for alternative control methodologies including host-targeted acaricides, vegetation management, host exclusion or eradication, as well as biological control agents and least toxic pesticides. This search for integrated pest management (IPM) approaches for Lyme disease prevention has been summarized by Hayes and Piesman, as well as Piesman and Eisen (Hayes and Piesman, 2003; Piesman and Eisen, 2008). Of particular interest are recent studies demonstrating that natural products applied to vegetation (Dolan et al., 2009) or acaricides applied directly to deer (Hoen et al., 2009) hold potential to reduce the risk of Lyme disease spirochete transmission.

Europe

Prevention of Lyme borreliosis in Europe amounts to avoiding tick bites. The avoidance of tick habitat is undoubtedly the best preventive strategy but may be unrealistic since woodlands and forests have always been and will continue to be frequently visited by people during recreational and occupational activities. Personal protection is actually the best way to minimize contacts. As in North America, protective clothing and properly used tick repellents can reduce risk of Lyme disease in Europe. In any case, a full-body inspection should be carefully undertaken after each visit in a tick-infested area. Ticks are very discreet arthropods: they can be undetectable when walking around on the skin for a suitable bite site, the bite is not painful, and ticks may attach on "hidden" parts of the body (armpit, groin, neck, head, behind joints, ears). Attached ticks should be removed as rapidly as possible: the quicker the removal occurs, the lower the risk of transmission of *Borrelia*. In Europe, efficient transmission of *B. burgdorferi* s.l. may already occur within 24 hours of tick attachment in the case of *I. ricinus*, and the risk of infection increases with the duration of tick attachment.(Kahl et al., 1998; Crippa et al., 2002) Dissemination to the salivary glands of European strains of *B. burgdorferi* s.l. has been shown to be dependent on genotype, strain, and the expression of OspC (Fingerle et al., 2002).

Residential areas in Europe are generally not very close to tick habitats, as is the case in North America. Peridomestic risk is consequently limited, but ticks may occasionally be found in gardens in close vicinity to woodlands. Regular mowing, removal of leaf litter, and cutting or removal of bushes close to the woodland edge would be sufficient to significantly reduce this threat.

For an optimal impact of preventive strategies in European countries, coordinated information on Lyme borreliosis, ticks, and adequate preventive measures should be dispersed as widely as possible. National public health agencies, specialized research institutions, physicians, and local communities have a key role in this concern, especially in highly endemic areas.

The control of Lyme borreliosis in nature is another aspect of prevention of this vector-borne disease. This implies strategies on a large scale to reduce risk of transmission to humans, by indirectly reducing either the tick population or the prevalence of infection in the tick population. Although many control strategies have already been developed in North America, such studies are almost nonexistent in Europe. An acaricide/repellent (permethrin) was used to treat small rodents to reduce the number of infesting *I. ricinus* larvae (Mejlon et al., 1995); a significant reduction was observed for *Clethrionomys* voles but not for *Apodemus* mice. Such an approach was not very conclusive given the diversity of reservoir species in Europe. No single strategy will provide an efficient tick control in Europe. As in North America, the best possible way for Lyme disease prevention is probably the development of integrated tick control, which combines diverse preventive measures. Initiatives in this direction should be strongly encouraged in Europe.

SUMMARY

Ixodes scapularis is the principal tick vector of Lyme disease spirochetes in North America, and *Ixodes ricinus* is the primary vector in Europe. In hyperendemic regions of North America, nymphal *I. scapularis* efficiently transmit *B. burgdorferi* s.s. to humans, whereas in Europe, *I. ricinus* transmits *B. burgdorferi* s.s., *B. afzelii*, and *B. garinii* serotypes to tick-bite victims. Both *I. scapularis* and *I. ricinus* are forest dwelling species that feed on a variety of small vertebrates as immatures and on deer as adults. Rodents are the principal reservoir for *B. burgdorferi* s.s. in North America, whereas the situation is more complex in Europe regarding reservoir hosts for the three major genospecies of *B. burgdorferi* s.l. that are commonly transmitted to humans. Personal protection remains the first line of defense against Lyme disease in both North America and Europe, although active research on novel tick control methods has made recent progress.

ACKNOWLEDGMENT

PFH was supported by the International Emerging Infectious Diseases (IEID) Fellowship Program administered by the Association of Public Health Laboratories (APHL) and funded by the Centers for Disease Control and Prevention (CDC).

REFERENCES

Aeschlimann A: *Ixodes ricinus*, Linné, 1758 (Ixodoidea; Ixodidae): Essai préliminaire de synthèse sur la biologie de cette espèce en Suisse. *Acta Trop* 29:321–340; 1972.

Anderson JF, Magnarelli LA, Mcaninch JB: New *Borrelia burgdorferi* antigenic variant isolated from *Ixodes dammini* from upstate New York. *J Clin Microbiol* 26:2209–2212; 1988.

Brisson D, Dykhuizen DE, Ostfeld RS: Conspicuous impacts of inconspicuous hosts on the Lyme disease epidemic. *Proc Biol Sci* 275:227–235; 2008.

Brownstein JS, Holford TR, Fish D: A climate-based model predicts the spatial distribution of the Lyme disease vector *Ixodes scapularis* in the United States. *Environ Health Perspect* 111:1152–1157; 2003.

Bunikis J, Tsao J, Garpmo U, Berglund J, Fish D, Barbour AG: Typing of *Borrelia* relapsing fever group strains. *Emerg Infect Dis* 10:1661–1664; 2004.

Burgdorfer W, Barbour AG, Hayes SF, Peter O, Aeschlimann A: Erythema chronicum migrans–a tickborne spirochetosis. *Acta Trop* 40:79–83; 1983.

Collares-Pereira M, Couceiro S, Franca I, Kurtenbach K, Schafer SM, Vitorino L, Goncalves L, Baptista S, Vieira ML., Cunha C: First isolation of *Borrelia lusitaniae* from a human patient. *J Clin Microbiol* 42:1316–1318; 2004.

Crippa M, Rais O, Gern L: Investigations on the mode and dynamics of transmission and infectivity of *Borrelia burgdorferi* sensu stricto and *Borrelia afzelii* in *Ixodes ricinus* ticks. *Vector Borne Zoonotic Dis* 2:3–9; 2002.

Dai J, Wang P, Adusumilli S, Booth CJ, Narasimhan S, Anguita J, Fikrig E: Antibodies against a tick protein, Salp15, protect mice from the Lyme disease agent. *Cell Host Microbe* 6:482–492; 2009.

De Michelis S, Sewell HS, Cillares-Pereira M, Santos-Reis M, Schouls LM, Benes V, Holmes EC, Kurtenbach K: Genetic diversity of *Borrelia burgdorferi* sensu lato in ticks from mainland Portugal. *J Clin Microbiol* 38:2128–2133; 2000.

Dennis DT, Nekomoto TS, Victor JC, Paul WS, Piesman J: Reported distribution of *Ixodes scapularis* and *Ixodes pacificus* (Acari: Ixodidae) in the United States. *J Med Entomol* 35:629–638; 1998.

Des Vignes F, Piesman J, Heffernan R, Schulze TL, Stafford KC, Fish D: Effect of tick removal on transmission of *Borrelia burgdorferi* and *Ehrlichia phagocytophila* by *Ixodes scapularis* nymphs. *J Infect Dis* 183:773–778; 2001.

Diuk-Wasser MA, Gatewood AG, Cortinas MR, Yaremych-Hamer S, Tsao J, Kitron U, Hickling G, Brownstein JS, Walker E, Piesman J, Fish D: Spatiotemporal patterns of host-seeking *Ixodes scapularis* nymphs (Acari: Ixodidae) in the United States. *J Med Entomol* 43:166–176; 2006.

Diza E, Papa A, Vezyri E, Tsounis S, Milonas I, Antoniadis A: *Borrelia valaisiana* in cerebrospinal fluid. *Emerg Infect Dis* 10:1692–1693; 2004.

Dolan MC, Jordan RA, Schulze TL, Schulze CJ, Manning MC, Ruffolo D, Schmidt JP, Piesman J, Karchesy JJ: Ability of two natural products, nootkatone and carvacrol, to suppress *Ixodes scapularis* and *Amblyomma americanum* (Acari: Ixodidae) in a Lyme disease endemic area of New Jersey. *J Econ Entomol* 102:2316–2324; 2009.

Falco RC, Fish D, Piesman J: Duration of tick bites in a Lyme disease-endemic area. *Am J Epidemiol* 143:187–192; 1996.

Fingerle V, Rauser S, Hammer B, Kahl O, Heimerl C, Schulte-Spechtel U, Gern L, Wilske B: Dynamics of dissemination and outer surface protein expression of different European *Borrelia burgdorferi* sensu lato strains in artificially infected *Ixodes ricinus* nymphs. *J Clin Microbiol* 40:1456–1463; 2002.

Fingerle V, Schulte-Spechtel UC, Ruzic-Sabljic E., Leonhard S, Hofmann H, Weber K, Pfister K, Strle F, Wilske B: Epidemiological aspects and molecular characterization of *Borrelia burgdorferi* s.l. from southern Germany with special respect to the new species *Borrelia spielmanii* sp. nov. *Int J Med Microbiol* 298:279–290; 2008.

Fraenkel CJ, Garpmo U, Berglund J: Determination of novel *Borrelia* genospecies in Swedish *Ixodes ricinus* ticks. *J Clin Microbiol* 40:3308–3312; 2002.

Gern L, Humair PF: Ecology of *Borrelia burgdorferi* sensu lato in Europe. *In* Gray J, Kahl O, Lane RS, Stanek G (eds): *Lyme Borreliosis: Biology, Epidemiology and Control.* New York, CAB International; 2002.

Gern L, Rouvinez E, Toutoungi LN, Godfroid E: Transmission cycles of *Borrelia burgdorferi* sensu lato involving *Ixodes ricinus* and/or *I. hexagonus* ticks and the European hedgehog, *Erinaceus europaeus*, in suburban and urban areas in Switzerland. *Folia Parasitol (Praha)* 44:309–314; 1997.

Gern L, Estrada-Pena A, Frandsen F, Gray JS, Jaenson TG, Jongejan F, Kahl O, Korenberg E, Mehl R, Nuttall PA: European reservoir hosts of *Borrelia burgdorferi* sensu lato. *Zentralbl Bakteriol* 287:196–204; 1998.

Gray JS: The development and seasonal activity of the tick *Ixodes ricinus*: A vector of Lyme borreliosis. *Rev Med Vet Entomol*, 79,323–333; 1991.

Gray JS, Kahl O, Janetzki C, Stein J: Studies on the ecology of Lyme disease in a deer forest in County Galway, *Ireland. J Med Entomol* 29:915–920; 1992.

Guerra M, Walker E, Jones C, Paskewitz S, Cortinas MR, Stancil A, Beck L, Bobo M, Kitron U: Predicting the risk of Lyme disease. Habitat suitability for *Ixodes scapularis* in the north central United States. *Emerg Infect Dis* 8:289–297; 2002.

Hanincova K, Schafer SM, Etti S, Sewell HS, Taragelova V, Ziak D, Labuda M, Kurtenbach K: Association of *Borrelia afzelii* with rodents in Europe. *Parasitology* 126:11–20; 2003a.

Hanincova K, Taragelova V, Koci J, Schafer SM, Hails R, Ullmann AJ, Piesman J, Labuda M, Kurtenbach K: Association of *Borrelia garinii* and *B. valaisiana* with songbirds in Slovakia. *Appl Environ Microbiol* 69:2825–2830; 2003b.

Hanincova K, Kurtenbach K, Diuk-Wasser M., Brei B, Fish D: Epidemic spread of Lyme borreliosis, northeastern United States. *Emerg Infect Dis* 12:604–611; 2006.

Hayes EB, Piesman J: How can we prevent Lyme disease? *N Engl J Med* 348:2424–2430; 2003.

Hoen AG, Rollend LG, Papero MA, Carroll JF, Daniels TJ, Mather TN, Schulze TL, Stafford K.C. III, Fish D: Effects of tick control by acaricide self-treatment of white-tailed deer on host-seeking tick infection prevalence and entomologic risk for *Ixodes scapularis*-borne pathogens. *Vector Borne Zoonotic Dis* 9:431–438; 2009.

Hubalek Z, Halouzka J: Prevalence rates of *Borrelia burgdorferi* sensu lato in host-seeking *Ixodes ricinus* ticks in Europe. *Parasitol Res* 84:167–172; 1998.

Huegli D, Hu CM, Humair PF, Wilske B, Gern L: Apodemus species mice are reservoir hosts of *Borrelia garinii* OspA serotype 4 in Switzerland. *J Clin Microbiol* 40:4735–4737; 2002.

Humair PF: Birds and *Borrelia. Int J Med Microbiol* 291(suppl 33): 70–74; 2002.

Humair PF, Gern L: Relationship between *Borrelia burgdorferi* sensu lato species, red squirrels (*Sciurus vulgaris*) and *Ixodes ricinus* in enzootic areas in Switzerland. *Acta Trop* 69:213–227; 1998.

Humair PF, Peter O, Wallich R, Gern L: Strain variation of Lyme disease spirochetes isolated from *Ixodes ricinus* ticks and rodents collected in two endemic areas in Switzerland. *J Med Entomol* 32:433–438; 1995.

Humair PF, Postic D, Wallich R, Gern L: An avian reservoir (*Turdus merula*) of the Lyme borreliosis spirochetes. *Zentralbl Bakteriol*, 287:521–538; 1998.

Humair PF, Rais O, Gern L: Transmission of *Borrelia afzelii* from *Apodemus* mice and *Clethrionomys* voles to *Ixodes ricinus* ticks. Differential transmission pattern and overwintering maintenance. *Parasitology* 118(pt 1): 33–42; 1999.

Jouda F, Perret JL, Gern L: *Ixodes ricinus* density, and distribution and prevalence of *Borrelia burgdorferi* sensu lato infection along an altitudinal gradient. *J Med Entomol* 41:162–169; 2004.

Kahl O, Knulle W: Water vapour uptake from subsaturated atmospheres by engorged immature ixodid ticks. *Exp Appl Acarol* 4:73–83; 1988.

Kahl O, Janetzki-Mittmann C, Gray JS, Jonas R, Stein J, De Boer R: Risk of infection with *Borrelia burgdorferi* sensu lato for a host in relation to the duration of nymphal *Ixodes ricinus* feeding and the method of tick removal. *Zentralbl Bakteriol* 287:41–52; 1998.

Korenberg EI, Gorelova NB, Kovalevskii YV: Ecology of *Borrelia burgdorferi* sensu lato in Russia. *In* Gray J, Kahl O, Lane RS, Stanek G (eds): *Lyme borreliosis. Biology, Epidemiology and Control.* New York, CAB International; 2002.

Kuo MM, Lane RS, Giclas PC: A comparative study of mammalian and reptilian alternative pathway of complement-mediated killing of the Lyme disease spirochete (*Borrelia burgdorferi*). *J Parasitol* 86:1223–1228; 2000.

Kurtenbach K, Carey D, Hoodless AN, Nuttall PA, Randolph SE: Competence of pheasants as reservoirs for Lyme disease spirochetes. *J Med Entomol* 35:77–81; 1998a.

Kurtenbach K, Peacey M, Rijpkema SG, Hoodless AN, Nuttall PA, Randolph SE: Differential transmission of the genospecies of *Borrelia burgdorferi* sensu lato by game birds and small rodents in England. *Appl Environ Microbiol* 64:1169–1174; 1998b.

Kurtenbach K, Sewell HS, Ogden NH, Randolph SE, Nuttall PA: Serum complement sensitivity as a key factor in Lyme disease ecology. *Infect Immun* 66:1248–1251; 1998c.

Liveris D, Varde S, Iyer R, Koenig S, Bittker S, Cooper D, McKenna D, Nowakowski J, Nadelman RB, Wormser GP, Schwartz I: Genetic diversity of *Borrelia burgdorferi* in lyme disease patients as determined by culture versus direct PCR with clinical specimens. *J Clin Microbiol* 37:565–569; 1999.

Marconi RT, Liveris D, Schwartz I: Identification of novel insertion elements, restriction fragment length polymorphism patterns, and discontinuous 23S rRNA in Lyme disease spirochetes. Phylogenetic analyses of rRNA genes and their intergenic spacers in *Borrelia japonica* sp. nov. and genomic group 21038 (*Borrelia andersonii* sp. nov.) isolates. *J Clin Microbiol* 33:2427–2434; 1995.

Margos G, Vollmer SA, Cornet M, Garnier M, Fingerle V, Wilske B, Bormane A, Vitorino L, Collares-Pereira M, Drancourt M, Kurtenbach K: A new *Borrelia* species defined by multilocus sequence analysis of housekeeping genes. *Appl Environ Microbiol* 75:5410–5416; 2009.

Maupin GO, Fish D, Zultowsky J, Campos EG, Piesman J: Landscape ecology of Lyme disease in a residential area of Westchester County, New York. *Am J Epidemiol* 133:1105–1113; 1991.

McCabe TR, McCabe RE: Recounting whitetails past. *In* McShea WJ, Underwood HB, Rappole JH (eds): *The Science of Overabundance. Deer Ecology and Population Management.* Washington DC, Smithsonian Institution Press; 1997.

Mejlon HA, Jaenson TG, Mather TN: Evaluation of host-targeted applications of permethrin for control of *Borrelia*-infected *Ixodes ricinus* (Acari: Ixodidae). *Med Vet Entomol* 9:207–210; 1995.

Norris DE, Johnson BJ, Piesman J, Maupin GO, Clark JL, Black WCT: Population genetics and phylogenetic analysis of Colorado *Borrelia burgdorferi*. *Am J Trop Med Hyg* 60:699–707; 1999.

Ogden NH, Lindsay LR, Hanincova K, Barker IK, Bigras-Poulin M, Charron DF, Heagy A, Francis CM, O'Callaghan CJ, Schwartz I, Thompson RA: Role of migratory birds in introduction and range expansion of *Ixodes scapularis* ticks and of *Borrelia burgdorferi* and *Anaplasma phagocytophilum* in Canada. *Appl Environ Microbiol* 74:1780–1790; 2008a.

Ogden NH, St-Onge L, Barker IK, Brazeau S, Bigras-Poulin M, Charron DF, Francis CM, Heagy A, Lindsay LR, Maarouf A, Michel P, Milord F, O'Callaghan CJ, Trudel L, Thompson RA: Risk maps for range expansion of the Lyme disease vector, *Ixodes scapularis*, in Canada now and with climate change. *Int J Health Geogr* 7:24; 2008b.

Oliver JJ, Owsley MR, Hutcheson HJ, James AM, Chen C, Irby WS, Dotson EM, McLain DK: Conspecificity of the ticks *Ixodes scapularis* and *I. dammini* (Acari: Ixodidae). *J Med Entomol* 30:54–63; 1993.

Olsen B, Duffy DC, Jaenson TG, Gylfe A, Bonnedahl J, Bergstrom S: Transhemispheric exchange of Lyme disease spirochetes by seabirds. *J Clin Microbiol* 33:3270–3274; 1995.

Olsen B, Jaenson TG, Noppa L, Bunikis J, Bergstrom S: A Lyme borreliosis cycle in seabirds and *Ixodes uriae* ticks. *Nature* 362:340–342; 1993.

Picken RN, Cheng Y, Strle F, Picken MM: Patient isolates of *Borrelia burgdorferi* sensu lato with genotypic and phenotypic similarities of strain 25015. *J Infect Dis* 174:1112–1115; 1996.

Piesman J: Transmission of Lyme disease spirochetes (*Borrelia burgdorferi*). *Exp Appl Acarol* 7:71–80; 1989.

Piesman J, Eisen L: Prevention of tick-borne diseases. *Annu Rev Entomol* 53:323–343; 2008.

Piesman J, Spielman A., Etkind P, Ruebush TK II, Juranek DD: Role of deer in the epizootiology of *Babesia microti* in Massachusetts, USA. *J Med Entomol* 15:537–540; 1979.

Postic D, Garnier M, Baranton G: Multilocus sequence analysis of atypical *Borrelia burgdorferi* sensu lato isolates. Description of *Borrelia californiensis* sp. nov., and genomospecies 1 and 2. *Int J Med Microbiol* 297:263–271; 2007.

Postic D, Ras NM, Lane RS, Hendson M, Baranton G: Expanded diversity among Californian *Borrelia* isolates and description of *Borrelia bissettii* sp. nov. (formerly *Borrelia* group DN127). *J Clin Microbiol* 36:3497–3504; 1998.

Qiu WG, Dykhuizen DE, Acosta MS, Luft BJ: Geographic uniformity of the Lyme disease spirochete (*Borrelia burgdorferi*) and its shared history with tick vector (*Ixodes scapularis*) in the Northeastern United States. *Genetics* 160:833–49; 2002.

Ramamoorthi N, Narasimhan S, Pal U, Bao F, Yang XF, Fish D, Anguita J, Norgard MV, Kantor FS, Anderson JF, Koski RA, Fikrig E: The Lyme disease agent exploits a tick protein to infect the mammalian host. *Nature* 436:573–577; 2005.

Rand PW, Holman MS, Lubelczyk C, Lacombe EH, Degaetano AT, Smith RP Jr.: Thermal accumulation and the early development of *Ixodes scapularis*. *J Vector Ecol* 29:164–176; 2004a.

Rand PW, Lubelczyk C, Holman MS, Lacombe EH, Smith RP Jr.: Abundance of *Ixodes scapularis* (Acari: Ixodidae) after the complete removal of deer from an isolated offshore island, endemic for Lyme Disease. *J Med Entomol* 41:779–784; 2004b.

Richter D, Matuschka FR: Perpetuation of the Lyme disease spirochete *Borrelia lusitaniae* by lizards. *Appl Environ Microbiol* 72:4627–4632; 2006.

Richter D, Postic D, Sertour N, Livey I, Matuschka FR, Baranton G: Delineation of *Borrelia burgdorferi* sensu lato species by multilocus sequence analysis and confirmation of the delineation of *Borrelia spielmanii* sp. nov. *Int J Syst Evol Microbiol* 56:873–881; 2006.

Richter D, Schlee DB, Allgower R, Matuschka FR: Relationships of a novel Lyme disease spirochete, *Borrelia spielmani* sp. nov., with its hosts in Central Europe. *Appl Environ Microbiol* 70:6414–6419; 2004.

Rudenko N, Golovchenko M, Grubhoffer L, Oliver JH Jr.: *Borrelia carolinensis* sp. nov., a new (14th) member of the *Borrelia burgdorferi* Sensu Lato complex from the southeastern region of the United States. *J Clin Microbiol* 47:134–141; 2009.

Schulze TL, Jordan RA, Hung RW: Suppression of subadult *Ixodes scapularis* (Acari: Ixodidae) following removal of leaf litter. *J Med Entomol* 32:730–733; 1995.

Schwan TG, Piesman J: Vector interactions and molecular adaptations of Lyme disease and relapsing fever spirochetes associated with transmission by ticks. *Emerg Infect Dis* 8:115–121; 2002.

Scoles GA, Papero M, Beati L, Fish D: A relapsing fever group spirochete transmitted by *Ixodes scapularis* ticks. *Vector Borne Zoonotic Dis* 1:21–34; 2001.

Spielman A: Lyme disease and human babesiosis: evidence incriminating vector and reservoir hosts. *In* Englund PT, Sher AE (eds): *Biology of Parasitism*. New York, AR Liss; 1988.

Telford SR III: The name *Ixodes dammini* epidemiologically justified. *Emerg Infect Dis* 4:132–134; 1998.

Terekhova D, Iyer R, Wormser GP; Schwartz I: Comparative genome hybridization reveals substantial variation among clinical isolates of *Borrelia burgdorferi* sensu stricto with different pathogenic properties. *J Bacteriol* 188:6124–6134; 2006.

Ullmann AJ, Lane RS, Kurtenbach K, Miller M, Schriefer ME, Zeldner N, Piesman J: Bacteriolytic activity of selected vertebrate sera for *Borrelia burgdorferi* sensu stricto and *Borrelia bissettii*. *J Parasitol* 89:1256–1257; 2003.

Van Dam AP, Kuiper H, Vos K, Al E: Different genospecies of *Borrelia burgdorferi* are associated with distinct clinical manifestations of Lyme borreliosis. *Clin Infec Dis* 17:708–717; 1993.

Varela AS, Luttrell MP, Howerth EW, Moore VA, Davidson WR, Stallknecht DE, Little SE: First culture isolation of *Borrelia lonestari*, putative agent of southern tick-associated rash illness. *J Clin Microbiol* 42:1163–1169; 2004.

Wang G, van Dam AP, Dankert J: Phenotypic and genetic characterization of a novel *Borrelia burgdorferi* sensu lato isolate from a patient with lyme borreliosis. *J Clin Microbiol* 37:3025–3028; 1999.

Wilske B, Preac MV, Gobel UB, Graf B, Jauris S, Soutschek E, Schwab E, Zumstein G: An OspA serotyping system for *Borrelia burgdorferi* based on reactivity with monoclonal antibodies and OspA sequence analysis. *J Clin Microbiol* 31:340–350; 1993.

3

EARLY LYME BORRELIOSIS

Vijay K. Sikand and Robert R. Müllegger

The early manifestations of Lyme borreliosis are best appreciated with an understanding of the protean nature of its presentation and clinical course. Initial descriptions of the disease in the United States categorized it in sequential stages. Stage 1 denoted erythema migrans (EM), a characteristic skin lesion appearing days to weeks after the bite of an infected tick and often accompanied by flu-like symptoms. Stage 2 primarily included cranial neuropathies, meningitis, and cardiac conduction abnormalities occurring weeks to months after infection. Stage 3 comprised rheumatologic and central nervous system pathologies presenting months to years later. However, with progressive clinical observation and increasing diagnostic acumen over the past three decades, it has become evident that there are no clear-cut junctures. For example, while the classic EM lesion is commonly the initial recognizable manifestation of the disease, it may present simultaneously with a cranial neuropathy such as Bell's palsy. By the same token, arthritis may occur early or late in the time course.

Consequently a more flexible descriptive terminology has evolved to describe the clinical presentation of Lyme borreliosis as early localized, early disseminated, and late disease. Any of these forms can be the initial manifestation of the disease. De novo presentation as late disease, which occurs in the minority of patients nowadays, represents a subclinical continuum of the original infection. Thus a broad understanding of its clinical features is essential for recognition of presenting syndromes, along with knowledge of diagnostic modalities that may be helpful or confirmatory at different time points. This

Lyme Borreliosis in Europe and North America: Epidemiology and Clinical Practice, First Edition.
Edited by Sunil K. Sood

chapter covers the early localized and disseminated skin lesion, the summer "flu-like illness," and asymptomatic seroconversion due to *Borrelia burgdorferi* sensu lato (*B. burgdorferi* sensu lato). All other manifestations including their early presentation are covered elsewhere in this volume.

In Europe the skin may be affected by three characteristic disease manifestations of Lyme borreliosis, EM, borrelial lymphocytoma, and acrodermatitis chronica atrophicans, which together account for about 80% of all cases of Lyme borreliosis. EM is the most common manifestation of Lyme borreliosis. The incidence of Lyme borreliosis is particularly high in the southern parts of Scandinavia (especially Sweden), the Netherlands, parts of Germany, Austria, Slovenia, and northern Italy, but the disease is found throughout Europe (O'Connell et al., 1998; Dennis, 2002). While EM is defined as the hallmark of early Lyme borreliosis, lymphocytoma is a subacute lesion, and acrodermatitis is the typical cutaneous manifestation of late Lyme borreliosis. In Europe at least three subtypes of the spirochete species group *B. burgdorferi* sensu lato can cause EM (van Dam et al., 1993; Picken et al., 1998; Wang et al., 1998). *Borrelia afzelii* infections are more prevalent than cases induced by *B. garinii* or *B. burgdorferi* sensu stricto (Müllegger, 2004). Other subtypes, such as *B. valaisiana* or *B. spielmanii* have occasionally been described to cause EM (Steere, 2006; Fingerle et al., 2008). In North America, *B. burgdorferi* sensu stricto is the only relevant subtype, which seems to be responsible for differences in clinical expression of EM between the continents. The spirochete is transmitted by ixodid ticks (Steere, 2001; Stanek and Strle, 2003; 2006). Although other insect bites are reported by about 5% of patients at the site of EM in Europe, these are likely coincidental (Strle et al., 1996a; Müllegger, 2001).

PATHOGENESIS

During the feeding process, spirochetes migrate to the tick's salivary glands from its midgut. They are then inoculated along with tick saliva into the skin at the site of attachment. Certain outer surface proteins play key roles in this transmission. OspA is expressed while the organism resides in the gut of the unfed tick, but as the tick gets attached, OspA is downregulated at the same time as OspC expression becomes detectable. This suggests that OspC is an essential factor allowing transmission from the tick to the mammalian host. Further, variability within OspC genetic sequences results in strain variability in *B. burgdorferi* sensu stricto, and this may be a major factor in dissemination, specifically whether a patient develops single or multiple EM (Seinost et al., 1999). The tick feeding process is much more complex, with the tick employing a "pharmacopoeia" of bioactive compounds, including salivary enzymes, cement, anticoagulants, and anti-inflammatory chemicals to ensure prolonged attachment and successful feeding. Further detail is beyond the scope of this chapter but can be found in the recent book *Tick-Borne Diseases of Humans* (Goodman et al., 2005).

Lyme borreliosis is an instructive example of a disease in which the clinical outcome is determined by interaction at several levels between the etiologic agent, *B*. burgdorferi sensu lato, its vector, and the host. On the part of the spirochete, different genospecies within the *B*. burgdorferi sensu lato complex have divergent pathogenic potential depending on their tissue tropism, binding to host proteins, cytokine induction, and susceptibility to complement-mediated lysis (Isogai et al., 1996; Kraiczy et al., 2004; Steere, 2006). These differences are clinically reflected by the fact that distinct clinical manifestations of

Lyme borreliosis are correlated with different subtypes of *B. burgdorferi* sensu lato (Wang et al., 1999).

The course of Lyme borreliosis is also greatly influenced by the host's immune response, which is mounted to eradicate *B. burgdorferi* sensu lato and is involved in the subsequent pathology, resulting in intense inflammatory reaction with perivascular accumulation of mononuclear leukocytes, and sometimes damage of infected tissues. In EM the immune response is concentrated at the site of infection in the skin and regional lymph nodes (Vaz et al., 2001). Its complex cellular and humoral reactions result from potent stimulatory effects of *B. burgdorferi* sensu lato on a variety of host cell types, including endothelial cells, macrophages, lymphocytes, and neutrophils, eliciting proliferation, cytokine and chemokine secretion, and upregulation of adhesion molecules (Müllegger, 2004; Steere, 2006).

After spirochetes have been transmitted from the tick to the skin, the following series of events ensues: Constituent cells secrete chemoattractants for neutrophils, dendritic cells, and macrophages as part of the innate immune response. Macrophages and dendritic cells engulf *B. burgdorferi* sensu lato and migrate to peripheral lymph nodes where they present processed spirochetal peptides to T cells, initiating the adaptive immune response (Filgueira et al., 1996; Sigal, 1997; Müllegger et al., 2000; Vaz et al., 2001). T cells have both cytotoxic potential and the ability to initiate specific antibody production by B cells for opsonization of *B. burgdorferi* sensu lato. This seems to be critically important for optimal killing of this large, extracellular pathogen in addition to the inflammatory innate immune response (Sigal, 1997; Müllegger et al., 2000; Steere, 2006). B cells, however, may also be primed directly by intact borrelial lipoproteins (McKisic and Barthold, 2000).

These immunologic mechanisms are well reflected by histologic, immunohistochemical, and molecular characteristics of the infection site. Macrophages, dendritic cells, neutrophils, and CD4+ as well as CD8+ T cells and their respective chemoattractants are all found in significant numbers or concentrations in EM lesions (Müllegger et al., 2000, 2007; Salazar et al., 2003). In addition smaller amounts of the B cell chemoattractant CXCL13 and B cells are regularly present (Müllegger et al., 2007). In a recent study using quantitative reverse transcription polymerase chain reaction to determine mRNA expression of chemokines, cytokines, and leukocyte markers in skin samples from EM patients (Müllegger et al., 2007), the IFN-γ-inducible Th1 chemokines, CXCL10 and CXCL9, which are strong chemoattractants for effector CD8+ and Th1-type CD4+ T cells, were found to be strongly expressed in EM lesions. T cells seem to be a source of IFN-γ, which helps activate, in a feedback loop, the IFN-γ-inducible Th1 chemokines and the IFN-γ-inducible macrophage chemokine CCL2, which results in the recruitment of more macrophages and effector CD8+ and Th1-type CD4+ T cells. This amplification mechanism may explain the discrepancy between the strong local inflammatory reaction and the generally low spirochetal load in EM lesions. Accordingly the cytokine expression in these skin lesions is primarily a proinflammatory pattern with particularly high amounts of IFN-γ, TNF-α, IL-1β, and IL-6, although some anti-inflammatory activity, mostly in the form of IL-10 production, is also found (Müllegger et al., 2000, 2007). Of interest, EM patients with associated extracutaneous symptoms produce more proinflammatory macrophage-derived cytokines (Müllegger et al., 2000).

Despite the innate and adaptive immune responses, *B. burgdorferi* sensu lato may disseminate to other organs and sometimes survive in certain sites, probably by downregulation of certain outer-surface proteins (Steere, 2006). The patient's immune response is influenced by several factors, including age and sex, inducing varying clinical expressions of Lyme borreliosis in children and adults (Müllegger, 2004; Bennet et al., 2006). Differences in tissue microenvironment, such as the presence of stromal cells in varying body sites and their interaction with infiltrating immune cells, as well as modulation of the immune response by ultraviolet radiation in sun-exposed surfaces, may be additional factors that influence the course of infection (Brown et al., 1995; Douglas et al., 2002).

CLINICAL MANIFESTATIONS

Erythema Migrans in North America

The characteristic early lesion of Lyme borreliosis in the United States is now termed EM. Clinicians in endemic areas and even patients themselves may readily recognize the familiar annular skin rash, but this pathognomonic clinical marker may occasionally manifest with atypical features that are diagnostically challenging. Since it appears in most patients at least one or two weeks before an identifiable immune response occurs, familiarity with the different appearances of EM is important in order to make an accurate clinical diagnosis and start antibiotic therapy before dissemination potentially takes place.

EM represents localized skin infection with *B. burgdorferi* sensu stricto, starting as a macule or papule, at a site where the person has been bitten by an *Ixodes* tick acquiring a blood meal. More often than not, patients do not remember a tick bite at this location. Indeed the history of a tick bite is only relevant if it was at the site of the skin rash, as other recalled tick bites may not be responsible for the presenting disease. More important is an awareness of the epidemiologic setting in which the rash has occurred. Because the likelihood of infection after the bite of an infected tick is directly related to duration of tick attachment (Sood et al., 1997), it is relevant that most lesions occur in hospitable intertriginous regions of the body, especially the inguinocrural areas, axillae and popliteal fossae, and the back, where ticks are less likely to be noticed thus allowing transmission of the spirochete. Other common sites, especially in children, are the retroauricular and nuchal areas.

The initial macule or papule enlarges centrifugally, resulting in a variety of types of well-circumscribed erythema, expanding in size as the duration of the lesion increases. For surveillance purposes, the Centers for Disease Control and Prevention in the United States has defined the size of EM to be at least 5 cm, although smaller lesions may be recognizable to experienced clinicians before they attain this diameter. While arbitrary, this criterion may be useful in clinical practice because tick bites often result in significant localized redness that may be mistaken for EM. This is an immediate inflammatory response or hypersensitivity reaction that may be minimal or occasionally enlarge to 4 or 5 cm in diameter. Patients usually relate that these rashes appeared within hours of the tick bite, unlike EM, which requires at least two or three days of spirochetal multiplication before it manifests. Although sometimes annular, local reactions to tick bites are less well circumscribed than EM, often with a somewhat patchy aspect and irregular borders. They are comparatively more pruritic, and progressively fade within two or three days without further expansion. The earliest appearance of EM may be somewhat difficult to differentiate with certainty from this type of localized reaction (see Differential Diagnosis).

Untreated EM typically enlarges and develops central clearing, a punctate area of scaly erythema and induration often remaining visible or palpable at the bite site. Lesions 20 to 30 cm or more in size are not uncommonly encountered. The early rash is more likely to present with homogeneous erythema that may be confluent or sometimes centrally dark red with a pale peripheral ring (Figure 3.1 and 3.2a). Central clearing is thus a chronological or

(a) (b)

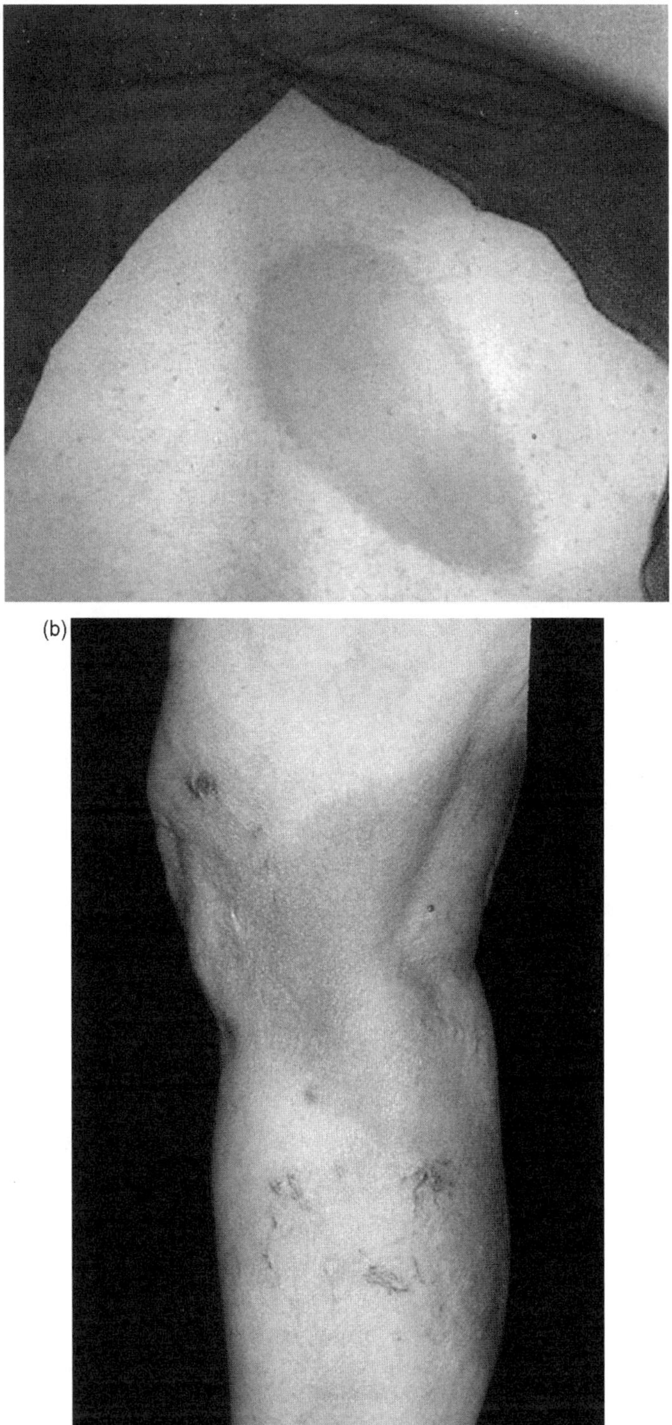

Figure 3.1 Solitary erythema migrans: (a) Plaque-like (United States—VKS), (b) large macular lesion (Europe—RRM). (*See insert for color representation*).

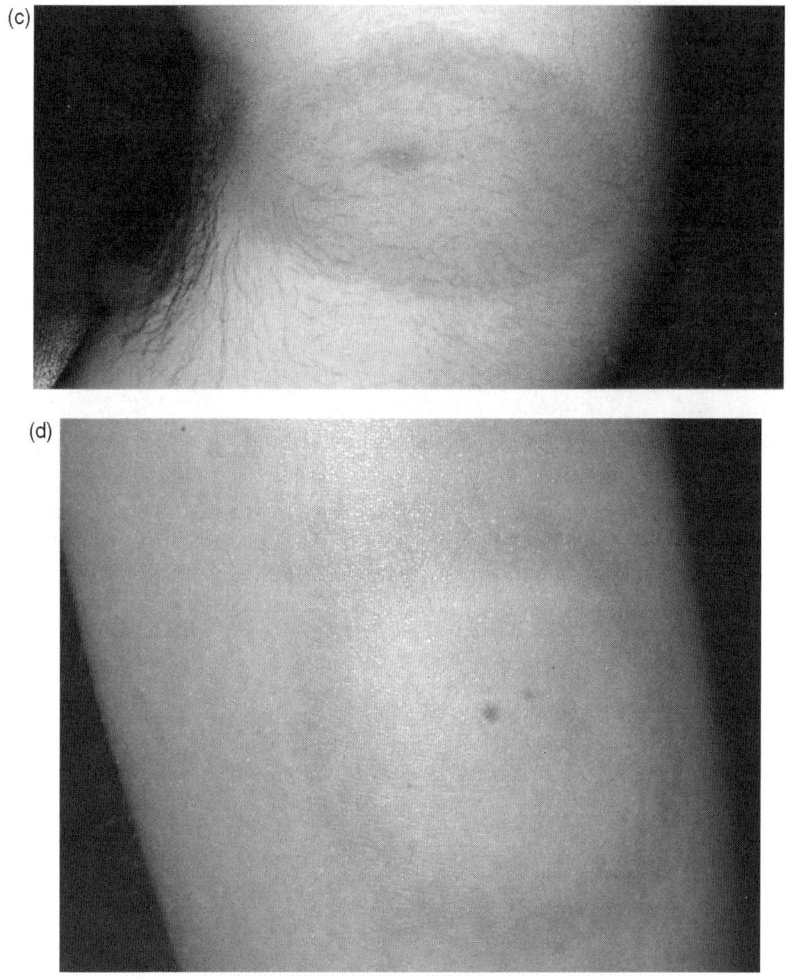

Figure 3.1 Solitary erythema migrans: (c) Dark annular (United States—VKS), (d) faint annular (Europe—RRM). (*See insert for color representation*).

evolutionary change in lesions seen later in their course with increasing duration and expansion in size (Nadelman et al., 1996; Smith et al., 2002). Untreated EM gradually clears within weeks or months after onset.

EM is usually slightly warm to the touch, although patients may not be aware of it. Many patients report a vague dysesthesia in the affected skin, while others describe a somewhat pruritic or burning sensation. Pain is much less common and more likely to be present with some of the intensely inflammatory lesions found in the popliteal fossa and axilla. In these locations, friction and occlusion of affected skin under mechanical tension from knee or shoulder movements exacerbate sensation and awareness of the rash, as well as predispose to necrosis or ulceration.

Atypical morphology may make the visual diagnosis more difficult. Depending on location, the shape may not be annular but instead conform to anatomical skin creases. Hence, in the inguinocrural area, popliteal fossa, axilla, shoulder, and adjacent mammary

(a)

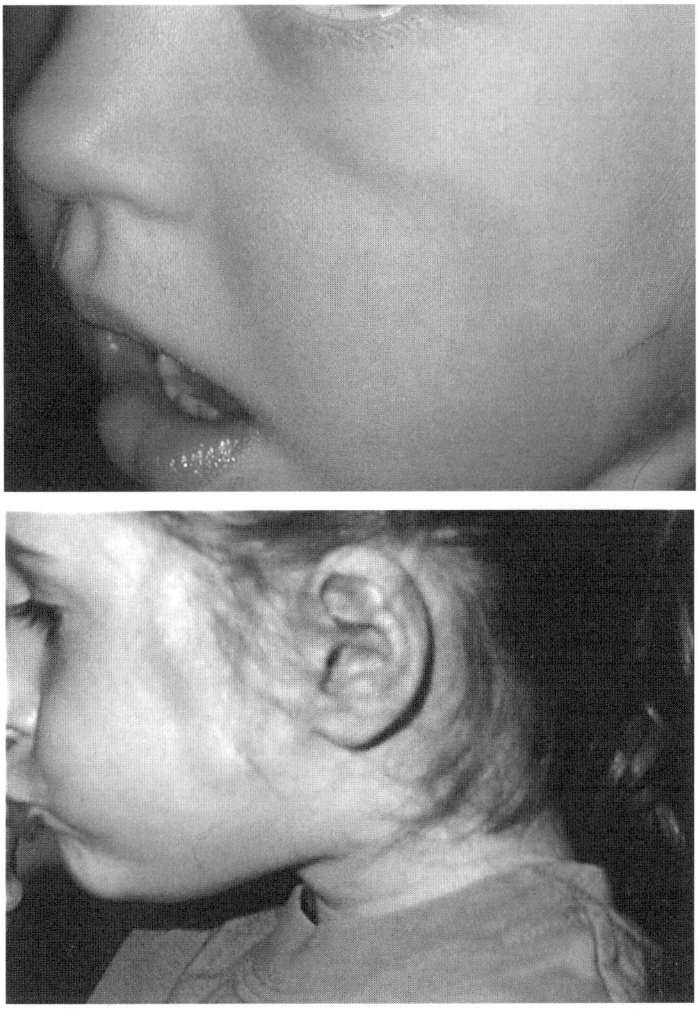

(b)

Figure 3.2 Erythema migrans on the head/face of a child: (a) On the face of a two-year-old girl (Europe—RRM); (b) scalp lesion only partially visible on the face (United States—VKS). (*See insert for color representation*).

locations, lesions may be found that are oval, triangular, or rhomboid in shape. EM presents occasionally on the scalp, especially in children, and in this location may be seen as a linear red streak emerging from the hairline onto the adjacent face or neck (Figure 3.2b). Although varying shades of red are the norm, coloration may occasionally be purpuric, with violaceous hues evolving to a yellow-brown. As with other erythematous skin rashes, the shade or tone of EM in dark-skinned individuals may vary according to the tint of the affected skin.

Besides differences in shape and color, other less common but well-documented morphological variations may present, including lesions with bullae, blistering, central vesiculation, pustule formation, ulceration, and necrosis (Nadelman et al., 1996) (Figure 3.3). Linear lesions are often found in the center of the popliteal fossa at the skin

(a)

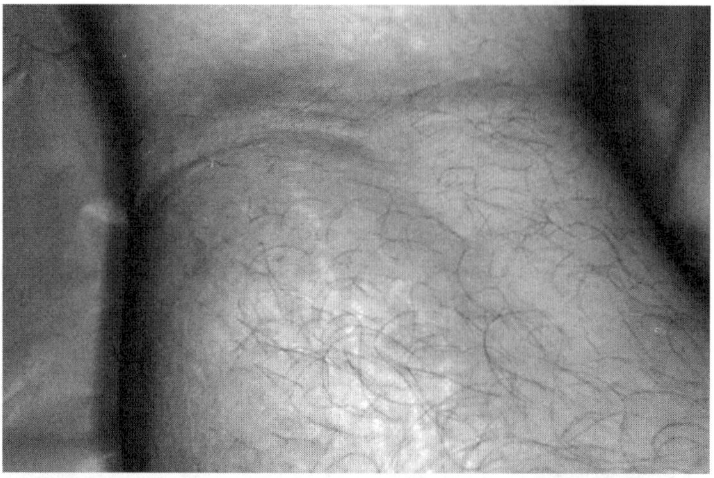

(b)

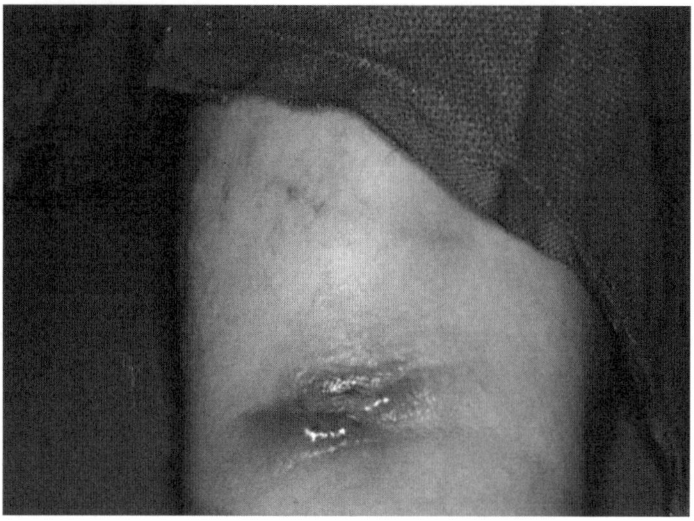

Figure 3.3 Atypical EM (United States—VKS): (a) Linear, (b) bullous. (*See insert for color representation*).

crease (Figure 3.3a). Patients are more likely to report localized pain or burning sensation when these atypical features are present. Indeed these atypical EM presentations may easily mimic similar lesions associated with viral etiology, other bacterial infections, and arthropod bites.[1]

Multiple Secondary Erythema Migrans

EM may also present in the United States with multiple secondary annular skin lesions, a sign of hematogenous or lymphatic dissemination of *B. burgdorferi* sensu stricto from the

[1] All figures by VKS *except 3.1(b)* are culture-proven lesions.

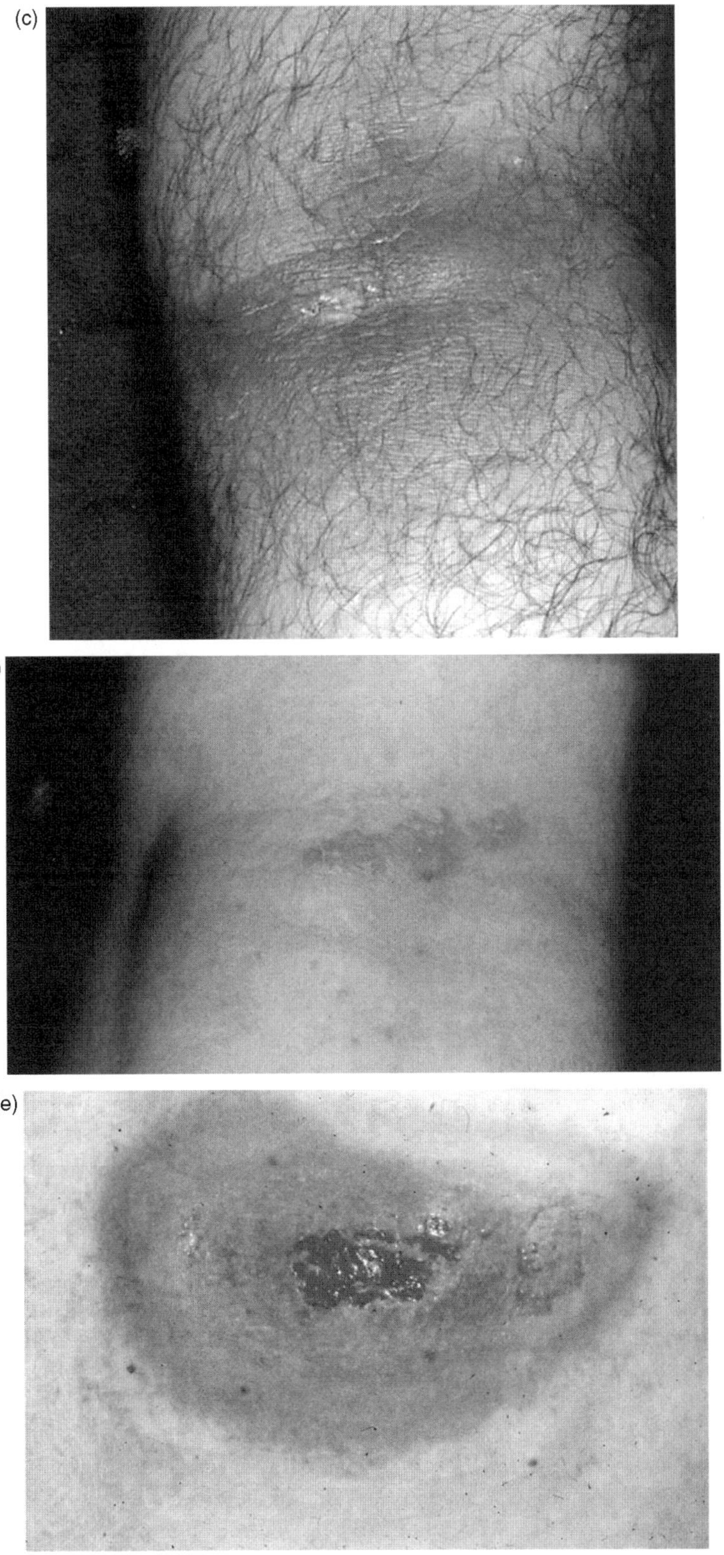

Figure 3.3 Atypical EM (United States—VKS): (c) Pustular, (d) vesicular, (e) ulcerated. (*See insert for color representation*).

tick bite site and primary lesion. This may occur days to weeks later and is related to duration of infection, host immunologic phenomena, and strain variation. With early diagnosis and treatment of primary EM lesions, less than 20% of patients present with secondary lesions (Smith et al., 2002), which are usually circular or oval in shape and uniformly red in color (Figure 3.4). Examination may reveal two or three satellite lesions or at times even dozens, appearing in quick succession in proximity to or very distant from the index lesion, sometimes fading evanescently and re-appearing. *Borrelia burgdorferi* sensu stricto can be cultured from punch biopsy specimens and aspirates from the leading margin (Berger et al., 1992; Wormser et al., 1992; Strle et al., 1996b).

Secondary EM lesions may be slightly warm to palpate, but they lack many of the characteristic morphologic features of primary EM. Since they are not associated with preceding tick bites, induration and scaling are not seen. Idiosyncratic features like vesicle formation, pustulation, hyperpigmentation, necrosis, and ulceration are not seen. Patients rarely report symptoms like local pain or itching. The most prominent attribute of multiple annular EM lesions is their dramatic presentation, with rather abrupt onset, rapid progression, and sporadic evanescence.

Symptoms and Signs Associated with Erythema Migrans

A nonspecific "flu-like" illness manifests as part of the presenting syndrome in about two-thirds of patients with EM in the United States (Berger, 1989; Nadelman et al., 1992). These constitutional symptoms and signs precede or accompany the appearance of the skin rash but occasionally occur days later. Symptoms include sub-acute onset of oligoarticular migratory arthralgias and myalgias, associated with headache, fatigue, neck stiffness, fever, chills, anorexia, nausea, and malaise. Less commonly, mild sore throat, back pain, and paresthesia or dysesthesia may be reported. Musculoskeletal symptoms of early Lyme borreliosis are typically migratory and intermittent. Headache, fatigue, and malaise may persist for several days or weeks. Coryza and gastrointestinal symptoms are notably absent.

Nonspecific physical signs like mild fever, meningismus, regional or generalized lymphadenopathy, and mild joint tenderness without swelling may be elicited in some patients. Less commonly, slight conjunctival and pharyngeal mucosal injection are seen, especially in febrile patients. Specific objective findings such as cranial neuritis are rarely encountered in association with EM. However, when present, seventh cranial nerve palsy is most common, followed by trigeminal paresthesia (Steere et al., 1998; Smith et al., 2002).

Erythema Migrans in Europe

EM is defined as an expanding round to oval, sharply demarcated, red to bluish-red skin lesion (Asbrink, 1985; Weber and Neubert, 1986; Asbrink and Hovmark, 1988; Asbrink, 1991; Stanek et al., 1996; Strle et al., 1996; Müllegger, 2001, 2004; Stanek and Strle, 2003). The average incubation period following a tick bite is two weeks, but ranges from three days to six months (Strle et al., 1996a,c; Müllegger, 2004). A history of tick bite is not elicited in up to two thirds of patients and should therefore not be used as a diagnostic criterion (Strle et al., 1996c; Arnez et al., 2001a). As ticks bite preferentially on areas of thinner skin in the warm bends of joints, EM in adults is most often located in the calf/knee, groin/buttock, or armpit/shoulder region, although they may be located anywhere on the

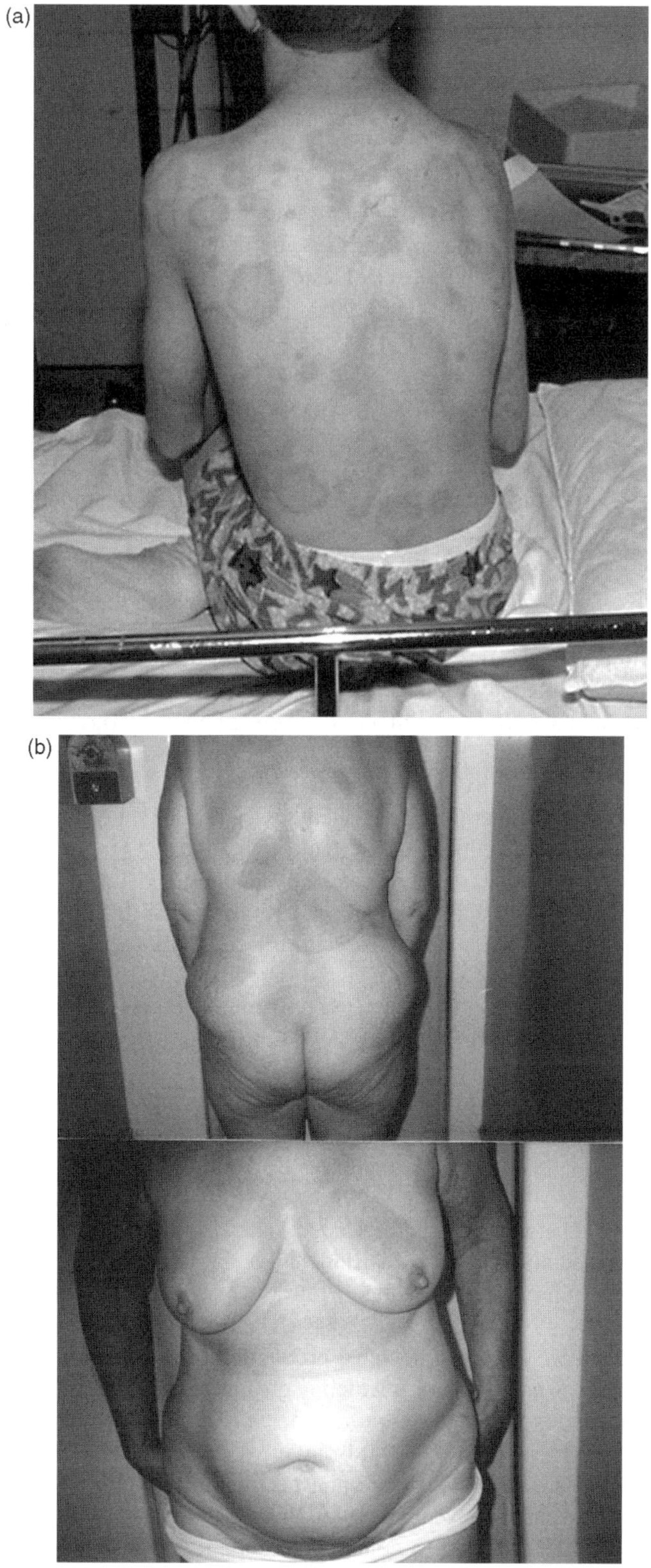

Figure 3.4 Disseminated erythema migrans: (a) Child (United States—Lorry Rubin), (b) adult (United States—VKS). (*See insert for color representation*).

body except for the palms and soles. In children the site of predilection is the head and neck region, due to their shorter height and play habits. EM in the head and neck region of children is sometimes followed by a peripheral facial palsy on the same side (Eiffert et al., 2004). The average diameter of EM is 15 cm, but varies widely from lesions beyond 80 cm to very small lesions, although these extreme sizes are rare (Stanek et al., 1996; Strle et al., 2002). A minimum diameter of 5 cm is, by definition, required for the diagnosis (Asbrink, 1991). Nevertheless, atypical EM lesions with a persistent small size occur in 1% to 3% of European patients (Müllegger, 2001). The term "mini(ature size) EM" has been coined for these lesions (Weber and Wilske, 2006), which are preferentially located on the lower extremities. For these to be recognized as EM, microbiologic confirmation of the presence of *B. burgdorferi* sensu lato or its DNA from the erythema should be obtained. The size of an EM lesion also depends considerably on disease duration. The average daily growth rate (largest diameter divided by disease duration) is 1.0 cm (Furst et al., 2006). Disease duration before the first visit ranges from one day to several months, with a median of 10 days.(Strle et al., 1999, 2002)

EM lesions can be classified clinically as solitary macular, solitary annular, or disseminated (multiple) lesions. Solitary macular EM, which remains homogeneously erythematous throughout the disease course (Figure 3.2b), is more frequent than solitary annular EM (~45:40%) (Müllegger, 2001). The latter displays a ring-like appearance with central clearing (Figure 3.2c). Recent studies have suggested that annular lesions are significantly more often associated with *B. afzelii* infection, whereas homogeneous lesions are caused by *B. garinii* infection (Carlsson et al., 2003). *Borrelia garinii*-associated macular EM is found in older patients, preferentially on the trunk, develops more rapidly and after a shorter incubation period, and is generally larger (Carlsson et al., 2003; Logar et al., 2004). These patients also more often have local and systemic symptoms and laboratory abnormalities (CRP, liver function tests) and are more frequently seropositive (Logar et al., 2004; Bennet et al., 2006). Thus *B. garinii* appears to induce a more virulent infection in European EM patients than does *B. afzelii*. A target-like appearance ("bull's eye" EM), which may be regarded as a variant of solitary annular EM, is observed in only 2% of European patients. In rare atypical cases the EM ring is interrupted or incomplete, or sometimes forms a C-like figure. A hemorrhagic or purpuric appearance is quite often seen in leg lesions, particularly in or distal to the popliteal fossa. Blistering and scaling may occasionally be observed (Asbrink, 1991; Weber, 1993). Local symptoms, such as itching or burning, which are reported by fewer than half of the patients, are generally mild, whereas regional neuritis that is present in a small number of patients may be painful for weeks (Asbrink, 1985; Strle et al., 2002).

Major differences between EM in the United States and Europe include shorter disease duration before presentation, faster expansion, higher frequency of abnormal liver function tests, and elevated erythrocyte sedimentation rate as well as seroreactivity to *Borrelia* in US patients (Arnez et al., 1999; Jones et al., 2008). The reason for these differences appears to be in part a *Borrelia* subtype-associated production of proinflammatory macrophage-associated chemokines and cytokines, which is greater in US lesions (Jones et al., 2008). Systemic extracutaneous signs and symptoms affect one-third to one-half of EM patients in Europe as opposed to at least two-thirds in the United States (Weber, 1993; Arnez et al., 1999; Jones et al., 2008). They are nonspecific, mild to moderate, and usually last only for a few days (Weber and Neubert, 1986; Weber, 1993; Nadelman et al., 1996; Arnez et al., 1999; Strle et al., 2002). Most common are fatigue, malaise, headache, arthralgias, myalgias, elevated temperature, and lymphadenopathy. It is important that other conditions be considered in the differential diagnosis of extracutaneous symptoms. These include concomitant manifestations such as neuroborreliosis, and co-infecting anaplasmosis or tick-borne encephalitis. In a serologic investigation of Austrian EM patients, co-infection with *Anaplasma phagocytophilum* was found in 12% of cases (RM, unpublished data). A significantly higher number of co-infected patients (64%) had extracutaneous symptoms.

Development of multiple EM lesions may result from hematogenous dissemination of the spirochete from a primary skin lesion (Asbrink and Hovmark, 1988; Arnez et al., 2001a; Maraspin et al., 2002). The disease course in this case involves a typical primary EM that is followed by secondary, often smaller and less intense, lesions after a latency period of a few days. According to our own observations (RM), multiple lesions may also be due to more than one tick bite or due to regional spread of the infection. The lesions in these cases are more clustered. Multiple EM lesions are described with varying frequency (range 4–>20% of EM patients) and are slightly less common in Europe (Weber and Neubert, 1986; Nadelman et al., 1996; Strle et al., 1999; Müllegger, 2001; Strle et al., 2002; Smith et al., 2002). The number of lesions per patient ranges from 2 to 70 (mean, 3–5) and is lower in Europe (Asbrink, 1985; Nadelman et al., 1996; Arnez et al., 2001a; Müllegger, 2001). Up to two-thirds of all patients with multiple EM lesions have extracutaneous symptoms or additional organ manifestations (Arnez et al., 2001a; Maraspin et al., 2002). EM may precede or accompany borrelial lymphocytoma in rare instances (Asbrink and Hovmark, 1988; Strle et al., 1992), and between <10% and 20% of patients with acrodermatitis chronica atrophicans had an EM lesion at the same body site months to years earlier (Asbrink et al., 1985; Müllegger, 2004)

Flu-like Illness of Early Lyme Borreliosis without Erythema Migrans

Early Lyme borreliosis may manifest in the United States with nonspecific systemic symptoms without the EM rash characteristic of localized infection (Feder et al., 1993; Steere et al., 2003a). There are no comparable data from Europe. These patients present in endemic areas during late spring, summer or early fall with a flu-like illness notable for the absence of respiratory or gastrointestinal symptoms. In some cases the EM might have been missed in a patient who has not completely undressed for a thorough examination of the skin. Others may have viral or different tick-borne infections, including *Babesia microti* and *Anaplasma* infection. The clinical picture in these patients is comparable to that encountered in the nonspecific flu-like illness typically seen in Lyme borreliosis associated with EM. Lest these symptoms and signs be dismissed as a "summer flu" by patient or clinician, the history of a tick bite in the preceding few days or weeks or recent outdoor activities in an endemic area should be elicited. Patients co-infected with other tick-borne pathogens will present with an even more severe form of this illness (see Chapter 8).

Patients who experience nonspecific systemic symptoms without a skin rash are less likely to seek early medical evaluation. As with EM, serology may be negative early in the course, but convalescent serum samples can establish the diagnosis.

Asymptomatic Infection with *Borrelia burgdorferi*

The occurrence of asymptomatic infection with *B. burgdorferi* is rare in the United States, but it has been well documented in a large controlled Lyme disease vaccine study of nearly

11,000 participants residing in 10 states where the disease is highly endemic (Steere et al., 1998, 2003b). Previous epidemiologic surveys on both continents have described groups of individuals with serological evidence of infection with *B. burgdorferi* who have no recollection of having experienced any symptoms of Lyme borreliosis (Hanrahan et al., 1984; Steere et al., 1986; Lastavica et al., 1989; Gustafson et al., 1990; Fahrer et al., 1991; Zhioua et al., 1998). Indeed clinicians in endemic areas often encounter seropositivity to *B. burgdorferi* in patients with no known history of this disease. Undoubtedly, some of these patients may have forgotten mild systemic symptoms or perhaps not noticed a skin rash in a difficult to visualize location that resolved without treatment. Nevertheless, their management could present a dilemma for primary care physicians in endemic areas.

The clinical significance of asymptomatic infection with *B. burgdorferi* is unclear and its management controversial. In the vaccine study Western blotting was performed with baseline sera that were stored and available to compare with sera obtained after two consecutive tick transmission seasons (Steere et al., 1998, 2003b). Most of the volunteers subsequently identified with asymptomatic IgG seroconversion were treated with antibiotics when laboratory results were available to the investigators about 4 to 6 months later in a protocol that encompassed two summers. They were followed for 4 to 14 months after treatment. Only one patient, a subject with asymptomatic seroconversion who was not treated with antibiotics, developed a late manifestation of Lyme borreliosis. This study volunteer presented with Lyme arthritis that was confirmed by polymerase chain reaction with synovial fluid aspirate.

Before the spirochetal etiology and antibiotic therapy of Lyme borreliosis were elucidated in the early 1980s, significant numbers of untreated patients with early symptoms of disease were observed to subsequently develop cardiac, neurologic, and rheumatologic manifestations weeks, months, or years later (Steere et al., 1987). Thus it would appear clinically prudent to treat patients identified with asymptomatic seroconversion empirically with a presumption of possible latent infection, as has long been the practice analogously in asymptomatic patients found to be seropositive for *Treponema pallidum*. Such an approach raises valid questions, however, such as whether to investigate these patients for possible latent central nervous system infection by cerebrospinal fluid analysis or radiologic imaging. If further studies are not done, should these patients be treated with oral or parenteral antibiotics and for what duration? In general, clinical practice in the highly endemic areas is to offer a one month course of oral antibiotics, after the potential benefits are discussed with the patient and weighed against the relatively low risk of adverse effects with treatment. While there is more art than science in this approach, it is favored by most patients over the relatively greater unpredictability of watchful waiting.

DIFFERENTIAL DIAGNOSIS

The differential diagnosis of a solitary EM lesion includes common arthropod bite reaction, cellulitis, circumscribed scleroderma (morphea), granuloma annulare, tinea, fixed drug eruption, erysipeloid, and contact dermatitis (Asbrink, 1985). Multiple EM may need to be distinguished from urticaria, multilocular fixed drug eruption, erythema annulare centrifugum, and erythema infectiosum.

With the exception of indoor spider bites, which occur throughout the year, insect bites are generally encountered during the same warm seasons and are also associated with outdoor activities. Differentiation between EM and a noninfectious arthropod bite reaction can usually be made by observing the progress of the lesion. A nonspecific reaction enlarges quickly after the bite and will clear from the edge within a few days without antibiotic therapy. In contrast, EM does not occur before a minimum incubation period of two to three days following the bite and progressively expands without treatment. The course of the lesion may be followed for a few days before committing to antibiotic treatment. When patients present early with lesions that are too small to confidently diagnose, the simple observational technique of drawing a line around the circumference of the rash and re-evaluating its evolution in one or two days is helpful in differentiating local reactions from EM. In Europe, because of the slower expansion of EM, patients are generally rechecked after four or five days. Also arthropod reactions usually itch or burn more intensely and often have an urticarial appearance. Constitutional symptoms commonly associated with early Lyme borreliosis are not reported with local hypersensitivity reactions.

Contact allergic dermatitis due to plant resins found in poison ivy, oak, sumac, and other foliage is frequently encountered during the same seasons as EM and may need to be differentiated from some atypical EM lesions. These inflammatory reactions present as erythematous plaques that can be readily distinguished by their severe and constant pruritus and significant epidermal changes (vesiculation, scaling). Plant contact dermatitis is more often found on exposed areas of skin, although the offending antigen may be transferred manually to other parts of the body, causing additional lesions. Erysipeloid is most typically found on the fingers or hands, is more violaceous, and expands much more slowly than EM.

Acute bacterial cellulitis may resemble EM early in its course, but commonly presents with acute onset of fever and chills, rapid progression, and pain. Underlying dermatoses or minor trauma may be noted as portals of bacterial skin entry. Cellulitis usually has irregular borders and plaque formation, and may be associated with lymphangitis and tender regional lymphadenopathy. Lymphadenopathy is uncommon in EM and is not associated with tenderness or overlying erythema when present. While EM is usually not found on the distal lower leg, this is the most common site for cellulitis.

Tinea corporis or "ringworm" presents as a well-demarcated annular erythematous plaque or patch with central clearing that may be confused with EM. However, its onset and progress are more insidious, with slow growth over a period of weeks or months. As with EM, ringworm may be slightly pruritic, but other defining differences like the presence of marginal scale and a slightly raised border usually make the diagnosis clear. Microscopic visualization of hyphae in potassium hydroxide preparations of scrapings obtained from the active border of the lesion supports the diagnosis. The annular bright red herald patch of pityriasis rosea may resemble the appearance of early EM, since it occasionally attains a size of 5 cm before the onset of highly characteristic secondary lesions on the trunk and proximal extremities.

The erythematous solitary and sometimes multiple patches that characterize fixed drug eruptions may mimic single or multiple secondary EM lesions. These start as macules and papules and can attain a size of 15 to 20 cm. Like EM, a fixed drug eruption is usually asymptomatic or may be slightly pruritic or have a burning sensation. However, a history of ingestion of a drug followed within minutes or hours by the rash is usually elicited, and the location is often on genital or facial skin or mucous membranes. If the drug is discontinued, these lesions resolve within days to weeks and will characteristically reappear at the same skin sites when the drug is taken again.

Erythema multiforme, which may also be accompanied by mild to moderate nonspecific constitutional symptoms like malaise and fever, may need to be differentiated from multiple secondary EM lesions. There is often a recent history of herpes simplex or drug ingestion. In this syndrome, acute erythematous vesicobullous or urticarial lesions occur typically on the extremities and involve the palms or soles, and at times mucous membranes, a distribution never seen in Lyme borreliosis. When present, target- or iris-shaped plaques are pathognomonic.

A tick-associated rash resembling EM, associated with mild systemic symptoms, including fever, headache, fatigue, and musculoskeletal pain, has been reported in the southeastern United States, a region where Lyme borreliosis is not known to occur (Campbell et al., 1995; Barbour, 1996; Kirkland et al., 1997). Almost all the affected patients have a history of a tick bite days to weeks earlier, identified in many of the cases as *Amblyomma americanum*, the Lone Star tick. Like EM, this rash occurs at the site of the tick bite, starting as a red papule that expands with central clearing and a somewhat annular appearance, occasionally associated with pain and pruritus. Its borders tend to be more irregular than typical EM. Acute and convalescent serological testing yield no antibody responses to *B. burgdorferi*, and cultures of skin biopsy specimens are negative for spirochetes. The organism causally related to this EM-like disease is still unknown, if this is an infectious illness at all. A 10-day course of doxycycline has been curative of the rash.

Determining the cause of a nonspecific febrile illness is clinically challenging in geographic areas where tick-borne diseases are endemic. In the absence of EM, differential diagnosis of early Lyme borreliosis centers on a careful consideration of other possible causes of flu-like illnesses. Nonspecific symptoms of common viral illnesses are usually associated with gastrointestinal or respiratory symptoms and signs. When these are clearly absent in an individual presenting during the late spring, summer, and early fall in an endemic area, and skin rash has been ruled out after a complete examination of the undressed patient, vector-borne diseases become a primary concern.

While tick-borne infections far outnumber other vector-borne illnesses in the United States and Europe, acute viral infections associated with mosquito bites, especially West Nile virus and eastern equine encephalitis in the United States, occur during the same seasons in the same geographic locations. As with infection caused by *B. burgdorferi*, symptoms of these mosquito-borne viral illnesses may be mild and self-limiting. In Europe and Asia, tick-borne encephalitis occurring in spring and summer is caused by a flavivirus transmitted by *I. ricinus* and *I. persulcatus* ticks. If prominent neurological symptoms are present in a North American patient who appears very ill, especially with severe headache and meningismus, a viral etiology should be considered along with Lyme borreliosis, Rocky Mountain Spotted Fever, anaplasmosis, ehrlichiosis, and babesiosis.

DIAGNOSIS

Despite the wealth of data accumulated in the research literature pertaining to serologic and microbiologic diagnosis of Lyme borreliosis, identification of early disease remains primarily a clinical diagnosis in practice (Nadelman et al., 1996; Smith et al., 2002). In France the recognition rate of EM by dermatologists was >90% (Lipsker et al., 2004). A somewhat delayed host antibody response during the first few weeks after infection severely limits the utility of serodiagnosis. Furthermore false-positive results by ELISA tests are commonly encountered in a wide array of patients, including viral infections such as infectious mononucleosis, autoimmune diseases, and human granulocytic anaplasmosis, as well as in healthy individuals. In addition baseline seropositivity is frequently encountered in endemic areas in individuals with previously treated Lyme borreliosis, untreated mild illness, or asymptomatic infection. For these reasons there is no role for diagnostic serology when a characteristic erythema migrans rash is present. Nevertheless, serologic analyses of IgG and IgM antibodies to *B. burgdorferi* sensu lato are frequently ordered in clinical practice on both continents. At the time of initial appearance of erythema migrans and flu-like illness (i.e., within about 7 days of onset of symptoms), antibody responses to *B. burgdorferi* can be detected in up to one-third of patients. This proportion is approximately two-thirds if the rash has been present for more than a week or is disseminated. All but about a fifth of EM patients will seroconvert as soon as 8 to 14 days after the initiation of antibiotic treatment. Thus testing of consecutive serum samples may be a diagnostic aid in selected situations, such as a very atypical rash. A detailed discussion of the role of serodiagnosis can be found in Chapter 10.

One other situation in which serodiagnosis may be warranted is the occurrence of summer flu-like symptoms without EM. In the United States many experienced clinicians in endemic areas treat such presentations empirically with doxycycline. This approach provides adequate coverage for Lyme borreliosis and human granulocytic anaplasmosis. However, if the patient appears very ill and has prominent fever, headache, and fatigue, infection with *Babesia* spp. should be ruled out, as doxycycline is not effective therapy for this tick-borne infection, and testing for Lyme borreliosis and *Anaplasma* infection should be considered. Confirmation of diagnosis for all these infections usually requires a convalescent serum sample to be tested.

The complete blood count (CBC) is an inexpensive and rapid test that can provide clues to the etiology of summer flu-like illnesses. White blood cell counts are usually normal in patients with Lyme borreliosis and babesiosis, but low in those with anaplasmosis. Significant thrombocytopenia is a common finding with babesiosis, and occasionally noted to a lesser extent in anaplasmosis, but is not generally seen in Lyme borreliosis alone. More severe babesial parasitemia may cause hemolytic anemia. When the CBC suggests a co-infection, the clinician should request peripheral smears to look for evidence of these other tick-borne organisms (see Chapter 8).

Diagnostic difficulty is often encountered in individuals bitten by ticks in endemic areas who subsequently present elsewhere for evaluation of symptoms and signs. As this disease is the most common vector-borne illness in North America and Europe, a large number of individuals fall into this category, including tourists, business travelers, and college students attending university in a distant state. A careful travel or residence history is thus essential for prompt diagnosis in non-endemic areas. In these circumstances, for the clinician unfamiliar with Lyme borreliosis, acute and convalescent serological evaluation may be warranted. Furthermore telediagnostic consultation with colleagues in endemic areas can be employed. The ready availability and instant transmission of digital photographs of skin lesions has revolutionized diagnostic capabilities in such settings. Telediagnostic recognition of EM in this manner is a pertinent example of how physicians can broaden their diagnostic armamentarium globally beyond the traditional laboratory.

Because of numerous practical limitations, at the present time culture or PCR for specific diagnosis of skin manifestation of LB are not recommended for use in routine clinical practice (see Chapter 9). With advances in automation in the molecular diagnostic

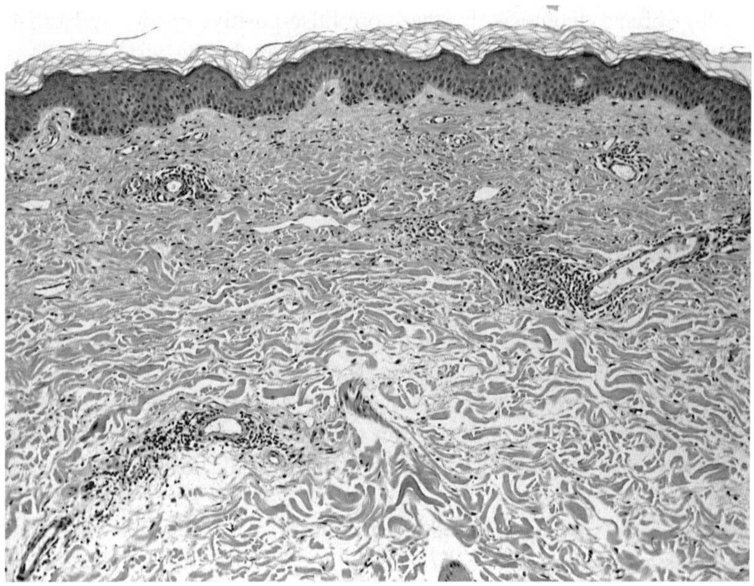

Figure 3.5 Histopathology of erythema migrans (hematoxylin/eosin, ×40) (RRM). (*See insert for color representation*).

microbiology laboratory, though, it is conceivable that real-time PCR will in the near future be used for laboratory diagnosis of Lyme borreliosis.

Histopathologic examination of the skin lesion can be helpful in clinically uncertain cases (Figure 3.5). The biopsy should be obtained from the leading edge of the erythema. The experienced dermatopathologist is able to diagnose EM with high probability in most cases or at least able to rule out most clinical differential diagnoses, such as tinea, granuloma annulare, and erysipelas. EM is characterized by a patchy lymphohistiocytic infiltrate accentuated around blood vessels, although it may also be found interstitially and surrounding adnexal structures (Figure 3.5). The infiltrate predominantly affects the superficial dermis but may spread into the deeper dermis and even the panniculus. Plasma cells are admixed in variable numbers, and a few eosinophils are sometimes present, particularly in early lesions (Weger and Müllegger, 2001). There is no salient difference in the histopathologic features of EM between European and US patients.

THERAPY

The natural history of untreated EM and associated symptoms of early disease is spontaneous gradual remission over weeks or months. Thus, in treating this infection, any measurement of antibacterial efficacy is problematic without a well-defined primary endpoint. Furthermore development of late manifestations of Lyme borreliosis is so uncommon after treatment at an early stage that purported failure of antibiotic therapy cannot be accurately defined by this criterion.

Early clinical trials of antibiotics, doses, and duration of therapy for EM were constrained by their reliance on physician clinical diagnosis rather than specific microbiologic evidence of infection as the basis for treatment. Although more recent controlled treatment studies have yielded more reliable data derived from culture and detection of *B. burgdorferi* sensu lato DNA by polymerase chain reaction, the majority of clinical trials have been handicapped by small sample sizes, lack of randomization, limited evaluation of medication compliance, and insufficient long-term follow-up.

Notwithstanding the shortcomings of research studies, a wealth of clinical experience has accumulated over the past three decades during which Lyme borreliosis has emerged as a well-recognized and even commonplace infectious disease in highly endemic regions. Indeed the initial excitement that accompanied the recognition and management of a newly emerging disease has waned, replaced by routine prescription of standard doses of generically available antibiotics.

Despite spontaneous clearance of EM in weeks to months in most cases (Weber and Neubert, 1986; Weber and Pfister, 1994), adequate treatment is mandatory in all patients, since viable *B. burgdorferi* sensu lato can remain in the skin in untreated patients (Kuiper et al., 1994), and secondary cutaneous or extracutaneous manifestations of Lyme borreliosis may result from reactivation and dissemination of the spirochete. Moreover it is not possible to predict the spontaneous course of the infection (e.g., dissemination to the central nervous system) from the clinical appearance or from the presence of absence of associated extracutaneous symptoms (Oksi et al., 2001; Maraspin et al., 2002) The goals of therapy are to eradicate the infection, to clear cutaneous and extracutaneous signs and symptoms, and to prevent progression of Lyme borreliosis. Treatment should be started based on clinical diagnosis, and it is most effective when initiated shortly after disease onset (Barsic et al., 2000).

EM is treated with oral antibiotics. There are three drugs for which efficacy has been demonstrated for treatment of localized and disseminated EM in large controlled prospective studies: doxycycline, amoxicillin, and cefuroxime axetil (Strle et al., 1992b; Nowakowski et al., 1995; Wormser et al., 2006). They are equally efficacious. Although only a few of these high-quality studies have been performed in European patients (Kuiper et al., 1994; Strle et al., 1992b, 1996b), it is reasonable to recommend the same antibiotics as medications of choice in Europe.

Doxycycline is the antibiotic of first choice in patients age 8 and over. It has superior penetration into the cerebrospinal fluid, which is advantageous given the potential of *B. burgdorferi* sensu lato to spread to the central nervous system in EM patients (Maraspin et al., 2002). Furthermore doxycycline is effective against occasionally co-transmitted *Anaplasma phagocytophilum*. It is important to inform the patient of the photosensitizing potential of doxycycline and to counsel appropriate skin protective measures. High-potency sunscreens that include ultraviolet A (UVA) and ultraviolet B (UVB) blocking factors may be helpful. Gastrointestinal adverse effects are more common with doxycycline.

When a patient is intolerant of doxycycline or when it is clinically impossible to differentiate between EM and cellulitis, amoxicillin (plus clavulanic acid in the latter case) or cefuroxime axetil (though more expensive) are the antibiotics of choice, unless MRSA is a consideration, in which instance an appropriate antibiotic would be added to the regimen.

Second-line antibiotics include the macrolide azithromycin that has been in particular tested in Europe (Strle et al., 1992b, 1996b; Weber et al., 1993; Barsic et al., 2000). When the use of macrolides is necessary, azithromycin is better tolerated and easier to comply with than erythromycin (500 mg four times a day for 14–21 days). In Slovenia and Croatia, its efficacy has been reported to be equivalent to doxycycline (Strle et al., 1992b, 1996b; Barsic et al., 2000), and greater than phenoxymethyl penicillin (Weber et al. 1993). In the

United States, azithromycin is inferior to amoxicillin (Luft et al., 1996). In Europe, it is administered in a dosage of 500 mg twice daily on the first day, followed by 500 mg daily for the next four days. In the United States, a daily dose of 500 mg for 7 to 10 days has been recommended. When macrolides are prescribed, careful follow-up is necessary to ensure that this therapy has been efficacious.

Parenteral antibiotic therapy is not indicated for treatment of EM. However, ceftriaxone (2 g once daily) may be used when EM presents in association with neurologic involvement or advanced atrioventricular heart block. For treatment of uncomplicated EM, parenteral antibiotic therapy is no more effective than first-line oral antibiotics (Weber et al., 1990) and is associated with a higher incidence of adverse reactions.

For many years it was recommended that EM be treated for three or four weeks, as antibiotics were given for this duration in most controlled trials. In the United States, a two to three-week course of treatment is now recommended for all first-line antibiotics (Wormser et al., 2006). Various studies have demonstrated equal success rates for two-week or three-week courses (Massarotti et al., 1992; Wormser et al., 2003). A three-week course is recommended for those with signs of dissemination such as prominent associated symptoms or multiple secondary skin lesions. However, a recent study in the United States has demonstrated that 10-day courses (of doxycycline) are sufficient to treat early Lyme borreliosis (Kowalski et al., 2010). In Europe, conflicting results have been published for the superiority of a either a two-week or a three-week regimen (Breier et al., 1996; Aberer et al., 2006), and current guidelines do not specify the optimum duration of therapy for EM.

For children younger than 8 years of age, amoxicillin is the first-line therapy (50 mg/kg/day, maximum 1500 mg in 3 divided doses). Alternatively, cefuroxime axetil (30 mg/kg/day, maximum 1000 mg in 2 divided doses), azithromycin (10 mg/kg/day, maximum 500 mg daily), or erythromycin (50 mg/kg/day in 4 divided doses, maximum 500 mg per dose) may be given.(Arnez et al., 2002; Eppes and Childs, 2002). Children age 8 or older may take doxycycline 4 mg/kg/day in two divided doses up to 100 mg per dose.

For pregnant or lactating women, the treatment of choice consists of amoxicillin or cefuroxime (Maraspin et al., 1999; Wormser et al., 2006), which are FDA category B medications and may be prescribed under stringent indication according to the German Red List. Doxycycline is contraindicated in Europe and the United States (FDA category D). If a patient is allergic to beta-lactam antibiotics, azithromycin can be given (FDA category B; stringent indication). In both Europe and the United States, EM in pregnancy has not been associated with an increased risk for the mother or the fetus after adequate treatment (Elliott et al., 2001; Maraspin et al., 1999). Although intravenous ceftriaxone is favored for pregnant women in Slovenia (Maraspin et al., 1999), current experience indicates that standard oral treatment is adequate during pregnancy. This practice is also recommended in recently developed German guidelines (Hofmann, 2005).

Antibiotics used for the treatment of EM are generally well tolerated and rarely produce severe adverse events. A small number of patients may experience a Jarisch–Herxheimer-type reaction shortly after initiation of antibiotic therapy. This is a transient aggravation of signs and symptoms that is manifested by fever, rigors, sweats, headache, and malaise, with temporary exacerbation of cutaneous lesions. It is associated with increased plasma concentrations of pro-inflammatory cytokines, including TNF-α, interleukin 6 and 8. Such a reaction seems to occur predominantly in blood-culture positive patients, with the use of amoxicillin or cefuroxime, and more often in the United States than in Europe (Luger et al., 1995; Arnez et al., 2001). When a Jarisch–Herxheimer-type reaction occurs, it is usually self-limited, resolves spontaneously in 12 to 24 hours, and may be treated with analgesics/antipyretics like paracetamol (acetaminophen) while continuing antibiotic therapy.

OUTCOME AND FOLLOW-UP

The outcome after adequate antibiotic treatment of adults and children is excellent, with complete clearance of the skin lesion(s) within a few weeks after initiation of therapy (Müllegger, 2004; Strle et al., 1996). Persistence or new development of mild to moderate extracutaneous signs and symptoms (most commonly arthralgias) are observed in less than 20% of patients; they are transient, may persist for weeks to months, and occur especially after a more severe initial presentation (Bennet et al., 2003; Müllegger, 2001, 2004; Aberer et al., 2006). In a recent study of 607 patients in the United States, it was demonstrated that treatment failure after appropriate antibiotic therapy is extremely rare. In a patient who has had prompt resolution of EM, yet prominent associated symptoms persist, tick-borne co-infections should be ruled out (Kowalski et al., 2010).

Objective treatment failures are extremely rare but have been reported anecdotally for almost every recommended antimicrobial agent. Retreatment is appropriate, preferably with a different antibiotic. Post–Lyme-disease syndrome or persistence of subjective symptoms such as fatigue, arthralgias, myalgias, and cognitive dysfunction, without objective findings or biological markers, has been described much less commonly in Europe than in the United States. It has been found that these symptoms are not *Borrelia* associated, and occur significantly more often in older patients and those with degenerative spine disease (Seidel et al., 2007).

Development of serum anti *B. burgdorferi* sensu lato antibodies following treatment of EM is variable and unpredictable. Antibody titers and bands on immunoblot (IgG as well as IgM) may decline, persist for months or years, or rise (Hammers-Berggren et al., 1994; Lomholt et al., 2000; Glatz et al., 2006). It is important to note that serologic test results do not correlate with type of therapy or clinical outcome and are therefore not suitable to assess efficacy (Lomholt et al., 2000; Glatz et al., 2006; Glatz et al., 2008). By the same token, retreatment is not indicated in case of persistent positive antibody titers unless there is a recurrence of clinical manifestations.

In contrast to patients who present with later manifestations, especially arthritis, patients do not develop protective antibodies after being treated for early infection. Therefore re-infection may occur after a subsequent tick bite.

ACKNOWLEDGEMENT

We thank our colleague Dr. Henry Feder for his guidance and suggestions for this manuscript.

REFERENCES

Aberer E, Kahofer P, Binder B, Kinaciyan T, Schauperl H, Berghold A: Comparison of a two- or three-week regimen and a review of treatment of erythema migrans with phenoxymethylpenicillin. *Dermatology* 212:160–167; 2006.

Arnez M, Pleterski-Rigler D, Luznik-Bufon T, Ruzic-Sabljic E, Strle F: Solitary erythema migrans in children: Comparison of treatment with azithromycin and phenoxymethylpenicillin. *Wien Klin Wochenschr* 114:498–504; 2002.

Arnez M, Pleterski-Rigler D, Ahcan J, Ruzic-Sabljic E, Strle F: Demographic features, clinical characteristics and laboratory findings in children with multiple erythema migrans in Slovenia. *Wien Klin Wochenschr* 113:98–101; 2001a.

Arnez M, Ruzic-Sabljic E, Ahcan J, Ransel-Medvescek A., Pleterski-Rigler D, Strle F: Isolation of *Borrelia burgdorferi* sensu lato from blood of children with solitary erythema migrans. *Pediatr Infect Dis J* 20:251–255; 2001b.

Arnez M, Radsel-Medvescek A, Pleterski-Rigler D, Ruzic-Sabljic E, Strle F: Comparison of cefuroxime axetil and phenoxymethyl penicillin for the treatment of children with solitary erythema migrans. *Wien Klin Wochenschr* 111:916–922; 1999.

Asbrink E: Erythema chronicum migrans Afzelius and acrodermatitis chronica atrophicans. Early and late manifestations of *Ixodes ricinus*-borne *Borrelia* spirochetes. *Acta Derm Venereol Suppl (Stockh)* 118:1–63; 1985.

Asbrink E: Cutaneous manifestations of Lyme borreliosis. Clinical definitions and differential diagnoses. *Scand J Infect Dis Suppl* 77:44–50; 1991.

Asbrink E, Hovmark A: Early and late cutaneous manifestations in *Ixodes*-borne borreliosis (erythema migrans borreliosis, Lyme borreliosis). *Ann N Y Acad Sci* 539:4–15; 1988.

Asbrink E, Hovmark A, Hederstedt B: Serologic studies of erythema chronicum migrans Afzelius and acrodermatitis chronica atrophicans with indirect immunofluorescence and enzyme-linked immunosorbent assays. *Acta Derm Venereol* 65:509–514; 1985.

Barbour AG: Does Lyme disease occur in the south?: A survey of emerging tick-borne infections in the region. *Am J Med Sci* 311:34–40; 1996.

Barsic B, Maretic T, Majerus L, Strugar J: Comparison of azithromycin and doxycycline in the treatment of erythema migrans. *Infection* 28:153–156; 2000.

Bennet L, Danell S, Berglund J: Clinical outcome of erythema migrans after treatment with phenoxymethyl penicillin. *Scand J Infect Dis* 35:129–131; 2003.

Bennet L, Fraenkel CJ, Garpmo U, Halling A, Ingman M, Ornstein K, Stjernberg L, Berglund J: Clinical appearance of erythema migrans caused by *Borrelia afzelii* and *Borrelia garinii.* Effect of the patient's sex. *Wien Klin Wochenschr* 118:531–537; 2006.

Berger BW: Dermatologic manifestations of Lyme disease. *Rev Infect Dis* 11 (suppl6): S1475–S1481; 1989.

Berger BW, Johnson RC, Kodner C, Coleman L: Cultivation of *Borrelia burgdorferi* from erythema migrans lesions and perilesional skin. *J Clin Microbiol* 30:359–361; 1992.

Breier F, Kunz G., Klade H, Stanek G, Aberer E: Erythema migrans: Three weeks treatment for prevention of late Lyme borreliosis. *Infection* 24:69–72; 1996.

Brown EL, Rivas JM, Ullrich SE, Young CR, Norris SJ, Kripke ML: Modulation of immunity to *Borrelia burgdorferi* by ultraviolet irradiation. Differential effect on Th1 and Th2 immune responses. *Eur J Immunol* 25:3017–3022; 1995.

Campbell GL, Paul WS, Schriefer ME, Craven RB, Robbins KE, Dennis DT: Epidemiologic and diagnostic studies of patients with suspected early Lyme disease, Missouri, 1990–1993. *J Infect Dis* 172:470–480; 1995.

Carlsson SA, Granlund H, Jansson C, Nyman D, Wahlberg P: Characteristics of erythema migrans in *Borrelia afzelii* and *Borrelia garinii* infections. *Scand J Infect Dis* 35:31–33; 2003.

Dennis DT: Epidemiology of Lyme borreliosis. *In* Gray J, Kahl O, Lane RS, Stanek G (eds): *Lyme Borreliosis. Biology, Epidemiology and Control.* New York, CAB International; 2002.

Douglas MR, Morrison KE, Salmon M, Buckley CD: Why does inflammation persist. A dominant role for the stromal microenvironment? *Expert Rev Mol Med* 4:1–18; 2002.

Eiffert H, Karsten A, Schlott T, Ohlenbusch A, Laskawi R, Hoppert M, Christen HJ: Acute peripheral facial palsy in Lyme disease. A distal neuritis at the infection site. *Neuropediatrics* 35:267–273; 2004.

Elliot DJ, Eppes SC, Klein JD: Teratogen update. Lyme disease. *Teratology* 64:276–281; 2001.

Eppes SC, Childs JA: Comparative study of cefuroxime axetil versus amoxicillin in children with early Lyme disease. *Pediatrics* 109:1173–1177; 2002.

Fahrer H, Van Der Linden SM, Sauvain MJ, Gern L, Zhioua E, Aeschlimann A: The prevalence and incidence of clinical and asymptomatic Lyme borreliosis in a population at risk. *J Infect Dis* 163:305–310; 1991.

Feder HM Jr, Gerber MA, Krause PJ, Ryan R, Shapiro ED: Early Lyme disease: A flu-like illness without erythema migrans. *Pediatrics* 91:456–459; 1993.

Filgueira L, Nestle FO, Rittig M, Joller HI, Groscurth P: Human dendritic cells phagocytose and process *Borrelia burgdorferi. J Immunol* 157:2998–3005; 1996.

Fingerle V, Schulte-Spechtel UC, Ruzic-Sabljic E, Leonhard S, Hofmann H, Weber K, Pfister K, Strle F, Wilske B: Epidemiological aspects and molecular characterization of *Borrelia burgdorferi* s.l. from southern Germany with special respect to the new species *Borrelia spielmanii* sp. nov. *Int J Med Microbiol* 298:279–290; 2008.

Furst B, Glatz M, Kerl H, Müllegger RR: The impact of immunosuppression on erythema migrans. A retrospective study of clinical presentation, response to treatment and production of *Borrelia* antibodies in 33 patients. *Clin Exp Dermatol* 31:509–514; 2006.

Glatz M, Golestani M, Kerl H, Müllegger RR: Clinical relevance of different IgG and IgM serum antibody responses to *Borrelia burgdorferi* after antibiotic therapy for erythema migrans. Long-term follow-up study of 113 patients. *Arch Dermatol* 142:862–868; 2006.

Glatz M, Fingerle V, Wilske B, Ambros-Rudolph C, Kerl H, Müllegger RR: Immunoblot analysis of the seroreactivity to recombinant *Borrelia burgdorferi* sensu lato antigens, including VlsE, in the long-term course of treated patients with erythema migrans. *Dermatology* 216:93–103; 2008.

Goodman JL, Dennis DT, Sonenshine DE: *Tick-Borne Diseases of Humans*. Washington, DC, American Society for Microbiology; 2005.

Gustafson R, Svenungsson B, Gardulf A, Stiernstedt G, Forsgren M: Prevalence of tick-borne encephalitis and Lyme borreliosis in a defined Swedish population. *Scand J Infect Dis* 22:297–306; 1990.

Hammers-Berggren S, Lebech AM, Karlsson M, Andersson U, Hansen K, Stiernstedt G: Serological follow-up after treatment of *Borrelia* arthritis and acrodermatitis chronica atrophicans. *Scand J Infect Dis* 26:339–347; 1994.

Hanrahan JP, Benach JL, Coleman JL, Bosler EM, Morse DL, Cameron DJ, Edelman R, Kaslow RA: Incidence and cumulative frequency of endemic Lyme disease in a community. *J Infect Dis* 150:489–496; 1984.

Hofmann H: [Lyme borreliosis. Cutaneous manifestation]. *Hautarzt* 56:783–795; quiz 796; 2005.

Isogai E, Isogai H, Kimura K, Hayashi S, Kubota T, Nishikawa T, Nakane A, Fujii N: Cytokines in the serum and brain in mice infected with distinct species of Lyme disease *Borrelia. Microb Pathog* 21:413–419; 1996.

Jones KL, Muellegger RR, Means TK, Lee M, Glickstein LJ, Damle N, Sikand VK, Luster AD, Steere AC: Higher mRNA levels of chemokines and cytokines associated with macrophage activation in erythema migrans skin lesions in patients from the United States than in patients from Austria with Lyme borreliosis. *Clin Infect Dis* 46:85–92; 2008.

Kirkland KB, Klimko TB, Meriwether RA, Schriefer M, Levin M, Levine J, MacKenzie WR, Dennis DT: Erythema migrans-like rash illness at a camp in North Carolina. A new tick-borne disease? *Arch Intern Med* 157:2635–2641; 1997.

Kowalski TJ, Tata S, Berth W, Mathiason MA, Agger WA: Antibiotic treatment duration and long-term outcomes of patients with early Lyme disease from a Lyme disease-hyperendemic area. *Clin Infect Dis* 50:512–520; 2010.

Kraiczy P, Hellwage J, Skerka C, Becker H, Kirschfink M, Simon MM, Brade V, Zipfel PF, Wallich R: Complement resistance of *Borrelia burgdorferi* correlates with the expression of BbCRASP-1, a novel linear plasmid-encoded surface protein that interacts with human factor H and FHL-1 and is unrelated to Erp proteins. *J Biol Chem* 279:2421–2429; 2004.

Kuiper H, Van Dam AP, Spanjaard L, De Jongh BM, Widjojokusumo A, Ramselaar T.C, Cairo I, Vos K, Dankert J: Isolation of *Borrelia burgdorferi* from biopsy specimens taken from healthy-looking skin of patients with Lyme borreliosis. *J Clin Microbiol* 32:715–720; 1994.

Lastavica CC, Wilson ML, Berardi VP, Spielman A, Deblinger RD: Rapid emergence of a focal epidemic of Lyme disease in coastal Massachusetts. *N Engl J Med* 320:133–137; 1989.

Lipsker D, Lieber-Mbomeyo A, Hedelin G: How accurate is a clinical diagnosis of erythema chronicum migrans? Prospective study comparing the diagnostic accuracy of general practitioners and dermatologists in an area where Lyme borreliosis is endemic. *Arch Dermatol* 140:620–621; 2004.

Logar M, Ruzic-Sabljic E, Maraspin V, Lotric-Furlan S, Cimperman J, Jurca T, Strle F: Comparison of erythema migrans caused by *Borrelia afzelii* and *Borrelia garinii. Infection* 32:15–19; 2004.

Lomholt H, Lebech AM, Hansen K, Brandrup F, Halkier-Sorensen L: Long-term serological follow-up of patients treated for chronic cutaneous borreliosis or culture-positive erythema migrans. *Acta Derm Venereol* 80:362–366; 2000.

Luft BJ, Dattwyler RJ, Johnson RC, Luger SW, Bosler EM, Rahn DW, Masters EJ, Grunwaldt E, Gadgil SD: Azithromycin compared with amoxicillin in the treatment of erythema migrans. A double-blind, randomized, controlled trial. *Ann Intern Med* 124:785–791; 1996.

Luger SW, Paparone P, Wormser GP, Nadelman RB, Grunwaldt E, Gomez G, Wisniewski M, Collins JJ: Comparison of cefuroxime axetil and doxycycline in treatment of patients with early Lyme disease associated with erythema migrans. *Antimicrob Agents Chemother* 39:661–667; 1995.

Maraspin V, Cimperman J, Lotric-Furlan S, Pleterski-Rigler D, Strle F: Erythema migrans in pregnancy. *Wien Klin Wochenschr* 111:933–940; 1999.

Maraspin V, Cimperman J, Lotric-Furlan S, Ruzic-Sabljic E, Jurca T, Strle F: Cerebrospinal fluid findings in adult patients with multiple erythema migrans. *Wien Klin Wochenschr* 114:505–509; 2002.

Massarotti EM, Luger SW, Rahn DW, Messner RP, Wong JB, Johnson RC, Steere AC: Treatment of early Lyme disease. *Am J Med* 92:396–403; 1992.

McKisic MD, Barthold SW: T-cell-independent responses to *Borrelia burgdorferi* are critical for protective immunity and resolution of Lyme disease. *Infect Immun*, 68:5190–5197; 2000.

Müllegger RR: Clinical aspects and diagnosis of erythema migrans and borrelial lymphocytoma. *Acta Dermatovenerol Alp Panonica Adriat* 10:152–158; 2001.

Müllegger RR: Dermatological manifestations of Lyme borreliosis. *Eur J Dermatol* 14:296–309; 2004.

Müllegger RR, McHugh G, Ruthazer R, Binder B, Kerl H, Steere AC: Differential expression of cytokine mRNA in skin specimens from patients with erythema migrans or acrodermatitis chronica atrophicans. *J Invest Dermatol* 115:1115–1123; 2000.

Müllegger RR, Means TK, Shin JJ, Lee M, Jones KL, Glickstein LJ, Luster AD, Steere AC: Chemokine signatures in the skin disorders of Lyme borreliosis in Europe. Predominance of CXCL9 and CXCL10 in erythema migrans and acrodermatitis and CXCL13 in lymphocytoma. *Infect Immun* 75:4621–4628; 2007.

Nadelman RB, Luger SW, Frank E, Wisniewski M, Collins JJ, Wormser GP: Comparison of cefuroxime axetil and doxycycline in the treatment of early Lyme disease. *Ann Intern Med* 117:273–280; 1992.

Nadelman RB, Nowakowski J, Forseter G, Goldberg NS, Bittker S, Cooper D, Aguero-Rosenfeld M, Wormser GP: The clinical spectrum of early Lyme borreliosis in patients with culture-confirmed erythema migrans. *Am J Med* 100:502–508; 1996.

Nowakowski J, Nadelman RB, Forseter G, McKenna D, Wormser GP: Doxycycline versus tetracycline therapy for Lyme disease associated with erythema migrans. *J Am Acad Dermatol* 32:223–227; 1995.

O'Connells S, Granstrom M, Gray JS, Stanek G: Epidemiology of European Lyme borreliosis. *Zentralbl Bakteriol* 287:229–240; 1998.

Oksi J, Marttila H, Soini H, Aho H, Uksila J, Viljanen MK: Early dissemination of *Borrelia burgdorferi* without generalized symptoms in patients with erythema migrans. *APMIS* 109:581–588; 2001.

Picken RN, Strle F, Picken MM, Ruzic-Sabljic E, Maraspin V, Lotric-Furlan S, Cimperman J: Identification of three species of *Borrelia burgdorferi* sensu lato (*B. burgdorferi* sensu stricto, *B. garinii,* and *B. afzelii*) among isolates from acrodermatitis chronica atrophicans lesions. *J Invest Dermatol* 110:211–214; 1998.

Salazar JC, Pope CD, Sellati TJ, Feder HM Jr, Kiely TG, Dardick KR, Buckman RL, Moore MW, Caimano MJ, Pope JG, Krause PJ, Radolf JD: Coevolution of markers of innate and adaptive immunity in skin and peripheral blood of patients with erythema migrans. *J Immunol* 171:2660–2670; 2003.

Seidel MF, Domene AB, Vetter H: Differential diagnoses of suspected Lyme borreliosis or post-Lyme-disease syndrome. *Eur J Clin Microbiol Infect Dis* 26:611–617; 2007.

Seinost G, Dykhuizen DE, Dattwyler RJ, Golde WT, Dunn JJ, Wang IN, Wormser GP, Schriefer ME, Luft BJ: Four clones of *Borrelia burgdorferi* sensu stricto cause invasive infection in humans. *Infect Immun* 67:3518–3524; 1999.

Sigal LH: Lyme disease: A review of aspects of its immunology and immunopathogenesis. *Annu Rev Immunol* 15:63–92; 1997.

Smith RP, Schoen RT, Rahn DW, Sikand VK, Nowakowski J, Parenti DL, Holman MS, Persing DH, Steere AC: Clinical characteristics and treatment outcome of early Lyme disease in patients with microbiologically confirmed erythema migrans. *Ann Intern Med* 136:421–428; 2002.

Sood SK, Salzman MB, Johnson BJ, Happ CM, Feig K, Carmody L, Rubin LG, Hilton E, Piesman J: Duration of tick attachment as a predictor of the risk of Lyme disease in an area in which Lyme disease is endemic. *J Infect Dis* 175:996–999; 1997.

Stanek G, O'Connell S, Cimmino M, Aberer E, Kristoferitsch W, Granstrom M, Guy E, Gray J: European Union Concerted Action on Risk Assessment in Lyme Borreliosis. Clinical case definitions for Lyme borreliosis. *Wien Klin Wochenschr* 108:741–747; 1996.

Stanek G, Strle F: Lyme borreliosis. *Lancet* 362:1639–1647; 2003.

Steere AC: Lyme disease. *N Engl J Med* 345:115–125; 2001.

Steere AC: Lyme borreliosis in 2005, 30 years after initial observations in Lyme Connecticut. *Wien Klin Wochenschr* 118:625–633; 2006.

Steere AC, Schoen RT, Taylor E: The clinical evolution of Lyme arthritis. *Ann Intern Med* 107:725–731; 1987.

Steere AC, Taylor E, Wilson ML, Levine JF, Spielman A: Longitudinal assessment of the clinical and epidemiological features of Lyme disease in a defined population. *J Infect Dis* 154:295–300; 1986.

Steere AC, Sikand VK, Meurice F, Parenti DL, Fikrig E, Schoen RT, Nowakowski J, Schmid CH, Laukamp S, Buscarino C, Krause DS: Vaccination against Lyme disease with recombinant *Borrelia burgdorferi* outer-surface lipoprotein A with adjuvant. Lyme Disease Vaccine Study Group. *N Engl J Med* 339:209–215; 1998.

Steere AC, Dhar A, Hernandez J, Fischer PA, Sikand VK, Schoen RT, Nowakowski J, McHugh G, Persing DH: Systemic symptoms without erythema migrans as the presenting picture of early Lyme disease. *Am J Med* 114:58–62; 2003a.

Steere AC, Sikand VK, Schoen RT, Nowakowski J: Asymptomatic infection with *Borrelia burgdorferi. Clin Infect Dis* 37:528–532; 2003b.

Strle F., Pleterski-Rigler D, Stanek G, Pejovnik-Pustinek A, Ruzic E, Cimperman J: Solitary borrelial lymphocytoma: report of 36 cases. *Infection* 20:201–206; 1992a.

Strle F., Ruzic E, Cimperman J: Erythema migrans: Comparison of treatment with azithromycin, doxycycline and phenoxymethylpenicillin. *J Antimicrob Chemother* 30:543–550; 1992b.

Strle F, Maraspin V, Lotric-Furlan S, Cimperman J: Epidemiological study of a cohort of adult patients with erythema migrans registered in Slovenia in 1993. *Eur J Epidemiol* 12:503–507; 1996a.

Strle F, Maraspin V, Lotric-Furlan S, Ruzic-Sabljic E, Cimperman J: Azithromycin and doxycycline for treatment of *Borrelia* culture-positive erythema migrans. *Infection* 24:64–68; 1996b.

Strle F., Nelson JA, Ruzic-Sabljic E, Cimperman J, Maraspin V, Lotric-Furlan S, Cheng Y, Picken MM, Trenholme GM, Picken RN: European Lyme borreliosis: 231 culture-confirmed cases involving patients with erythema migrans. *Clin Infect Dis* 23:61–65; 1996c.

Strle F., Nadelman RB, Cimperman J, Nowakowski J, Picken RN, Schwartz I, Maraspin V, Aguero-Rosenfeld ME, Varde S, Lotric-Furlan S, Wormser GP: Comparison of culture-confirmed erythema migrans caused by *Borrelia burgdorferi* sensu stricto in New York State and by *Borrelia afzelii* in Slovenia. *Ann Intern Med* 130:32–36; 1999.

Strle F., Videcnik J, Zorman P, Cimperman J, Lotric-Furlan S, Maraspin V: Clinical and epidemiological findings for patients with erythema migrans. Comparison of cohorts from the years 1993 and 2000. *Wien Klin Wochenschr* 114:493–497; 2002.

Van Dam AP, Kuiper H, Vos K, Widjojokusumo A, De Jongh BM, Spanjaard L., Ramselaar AC, Kramer MD, Dankert J: Different genospecies of *Borrelia burgdorferi* are associated with distinct clinical manifestations of Lyme borreliosis. *Clin Infect Dis* 17:708–717; 1993.

Vaz A, Glickstein L, Field JA, McHugh G, Sikand VK, Damle N, Steere AC: Cellular and humoral immune responses to *Borrelia burgdorferi* antigens in patients with culture-positive early Lyme disease. *Infect Immun* 69:7437–444; 2001.

Wang G, van Dam AP, Schwartz I, Dankert J: Molecular typing of *Borrelia burgdorferi* sensu lato: Taxonomic, epidemiological, and clinical implications. *Clin Microbiol Rev* 12:633–653; 1999.

Wang G, van Dam AP, Spanjaard L, Dankert J: Molecular typing of *Borrelia burgdorferi* sensu lato by randomly amplified polymorphic DNA fingerprinting analysis. *J Clin Microbiol* 36:768–776; 1998.

Weber K: Erythema migrans and early signs and symptoms. *In* Weber K, Burgdorfer W (eds): *Aspects of Lyme Borreliosis*. Berlin: Springer; 1993.

Weber K, Neubert U: Clinical features of early erythema migrans disease and related disorders. *Zentralbl Bakteriol Mikrobiol Hyg [A]* 263:209–228; 1986.

Weber K, Pfister HW: Clinical management of Lyme borreliosis. *Lancet* 343:1017–1020; 1994.

Weber K, Wilske B: Mini erythema migrans. A sign of early Lyme borreliosis. *Dermatology* 212:113–116; 2006.

Weber K, Preac-Mursic V, Wilske B, Thurmayr R, Neubert U, Scherwitz C: A randomized trial of ceftriaxone versus oral penicillin for the treatment of early European Lyme borreliosis. *Infection* 18:91–96; 1990.

Weber K, Wilske B, Preac-Mursic V, Thurmayr R: Azithromycin versus penicillin V for the treatment of early Lyme borreliosis. *Infection* 21:367–372; 1993.

Weger W, Müllegger RR: Histopathology and immunohistochemistry of dermatoborreliosis. *Acta Derm Venereol APA* 10:135–142; 2001.

Wormser GP, Forseter G, Cooper D, Nowakowski J, Nadelman RB, Horowitz H, Schwartz I, Bowen SL, Campbell GL, Goldberg NS: Use of a novel technique of cutaneous lavage for diagnosis of Lyme disease associated with erythema migrans. *JAMA* 268:1311–1313; 1992.

Wormser GP, Ramanathan R, Nowakowski J, McKenna D, Holmgren D, Visintainer P, Dornbush R, Singh B, Nadelman RB: Duration of antibiotic therapy for early Lyme disease. A randomized, double-blind, placebo-controlled trial. *Ann Intern Med* 138:697–704; 2003.

Wormser GP, Dattwyler RJ, Shapiro ED, Halpern JJ, Steere AC, Klempner MS, Krause PJ, Bakken JS, Strle F, Stanek G, Bockenstedt L, Fish D, Dumler JS, Nadelman RB: The clinical assessment, treatment, and prevention of Lyme disease, human granulocytic anaplasmosis, and babesiosis. Clinical practice guidelines by the Infectious Diseases Society of America. *Clin Infect Dis* 43:1089–1134; 2006.

Zhioua E, Gern L, Aeschlimann A, Sauvain MJ, van der Linden S, Fahrer H: Longitudinal study of Lyme borreliosis in a high risk population in Switzerland. *Parasite* 5:383–386; 1998.

4

LYME CARDITIS

Fadi A. Haddad and Sunil K. Sood

Carditis is a rare manifestation of Lyme borreliosis, one that occurs concurrently with the more frequent cutaneous, rheumatologic, or neurologic manifestations (Nadelman and Wormser, 1998; Haddad and Nadelman, 2003). There are three described clinical entities within Lyme carditis: intermittent atrioventricular (AV) block, myopericarditis, and cardiomyopathy.

In the early 1980s cases of Lyme carditis were reported among untreated patients in whom the disease had taken its natural course (Steere et al., 1980). Nowadays the presentation and the severity of Lyme carditis are likely to be different because of early recognition and treatment of early Lyme borreliosis. In this chapter we review specific cardiac manifestations of Lyme borreliosis, and the notable variance between Lyme carditis in Europe and North America with special reference to cardiomyopathy. All published reports are subject to one of more of the following caveats: false-positive serology, especially in earlier reports unconfirmed by immunoblot, unconfirmed spirochete-like structures given the limitations of staining techniques, and the presence of co-morbidities that could alternatively explain the cardiac manifestation. The data summarized herein are based on a critical review of the literature.

Lyme Borreliosis in Europe and North America: Epidemiology and Clinical Practice, First Edition.
Edited by Sunil K. Sood

HISTORICAL PERSPECTIVE AND EPIDEMIOLOGY

The first cases of Lyme carditis were reported in the United States in 1980 (Steere et al., 1980). In 1982 a patient with Lyme carditis was reported in Australia followed by European cases in 1984 (Stewart et al., 1982; Houwerzyl et al., 1984). The reported proportion of Lyme carditis ranges between 0.5% and 8% of Lyme borreliosis in the United States (Rubin et al., 1992) and in Europe it has been estimated to be 1% to 4% (Sigal, 1995; O'Connell et al., 1998). These numbers from earlier observations may not be applicable today. From 1992 to 2004 heart block was reported to the Centers for Disease Control and Prevention (CDC) in < 1% of 119,965 patients for whom at least one symptom was reported. It is unclear if all these patients had received antibiotic treatment. In addition two studies, one prospective, the other retrospective, found that antimicrobial therapy for early Lyme borreliosis reduces the incidence of cardiac manifestations (Rubin et al., 1992; Sangha et al., 1998). In the prospective efficacy studies of recombinant OspA vaccines, no evidence of carditis was found among 233 patients diagnosed with definite Lyme borreliosis (Sigal et al., 1998; Steere et al., 1998). In a prospective study of children diagnosed with Lyme borreliosis in southeastern Connecticut, 1 of 201 (0.5%) of children had carditis (Gerber et al., 1996). Thus recent data suggest that the current prevalence of carditis is less than 1%. A 14-year review of 207 children with early disseminated Lyme disease seen at a children's hospital emergency department or hospitalized identified 33 (16%) cases of carditis. This high incidence was attributed to referral and selection biases (Costello et al., 2009).

In published studies, the incidence, manifestations, and sequelae of Lyme carditis are different on the North American and European continents. This could be explained by the difference in genospecies, selection bias, or case definition. Only two genospecies of *Borrelia* (*Borrelia burgdorferi* sensu stricto and *B. garinii*) have been definitively implicated in Lyme carditis, by isolation on blood culture, with *B. garinii* in a single case only, where the patient had arthritis as well (van Dam et al., 1993). This does not exclude *B. afzelii* as a causative genospecies, as most confirmed cases of Lyme borreliosis are not culture proved. However, *B. afzelii* is the most commonly isolated species in Slovenia (Ruzic-Sabljic et al., 2005), and carditis is not commonly seen in cases of disseminated Lyme borreliosis due to this species (Strle et al., 1999). Wormser et al. found that specific genetic subtypes of *B. burgdorferi* sensu stricto influence disease pathogenesis, thus contributing to different clinical manifestations (Wormser et al., 1999). A mouse model was used to study such an effect. Using polymerase chain reaction (PCR), restriction fragment length polymorphism (RFLP) carditis was observed to be more frequently associated with one RFLP type, which also caused more severe carditis and arthritis (Wang et al., 2002). RFLP typing of the isolate was performed in two patients in Westchester County, New York; the clinical features of one are depicted in Figure 4.1.

The incidence of Lyme carditis is variable within Europe. A prospective, population-based survey of cases of Lyme borreliosis in southern Sweden found that carditis was rare. There were five cases of Lyme carditis among 1471 patients. The case definition of carditis excluded palpitations, bradycardia, bundle-branch block, or myocarditis occurring as single symptoms (Berglund et al., 1995). A Norwegian study during the period 1995 to 2004 reported a total of 1506 cases of disseminated and chronic Lyme borreliosis (Nygard et al., 2005). The most common clinical presentation in the study was neuroborreliosis, reported in 1070 (71%) of the patients, most commonly facial palsy. Ten cases (0.7%) had cardiac manifestations as a main or concomitant finding. In the United Kingdom, conduction disturbances have been described, but there has been no confirmed case of *Borrelia* cardiomyopathy (Haywood et al., 1993). In the Würzburg region of Germany, only one case

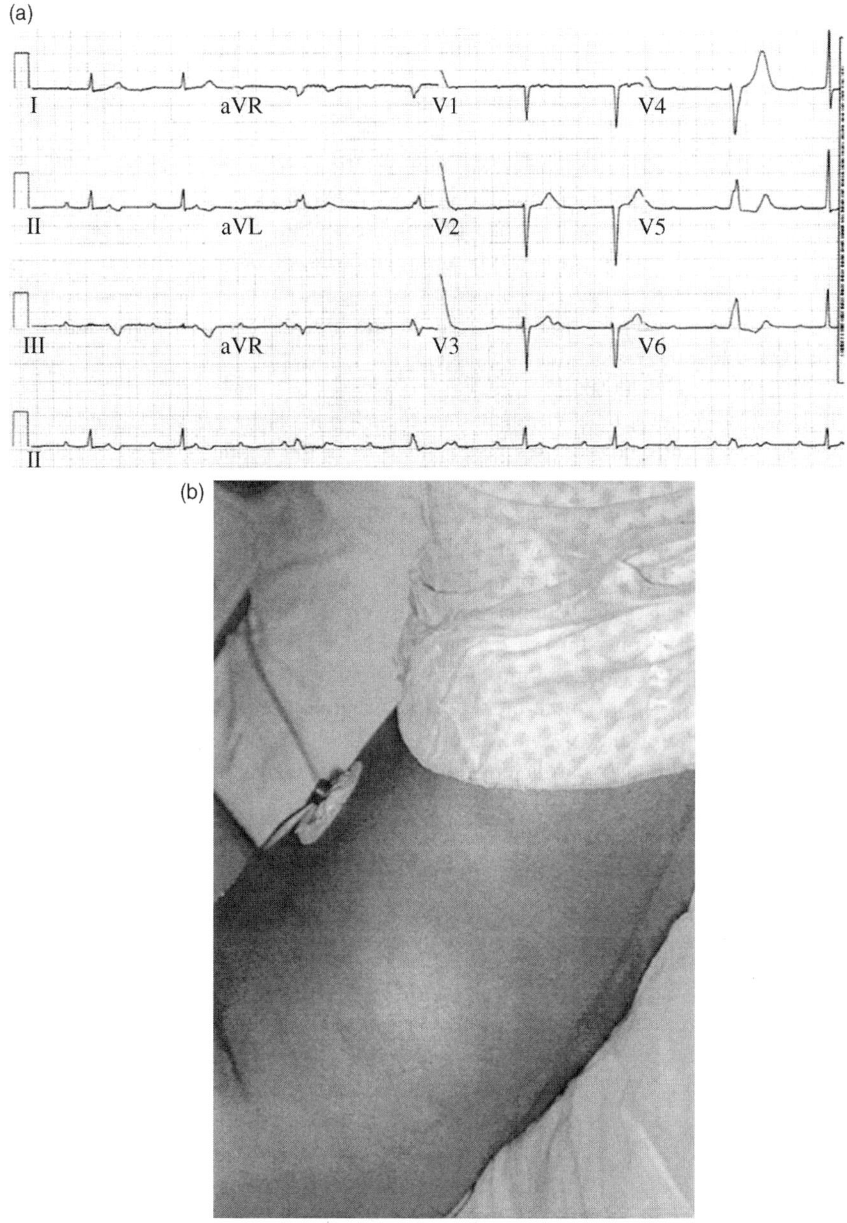

Figure 4.1 (a) ECG showing complete AV block in patient with *B. burgdorferi* RFLP type 2 isolated on blood culture. (b) Erythema migrans rash of same patient. Source: Haddad FA, Nadelman RB: Lyme disease and the heart. *Front Biosci* 8: s769–s782; 2003. (*See insert for color representation of* (*b*)).

of carditis occurred among 313 patients diagnosed with Lyme borreliosis over 12 months in a prospective, population-based surveillance study (Huppertz et al., 1999). The proportion of carditis in Lyme borreliosis was estimated as 4% in Poland, and zero in northeastern France (Lipsker et al., 2001, Grzesik et al., 2004). In a serological survey in Spain, 101 of 499 seropositive patients had carditis, but the specificity of the serologic assay used can be questioned, especially since cross-reactivity with relapsing fever could not be ruled out (Anda et al., 1993).

CLINICAL MANIFESTATIONS

Atrioventricular Block and Arrhythmias

AV block was the original reported cardiac manifestation (Steere et al., 1980). A fluctuating degree of AV block was the most common form, observed in 18 of their 20 patients. Two progressed to Wenckebach-type second-degree block, and 8 developed complete heart block, and therefore syncope was a common symptom. No patients had bundle branch blocks (Steere et al., 1980). Forty-eight percent of 33 children in the Boston series had first-degree heart block, and 42% had advanced-degree block; 18% had prolongation of the corrected QT interval, and 6% had only ST-T wave changes. In one child the EKG was normal (Costello et al., 2009).

Van der Linde reviewed and compared cases of Lyme carditis in the United States and Europe, comprising 66 and 39 cases, respectively (van der Linde, 1991). Complete heart block was the most common form of arrhythmia in both groups, but patients with complete heart block are more likely to come to clinical attention because patients with first- and second-degree heart block can be asymptomatic. Patients on both continents had concomitant neurological illness. Using electrophysiological studies, the origin of the block was supraventricular in 68% of the patients, but diffuse conduction extending to His-ventricular pathway was present in one third of the patients. Infra-His location of the block was not documented. In separate studies sinus node dysfunction, blocks above the His bundle and fluctuating left or right bundle branch lock, was observed (Reznick et al., 1986; Rey et al., 1991; Berglund et al., 1995; Midttun et al., 1997, 1990; van der Linde et al.,1990) (Figure 4.2) . Fascicular tachycardia, episodic asystole, and atrial fibrillation have also been

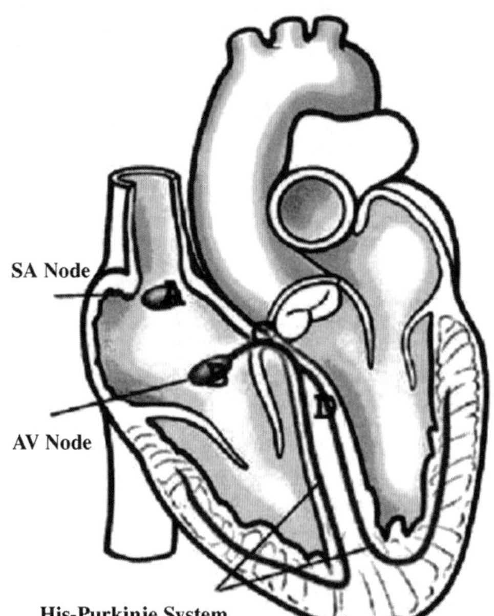

Figure 4.2 Potential locations (A–D) for conduction disturbances from various electrocardiographic studies in Lyme carditis. Source: Haddad FA, Nadelman RB: Lyme disease and the heart. *Front Biosci* 8:s769–s782; 2003.

reported in several patients with Lyme borreliosis, although these rhythm disturbances could have resulted from unrelated structural heart disease (Steere et al., 1980; Vlay et al., 1991; Rosenfeld et al., 1999).

Although AV block has been reported in the absence of other manifestations of Lyme borreliosis (Kimball et al., 1989; Baylac-Domengetroy et al., 1991), it is more likely that erythema migrans occurred unnoticed or else resolved before the arrhythmia manifested (Haddad and Nadelman, 2003). In the series of pediatric carditis patients in Boston, 97% had concurrent manifestations of early Lyme disease (Costello et al., 2009). Arthralgias and cardiopulmonary symptoms were independent predictors of Lyme carditis in these children, as was age older than 10 years.

Asymptomatic patients seropositive for Lyme borreliosis have been studied for electrocardiographic abnormalities. In an endemic area in the United States, healthy individuals with positive serology for Lyme borreliosis had bradycardia more often compared to controls (Vidaillet et al., 1993). An important limitation was that the diagnosis of past Lyme borreliosis was not confirmed by immunoblot. Moreover the study failed to control for physical fitness or amount of outdoor activity. In Slovenia short Q wave duration and deep S wave, nonspecific findings that may be seen in healthy individuals, were observed in patients with Lyme borreliosis manifesting with solitary erythema migrans, and AV block was observed as often as in healthy controls (Pikelj-Pecnik et al., 2002). Mravljak et al. compared electrocardiographic findings in children with solitary or multiple erythema migrans with findings in healthy controls of comparable age and sex distribution. Abnormal electrocardiographic findings were detected more often in healthy children (14% vs. 5%, $P = 0.03$). AV block (first-degree) occurred in only one patient with erythema migrans (Mravljak et al., 2006). Given these observations, the presence of relatively common ECG abnormalities should not be ascribed to Lyme borreliosis in the absence of strong clinical and epidemiologic evidence.

Myocarditis, Pericarditis, and Endocarditis

Acute myocarditis and myopericarditis have been reported in the United States and Europe (Jacobs et al., 1984; Gasser et al., 1992, Globits et al., 1994; Wormser et al., 2000; Munk et al., 2007; Wormser et al., 2006). These were defined by ST segment and T wave changes, and additionally by nuclear imaging in some cases (Steere et al., 1980, Klein et al., 1991; Suedkamp et al., 1999). Myocarditis occurred in less than 15% of 84 US patients with Lyme carditis as reported to the CDC (Ciesielski et al., 1989). The frequency of pericarditis in Lyme carditis cases in Europe was reported to be four times the US rate (23% vs. 5% of patients; van der Linde, 1991). This is difficult to explain given the apparent lower incidence of Lyme carditis in Europe, so the difference may relate to the case definition of pericarditis used, or possibly to differences in genospecies. Four (9%) of 33 children in the Boston series had severe depression of ventricular systolic function. Three of these children presented in cardiogenic shock, and all had endomyocardial biopsy evidence of lymphocytic myocarditis.

The vast majority of reported Lyme myo/pericarditis patients, although they may present with congestive heart failure, had a mild illness and a short course. Cardiac tamponade has been reported in one case of Lyme pericarditis in the Netherlands (Bruyn et al., 1994). The evidence for *B. burgdorferi* infection was visualization of spirochetes on two immunostaining methods, and seropositive status (by indirect immunofluorescence, an assay considered subject to false-positive readings). Recurrent pericardial effusion in a patient was attributed to Lyme borreliosis, based on a history of EM, positive serologic tests of unspecified methods in serum and pericardial fluid, and response to ceftriaxone (Gasser et al., 1998).

Borrelia burgdorferi has been implicated in the etiology of valvular degeneration, myocardial infarction, and subacute bacterial endocarditis based on elevated IgG antibody levels to *B. burgdorferi* (Kaell et al., 1990; Oksi et al., 1997; Canver et al., 2000). However, in none of these cases were spirochetes identified pathologically, and the evidence for Lyme borreliosis was not compelling in any of these reports. Moreover positive antibodies (both by ELISA and immunoblot) to *B. burgdorferi* can be present in patients with nonspirochetal subacute bacterial endocarditis.

Pancarditis was evident on autopsy of a patient with Lyme carditis and simultaneous babesiosis. There was a diffuse lymphoplasmacytic infiltration, and spirochetes were demonstrated in the myocardium by Dieterle silver staining (Marcus et al., 1985). In another patient presented as dying of Lyme pancarditis in the United Kingdom, the role of *Borrelia* infection is questionable, with only IgG antibodies present and a negative Warthin–Starry stain for spirochetes on autopsy (Cary et al., 1990). Sudden death in a 37-year-old American man with second-degree AV-block, fever, and rash was attributed to *B. burgdorferi* infection, confirmed by serum immunoblot and myocardial PCR for OspA. Post-mortem pathology revealed diffuse carditis with interstitial, endocardial, and perivascular infiltrates of lymphocytes, macrophages, plasma cells, and eosinophils and areas of myocyte necrosis (Tavora et al., 2008).

Cardiomyopathy

Borrelia burgdorferi has been cultivated from the myocardium of a few patients with dilated cardiomyopathy in Europe (Stanek et al., 1990; Lardieri et al., 1993). A diagnosis of cardiomyopathy has been attributed to Lyme borreliosis based on spirochete-like forms seen in cardiac tissue in several other reports (Haddad and Nadelman, 2003). In a small study in Austria, 11 (24%) of 46 patients with dilated cardiomyopathy, defined by a mean left ventricular ejection fraction of 30% by cardiac catheterization and echocardiography, were seropositive for *B. burgdorferi* (Gasser et al., 1996). Nine of 11 had a history of a tick bite followed by erythema migrans or a manifestation of disseminated Lyme borreliosis. No endomyocardial biopsy results were reported. Nine patients had improved or normalized left ventricular function six months after completion of a two-week course of ceftriaxone.

Similar findings have not been demonstrated in the United States. On the contrary, a study was unable to link heart failure to *B. burgdorferi* infection in an endemic area. Among 175 patients with cardiomyopathy in Minnesota, 14 had borderline or seropositive reactivity to *B. burgdorferi* by EIA, and of 13 who had immunoblots performed on their sera, 1 was positive by the then standard criteria of Dressler et al. (Dressler et al., 1993). Six seropositive patients were treated with ceftriaxone or doxycycline because at least circumstantial evidence of possible Lyme borreliosis was ascertained, although two had documented ischemic heart disease. A mild improvement of ejection fraction and of fatigue and arthralgias were observed in one case. The authors concluded that Lyme borreliosis was not a common cause of idiopathic heart failure in the midwestern United States (Sonnesyn et al., 1995).

It is important to note that the association of *B. burgdorferi* infection with cardiomyopathy is largely anecdotal. Collagen fibrils in cardiac tissue could mimic the helical form of a spirochete, giving rise to false-positive results on silver staining used to detect *Borrelia*. In Germany a retrospective study used PCR to detect *B. burgdorferi* recombinant outer surface protein A (OspA) gene in myocardial tissue from 68 patients who had undergone heart transplantation for dilated cardiomyopathy, 3 of whom were *B. burgdorferi* antibody positive. *Borrelia burgdorferi* DNA was not detected in any of the 68 hearts (Suedkamp et al., 1999). It is still unclear if the observations of cardiomyopathy in Europe can be ascribed to the different genospecies of *Borrelia* or to an agent–host phenomenon that is not completely understood. There are presently insufficient data to address this possibility, mainly because of the rarity with which *B. burgdorferi* has been isolated from heart tissue.

PATHOLOGY

Humans

Among the few human cases with pathologic findings of Lyme carditis reported, no characteristic pathologic hallmarks have emerged. Among features observed are dense band-like infiltrates of lymphocytes (mixed T and B cells with the latter predominating) and plasma cells in the endomyocardium, interstitial myocarditis, myocyte necrosis, pericarditis, perivascular inflammation, and small vessel vasculitis (Reznick et al., 1986; Duray, 1989; de Koning et al., 1989; Cox and Krajden, 1991; Tavora et al., 2008; Costello et al., 2009). Endomyocardial biopsy of a patient with dilated cardiomyopathy in Austria showed infiltrates consisting of lymphocytes and plasma cells in the endomysium and endomysial vessels, and spirochete-like structures were seen in the myocardium using silver staining (Stanek et al., 1990).

Animal Models

In a mouse model, 10 days after needle inoculation with *B. burgdorferi* both susceptible (C3H) and resistant (B6) mice developed evidence of carditis, but the susceptible mice had more severe disease (Armstrong et al., 1992). Mixed leukocyte infiltration and fibroblastic proliferation were detected, and spirochete infiltration was maximal 15 days after infection. After 30 days lymphocytes and macrophages replaced neutrophils as the predominant cell type. Although ECG evidence of conduction disturbances was not noted, some infected mice developed transient tachycardia or bradycardia, without an elevation of cardiac enzymes. Following subsidence of cardiac inflammation after 2 weeks, a residual periaortic lymphoplasmacytic infiltrate persisted until the end of the experiment at day 90. Lyme carditis was postulated to result from the direct interaction of spirochetes with macrophages, which predominated in cardiac infiltrates. In addition wider QRS complexes were observed in a murine model of Lyme carditis (Saba et al., 2001). In the latter model the ECG abnormalities appeared 2 weeks after infection and resolved at 8 weeks without intervention, and mimicked the electrophysiologic course seen in humans.

APPROACH TO DIAGNOSIS

Lyme carditis is considered an early manifestation of disseminated *Borrelia* infection. It occurs within weeks of initial infection in most cases, with a median of three weeks after the onset of erythema migrans estimated in one cohort (Steere et al., 1980). In Europe cases of

Borrelia associated cardiomyopathy have been reported where infection had taken place years previously (Stanek et al., 1991; Klein et al., 1991).

A tick bite and the history or finding of erythema migrans rash on examination may go unnoticed by the patient and could be missed by the physician. Therefore the presentation of cardiac conduction disturbances in a patient who lives in an endemic area is adequate to include Lyme carditis in the differential diagnosis. Symptoms of Lyme carditis include general symptoms such as malaise, fatigue, headache, stiff neck, fever, myalgias, and sore throat. Specific symptoms include syncope, chest pain, palpitations, and/or dyspnea. Patients with cardiomyopathy present with chronic dyspnea with or without lower extremity edema. Physical examination should include a complete skin inspection to look for single or multiple erythema migrans skin lesions, bradycardia or tachycardia, pericardial rub, murmurs, rales, hepatojugular reflux, and gallop rhythms. It is the practice of one of the authors (SS) to perform an ECG when a patient presents with any of the other manifestations of early disseminated Lyme borreliosis.

Laboratory Diagnosis

As in most bacterial infections, isolation of agent in culture is the gold standard for diagnosis. This is difficult in Lyme carditis because of the impracticality of maintaining the culture technique in most clinical laboratories and because of the invasive procedures necessary to obtain myocardial tissue for culture. Therefore the supportive evidence for Lyme carditis is usually a serologic assay, most commonly an enzyme linked immunosorbent assay (ELISA) as a first-step followed by an immunoblot when the ELISA is positive or equivocal (see Chapter 10). Because of the short duration of infection in some patients who develop cardiac manifestations, they may have negative serology initially and convalescent serum samples should be drawn if an alternate diagnosis has not been established in the interim. As with other manifestations, IgM and IgG antibodies could remain positive indefinitely after infection and should not be used as a tool for therapy (Wormser et al., 1999a). Careful interpretation of test results is crucial when evaluating patients in non-endemic areas as the positive predictive value of the test is directly proportional to the prevalence of disease.

Radiographic and Other Diagnostic Modalities

Radiographic imaging and 2D echocardiography have been employed to support the diagnosis (Rienzo et al., 1987; Veluvolu et al., 1992). Transient cardiomegaly, pericardial effusions, and decreased ejection fraction have been described. Gallium scanning, magnetic resonance imaging, and indium scanning have been used to demonstrate inflammation. Increased radionuclide uptake is noted with gallium and indium scanning (Veluvolu et al., 1992; Bergler-Klein et al., 1993). In one recent report MRI showed persistent epicardial enhancement after gadolinium injection at four month follow-up (Munk et al., 2007). Obviously these modalities are not specific for inflammation caused by *Borrelia* infection.

MANAGEMENT AND ANTIMICROBIAL THERAPY

There are no controlled comparative trials in the treatment of Lyme carditis. Most cases of Lyme carditis resolve spontaneously within weeks of the infection, and there is no evidence that antibiotic therapy hastens the resolution of abnormalities. Nevertheless, therapy is recommended for all patients and will prevent later manifestations of Lyme borreliosis (Wormser et al., 2006). Treatment with parenteral and oral regimens is equivalent and is recommended for 14 days for AV block with or without myopericarditis. Hospitalization for cardiac monitoring is recommended for symptomatic patients with cardiovascular symptoms, second- or third-degree AV block, or first-degree AV block with prolonged PR interval (>30 milliseconds). Although not supported by clinical trials (IDSA-USPHS Evidence Level B-III), it is recommended that hospitalized patients receive an intravenous antibiotic such as ceftriaxone followed by oral antibiotic regimen as outpatients to finish the treatment course. Temporary pacing may be required and can be discontinued when the advanced block has resolved.

Carditis with concurrent central nervous system manifestations or peripheral neuropathy due to Lyme borreliosis should be treated with intravenous antibiotics, regardless of the degree of AV block. There is no evidence that the sole use of intravenous antimicrobials can reverse end-stage dilated cardiomyopathy putatively caused by Lyme borreliosis. In one uncontrolled trial from Europe, 46 patients with end-stage dilated cardiomyopathy reported subjective improvement after intravenous antimicrobial therapy (Gasser et al., 1996). Antibiotics were given in conjunction with cardiac medications that could have improved cardiac output. The IDSA guidelines do not address the treatment of such patients because of the controversial evidence for Lyme borreliosis as a cause of chronic cardiomyopathy.

Lyme carditis has an excellent outcome, with the conduction abnormalities usually resolving in one to six weeks, althoguh persistent second-degree AV block occurred in one child (Costello et al., 2009). Case reports of fatality should be interpreted with caution as the role of co-morbidities is difficult to exclude.

REFERENCES

Anda P, Rodriguez I, De la Loma A, Fernandez MV, Lozano A: A serological survey and review of clinical Lyme borreliosis in Spain. *Clin Infect Dis* 16:310–319; 1983.

Armstrong AL, Barthold SW, Persing DH, Beck DS: Carditis in Lyme disease susceptible and resistant strains of laboratory mice infected with *Borrelia burgdorferi. Am J Trop Med Hyg* 47:249–258; 1992.

Baylac-Domengetroy F, Vieyres C, Barraine R: Complete heart block as the sole presentation of Lyme disease. *Arch Intern Med* 151:1240; 1991.

Bergler-Klein J, Sochor H, Stanek G, Globits S, Ullrich R, Glogar D: Indium 111-monoclonal antimyosin antibody and magnetic resonance imaging in the diagnosis of acute Lyme myopericarditis. *Arch Intern Med* 153:2696–2700; 1993.

Berglund J, Eitrem R, Ornstein K, Lindberg A, Ringer A, Elmrud H, Carlsson M, Runehagen A, Svanborg C, Norrby R: An epidemiologic study of Lyme disease in southern Sweden. *N Engl J Med* 333:1319–1327; 1995.

Bruyn GA, De Koning J, Reijsoo FJ, Houtman PM, Hoogkamp-Korstanje JA: Lyme pericarditis leading to tamponade. *Br J Rheumatol* 33:862–866; 1994.

Canver CC, Chanda J, Debellis DM, Kelley JM: Possible relationship between degenerative cardiac valvular pathology and Lyme disease. *Ann Thorac Surg* 70:283–285; 2000.

Cary NR, Fox B, Wright DJ, Cutler SJ, Shapiro LM, Grace AA: Fatal Lyme carditis and endodermal heterotopia of the atrioventricular node. *Postgrad Med J* 66:134–136; 1990.

Ciesielski CA, Markowitz LE, Horsley R, Hightower AW, Russell H, Broome CV: Lyme disease surveillance in the United States, 1983–1986. *Rev Infect Dis* 11(suppl 6): S1435–S1441; 1989.

Costello JM, Alexander ME, Greco KM, Perez-Atayde AR, Laussen PC: Lyme carditis in children. Presentation, predictive factors, and clinical course. *Pediatrics* 123:e835–e841; 2009.

Cox J, Krajden M: Cardiovascular manifestations of Lyme disease. *Am Heart J* 122:1449–1455; 1991.

de Koning J, Hoogkamp-Korstanje JA, van der Linde MR, Crijns HJ: Demonstration of spirochetes in cardiac biopsies of patients with Lyme disease. *J Infect Dis* 160:150–153; 1989.

Dressler F, Whalen JA, Reinhardt BN, Steere AC: Western blotting in the serodiagnosis of Lyme disease. *J Infect Dis* 167:392–400; 1993.

Duray PH: Clinical pathologic correlations of Lyme disease. *Rev Infect Dis* 11(suppl 6): S1487–S1493; 1989.

Gasser R, Dusleag J, Reisinger E, Stauber R, Feigl B, Pongratz S, Klein W, Furlan C, Pierer K: Reversal by ceftriaxone of dilated cardiomyopathy *Borrelia burgdorferi* infection. *Lancet* 339:1174–1175; 1992.

Gasser R, Fruhwald F, Schumacher M, Seinost G, Reisinger E, Eber B, Keplinger A, Horvath R, Sedaj B, Klein W, Pierer K: Reversal of *Borrelia burgdorferi* associated dilated cardiomyopathy by antibiotic treatment? *Cardiovasc Drugs Ther* 10:351–360; 1996.

Gasser R, Horn S, Reisinger E, Fischer L, Pokan R, Wendelin I, Klein W: First description of recurrent pericardial effusion associated with *Borrelia burgdorferi* infection. *Int J Cardiol* 64:309–310; 1998.

Gerber MA, Shapiro ED, Burke GS, Parcells VJ, Bell GL: Lyme disease in children in southeastern Connecticut. Pediatric Lyme Disease Study Group. *N Engl J Med* 335:1270–1274; 1996.

Globits S, Bergler-Klein J, Stanek G, Ullrich R, Glogar D: Magnetic resonance imaging in the diagnosis of acute Lyme carditis. *Cardiology* 85:415–417; 1994.

Grzesik P, Oczko-Grzesik B, Kepa L: [Cardiac manifestations of Lyme borreliosis]. *Przegl Epidemiol* 58:589–596; 2004.

Haddad FA, Nadelman RB: Lyme disease and the heart. *Front Biosci* 8:s769–s782; 2003.

Haywood GA, O'Connell S, Gray HH: Lyme carditis. A United Kingdom perspective. *Br Heart J* 70:15–16; 1993.

Houwerzyl J, Root JJ, Hoogkamp-Korstanje JA: A case of Lyme disease with cardiac involvement in the Netherlands. *Infection* 12:358; 1984.

Huppertz HI, Bohme M, Standaert SM, Karch H, Plotkin SA: Incidence of Lyme borreliosis in the Wurzburg region of Germany. *Eur J Clin Microbiol Infect Dis* 18:697–703; 1999.

Jacobs JC, Rosen JM, Szer IS: Lyme myocarditis diagnosed by gallium scan. *J Pediatr* 105:950–952; 1984.

Kaell AT, Volkman DJ, Gorevic PD, Dattwyler RJ: Positive Lyme serology in subacute bacterial endocarditis. A study of four patients. *JAMA* 264:2916–2918; 1990.

Kimball SA, Janson PA, Laraia PJ: Complete heart block as the sole presentation of Lyme disease. *Arch Intern Med* 149:1897–1898; 1989.

Klein J, Stanek G, Bittner R, Horvat R, Holzinger C, Glogar D: Lyme borreliosis as a cause of myocarditis and heart muscle disease. *Eur Heart J* 12(suppl D): 73–75; 1991.

Lardieri G, Salvi A, Camerini F, Cinco M, Trevisan G: Isolation of *Borrelia burgdorferi* from myocardium. *Lancet* 342:490; 1993.

Lipsker D, Hansmann Y, Limbach F, Clerc C, Tranchant C, Grunenberger F, Caro-Sampara F, Attali P, Frey M, Kubina M, Piemont Y, Sibilia J, Jaulhac B: Disease expression of Lyme borreliosis in northeastern France. *Eur J Clin Microbiol Infect Dis* 20:225–230; 2001.

Marcus LC, Steere AC, Duray PH, Anderson AE, Mahoney EB: Fatal pancarditis in a patient with coexistent Lyme disease and babesiosis. Demonstration of spirochetes in the myocardium. *Ann Intern Med* 103:374–376; 1985.

Midttun M, Lebech AM, Hansen K, Videbaek J: Lyme carditis. A clinical presentation and long time follow-up. *Scand J Infect Dis* 29:153–157; 1997.

Mravljak M, Velnar T, Bricelj V, Ruzic-Sabljic E, Arnez M: Electrocardiographic findings in children with erythema migrans. *Wien Klin Wochenschr* 118:691–695; 2006.

Munk PS, Orn S, Larsen AI: Lyme carditis: persistent local delayed enhancement by cardiac magnetic resonance imaging. *Int J Cardiol* 115:e108–e110; 2007.

Nadelman RB, Wormser GP: Lyme borreliosis. *Lancet* 352:557–565; 1998.

Nygard K, Brantsaeter AB, Mehl R: Disseminated and chronic Lyme borreliosis in Norway, 1995–2004. *Euro Surveill* 10:235–238; 2005.

O'Connell S, Granstrom M, Gray JS, Stanek G: Epidemiology of European Lyme borreliosis. *Zentralbl Bakteriol* 287:229–240; 1998.

Oksi J, Voipio-Pulkki LM, Uksila J, Pulkki K, Laippala P, Viljanen MK: *Borrelia burgdorferi* infection in patients with suspected acute myocardial infarction. *Lancet* 350:1447–1448; 1997.

Pikelj-Pecnik A, Lotric-Furlan S, Maraspin V, Cimperman J, Logar M, Jurca T, Strle F: Electrocardiographic findings in patients with erythema migrans. *Wien Klin Wochenschr* 114:510–514; 2002.

Rey MJ, Zimmermann M, Adamec R, Fleisch M, Viquerat C, De Freudenreich J: Intra-hisian 2:1 atrioventricular block secondary to Lyme disease. *Eur Heart J* 12:1048–1051; 1991.

Reznick JW, Braunstein DB, Walsh RL, Smith CR, Wolfson PM, Gierke LW, Gorelkin L, Chandler FW: Lyme carditis. Electrophysiologic and histopathologic study. *Am J Med* 81:923–927; 1986.

Rienzo RJ, Morel DE, Prager D, Barron L, Post R: Gallium avid Lyme myocarditis. *Clin Nucl Med* 12:475–476; 1987.

Rosenfeld ME, Beckerman B, Ward MF, Sama A: Lyme carditis. Complete AV dissociation with episodic asystole presenting as syncope in the emergency department. *J Emerg Med* 17:661–664; 1999.

Rubin DA, Sorbera C, Nikitin P, MaAllister A, Wormser GP, Nadelman RB: Prospective evaluation of heart block complicating early Lyme disease. *Pacing Clin Electrophysiol* 15:252–255; 1992.

Ruzic-Sabljic E, Arnez M, Logar M, Maraspin V, Lotric-Furlan S, Cimperman J, Strle F: Comparison of *Borrelia burgdorferi* sensu lato strains isolated from specimens obtained simultaneously from two different sites of infection in individual patients. *J Clin Microbiol* 43:2194–2200; 2005.

Saba S, Vanderbrink BA, Perides G, Glickstein LJ, Link MS, Homoud MK, Bronson RT, Estes M III, Wang PJ: Cardiac conduction abnormalities in a mouse model of Lyme borreliosis. *J Interv Card Electrophysiol* 5:137–143; 2001.

Sangha O, Phillips CB, Fleischmann KE, Wang TJ, Fossel AH, Lew R, Liang MH, Shadick NA: Lack of cardiac manifestations among patients with previously treated Lyme disease. *Ann Intern Med* 128:346–353; 1998.

Sigal LH: Early disseminated Lyme disease: cardiac manifestations. *Am J Med* 98:25S–28S; discussion 28S–29S; 1995.

Sigal LH. Zahradnik JM, Lavin P, Patella SJ, Bryant G, Haselby R, Hilton E, Kunkel M, Adler-Klein D, Doherty T, Evans J, Molloy PJ, Seidner AL, Sabetta JR, Simon HJ, Klempner MS, Mays J, Marks D, Malawista SE: A vaccine consisting of recombinant *Borrelia burgdorferi* outer-surface protein A to prevent Lyme disease. Recombinant Outer-Surface Protein A Lyme Disease Vaccine Study Consortium. *N Engl J Med* 339:216–222; 1998.

Sonnesyn SW, Diehl SC, Johnson RC, Kubo SH, Goodman JL: A prospective study of the seroprevalence of *Borrelia burgdorferi* infection in patients with severe heart failure. *Am J Cardiol* 76:97–100; 1995.

Stanek G, Klein J, Bittner R, Glogar D: Isolation of *Borrelia burgdorferi* from the myocardium of a patient with longstanding cardiomyopathy. *N Engl J Med* 322:249–252; 1990.

Stanek G, Klein J, Bittner R, Glogar D: *Borrelia burgdorferi* as an etiologic agent in chronic heart failure? *Scand J Infect Dis Suppl* 77:85–87; 1991.

Steere AC, Batsford WP, Weinberg M, Alexander J, Berger HJ, Wolfson S, Malawista SE: Lyme carditis. Cardiac abnormalities of Lyme disease. *Ann Intern Med* 93:8–16; 1980.

Steere AC, Sikand VK, Meurice F, Parenti DL, Fikrig E, Schoen RT, Nowakowski J, Schmid CH, Laukamp S, Buscarino C, Krause DS: Vaccination against Lyme disease with recombinant *Borrelia burgdorferi* outer-surface lipoprotein A with adjuvant. Lyme Disease Vaccine Study Group. *N Engl J Med* 339:209–215; 1998.

Stewart A, Glass J, Patel A, Watt G, Cripps A, Clancy R: Lyme arthritis in the Hunter Valley. *Med J Aust* 1:139; 1982.

Strle F, Nadelman RB, Cimperman J, Nowakowski J, Picken RN, Schwartz I, Maraspin V, Aguero-Rosenfeld ME, Varde S, Lotric-Furlan S, Wormser GP: Comparison of culture-confirmed erythema migrans caused by *Borrelia burgdorferi* sensu stricto in New York State and by *Borrelia afzelii* in Slovenia. *Ann Intern Med* 130:32–36; 1999.

Suedkamp M, Lissel C, Eiffert H, Flesch M, Boehm M, Mehlhorn U, Thomssen R, De Vivie ER: Cardiac myocytes of hearts from patients with end-stage dilated cardiomyopathy do not contain *Borrelia burgdorferi* DNA. *Am Heart J* 138:269–272; 1999.

Tavora F, Burke A, Li L, Franks TJ, Virmani R: Postmortem confirmation of Lyme carditis with polymerase chain reaction. *Cardiovasc Pathol* 17:103–107; 2008.

Van Dam AP, Kuiper H, Vos K, Widjojokusumo A, De Jongh BM, Spanjaard L, Ramselaar AC, Kramer MD, Dankert J: Different genospecies of *Borrelia burgdorferi* are associated with distinct clinical manifestations of Lyme borreliosis. *Clin Infect Dis* 17:708–717; 1993.

Van der Linde MR: Lyme carditis: clinical characteristics of 105 cases. *Scand J Infect Dis Suppl* 77:81–84; 1991.

Van der Linde MR, Crijns HJ, De Koning J, Hoogkamp-Korstanje JA, De Graaf JJ, Piers DA, van der Galien A, Lie KI: Range of atrioventricular conduction disturbances in Lyme borreliosis: a report of four cases and review of other published reports. *Br Heart J* 63:162–168; 1990.

Veluvolu P, Balian AA, Goldsmith R, Gallant TE, Barthel L, Vidaillet HJ, Melski JW: Lyme carditis. Evaluation by Ga-67 and MRI. *Clin Nucl Med* 17:823; 1992.

Vidaillet HJ Jr, Broste SK, Marx JJ Jr, McCarty PA, Layde PM, Mitchell PD, Dlesk A: The 12-lead electrocardiogram of "healthy" ambulatory subjects with positive Lyme immunoserology. *Am J Cardiol* 71:1249–1251; 1993.

Vlay SC, Dervan JP, Elias J, Kane PP, Dattwyler R: Ventricular tachycardia associated with Lyme carditis. *Am Heart J* 121:1558–1560; 1991.

Wang G, Ojaimi C, Wu H, Saksenberg V, Iyer R., Liveris D, McClain SA, Wormser GP, Schwartz I: Disease severity in a murine model of Lyme borreliosis is associated with the genotype of the infecting *Borrelia burgdorferi* sensu stricto strain. *J Infect Dis* 186:782–791; 2002.

Wormser GP, Aguero-Rosenfeld ME, Nadelman RB: Lyme disease serology: problems and opportunities. *JAMA* 282:79–80; 1999a.

Wormser GP, Liveris D, Nowakowski J, Nadelman RB, Cavaliere LF, McKenna D, Holmgren D, Schwartz I: Association of specific subtypes of *Borrelia burgdorferi* with hematogenous dissemination in early Lyme disease. *J Infect Dis* 180:720–725; 1999b.

Wormser GP, Nadelman RB, Dattwyler RJ, Dennis DT, Shapiro ED, Steere AC, Rush TJ, Rahn DW, Coyle PK, Persing DH, Fish D, Luft BJ: Practice guidelines for the treatment of Lyme disease. The Infectious Diseases Society of America. *Clin Infect Dis* 31(suppl 1):1–14; 2000.

Wormser GP, Dattwyler RJ, Shapiro ED, Halperin JJ, Steere AC, Klempner MS, Krause PJ, Bakken JS, Strle F, Stanek G, Bockenstedt L, Fish D, Dumler JS, Nadelman RB: The clinical assessment, treatment, and prevention of Lyme disease, human granulocytic anaplasmosis, and babesiosis. Clinical practice guidelines by the Infectious Diseases Society of America. *Clin Infect Dis* 43:1089–1134; 2006.

5

NERVOUS SYSTEM LYME BORRELIOSIS

John J. Halperin and Leif Dotevall

How does Lyme disease (Lyme borreliosis, Lyme neuroborreliosis), the result of *Borrelia burgdorferi* infection (in the United States) involve the nervous system? Is it fundamentally similar to, or different from, the disorder caused by its very closely related European "cousins," *B garinii* and *B afzelii*? If similar, how can the European experience inform US diagnosis and treatment? If not, what accounts for the differences? For that matter, what do we mean by "nervous system involvement"? Such seemingly simple questions have led to tremendous confusion among both clinicians and patients, and probably more than anything else account for the wide divergence of opinion about what constitutes the clinical spectrum of Lyme disease and its appropriate treatment.

Early in the history of Lyme disease, Reik (Reik et al., 1979) and Pachner (Pachner and Steere, 1984) described neurologic manifestations remarkably similar to those seen in neuroborreliosis in Europe. Despite this, it has been commonplace to stress the clinical differences between European and US disease—with joint involvement felt to be far more prominent in the United States, and nervous system disorders much more common in Europe. Microbiologic studies have shown that the two predominant genospecies of *B. burgdorferi* present in Europe do not occur in the United States, where only *B. burgdorferi* sensu stricto (which is also present in Europe) is found (although *B. garinii* has been found in seabirds in Newfoundland) (Smith et al., 2006). All three major Lyme *Borrelia* genospecies have been identified by PCR in cerebrospinal fluid in European patients, although *B. garinii* has been found to be the most frequent etiological agent (Ornstein et al., 2002;

Lyme Borreliosis in Europe and North America: Epidemiology and Clinical Practice, First Edition. Edited by Sunil K. Sood

Lebech, 2002). Two other subspecies of *B. burgdorferi* sensu lato, *B. valaisiana* (Diza et al., 2004) and *B. bissettii* (Fingerle et al., 2008) have been reported in CSF in one patient each with Lyme neuroborreliosis. The only subspecies found in American patients, *B. burgdorferi* sensu stricto, seems to have a lower neurotropism than *B. garinii* (van Dam et al., 1993). Most authors suggest that the clinical differences between European and American disease are a result of these strain differences.

Neurological abnormalities of any kind have been reported to occur in 10% to 20% of all untreated patients with Lyme borreliosis in Europe (Weber and Pfister, 1993; Berglund et al., 1995), and about 12% in North America (CDC, 2007).

Lyme neuroborreliosis most often presents with all or part of the triad of radiculoneuritis with intense radicular pain, cranial neuropathies (most often facial nerve palsy), and lymphocytic meningitis, as described in 1922 by the French physicians Garin and Bujadoux in the earliest published case report of neuroborreliosis (Garin and Bujadoux, 1922). Pfister et al. later found in a European study that 78% of adults with neurological borreliosis showed this typical clinical pattern. This clinical triad was further described in 1941 by the German neurologist Bannwarth (Bannwarth, 1941) in his comprehensive clinical report of 14 patients with lymphocytic meningitis. He observed that patients suffered from severe neuralgic, migrating radicular pain in the extremities and on the trunk, often most evident at night. Bannwarth described unilateral facial nerve palsy in two patients and bilateral palsy in four. He also noted recurrences with intense multifocal pain even after the CSF cell counts had normalized. Numerous subsequent case reports have emphasized that severe pain is a typical symptom of this clinical entity.

In 1945 Gelbjerg-Hansen reported another patient with lymphocytic meningitis that appeared after tick bite. During the following years many additional case reports of tick-borne meningoradiculitis were published. Schaltenbrand described eight patients with subacute meningitis after tick bites in 1949 (Schaltenbrand, 1949) and another three cases in 1962 (Schaltenbrand, 1962). He was the first author to speculate on the relationship between the topographical location of the tick bite and the subsequent neurological manifestations. He postulated that a tick-borne infectious agent was "migrating" along the nerves and lymphatics to the central nervous system. He also described prompt improvement after treatment with corticosteroids and tetracycline. In 1951 Hellerström reported the first case of successful penicillin treatment of one patient with meningitis and erythema migrans (Hellerstrom, 1951).

Shortly after Steere began describing clusters of cases of what appeared to be juvenile arthritis in Connecticut, he, Reik, and Pachner recognized that in addition to the clinical findings of erythema migrans, arthritis, and carditis, these patients also often experienced neurological difficulties (Steere et al., 1977).

APPROACH TO DIAGNOSIS

To define the spectrum of nervous system involvement in Lyme disease, or neuroborreliosis, regardless of geographical locale it is first essential to agree on the minimum requirements needed to identify a particular clinical problem as a true neurologic manifestation of this infection. Three key elements seem logically unavoidable: affected patients must have nervous system disease, they must have Lyme disease, and the two disorders must be causally related.

Much of the current controversy—and public anxiety—about Lyme disease relates to several widely held misperceptions. These are (1) that a variety of nonspecific symptoms are indicative of nervous system damage; (2) that the presence of such symptoms, in isolation, is diagnostic of nervous system Lyme disease; (3) that neurologic disease is inherently very difficult to diagnose; and (4) that nervous system involvement leads to untreatable, irreversible neurologic impairment.

Contrary to these assumptions, the diagnosis of nervous system disease is, in general, straightforward. An essential prerequisite is the presence of objective evidence of damage to the peripheral nervous system (PNS) or central nervous system (CNS). Simply feeling tired, suffering from headaches, feeling memory or cognition to be suboptimal, or feeling depressed do not constitute evidence of neurologic disease. A core tenet of clinical neurology is that damage to the nervous system causes objectively demonstrable deficits on clinical neurologic evaluation, that can, as appropriate, be augmented by formal neuropsychologic testing, or by other objective laboratory techniques such as brain imaging (primarily MRI) if the CNS is involved, or neurophysiologic tests (electromyography, EMG) when the PNS is affected. Moreover, when dealing with any CNS infection, there are almost invariably changes in the cerebrospinal fluid—at a minimum a reactive inflammatory cell response or increase in CSF protein concentration. In CNS *Borrelia* infections an increase in CSF immunoglobulin production (intrathecal antibody production) occurs frequently, typically quantifiable as increased CSF immunoglobulin G (IgG) synthesis rate or an increase in the calculated IgG index. When, as in neuroborreliosis, this increase in CSF immunoglobulin is in response to a specific infectious organism, it is often possible to demonstrate that antibody specific to that organism is preferentially elevated in the CSF. In the absence of any abnormality on clinical exam, or, for CNS disease, imaging studies or CSF examination, or, for PNS disease, neurophysiologic testing, it is quite unlikely that neurologic disease is present.

Similarly, although the diagnosis of Lyme disease is often described as controversial and challenging, this controversy is irrelevant to clinical diagnosis and treatment. Again, a simple logical approach typically suffices. First, there must be a reasonable likelihood of exposure. Lyme disease is spread exclusively by the bites of *Ixodes* ticks—*I. scapularis* in most of the United States, *I. ricinus* in Europe. The tick must have fed on an infected reservoir host—typically a small mammal, such as a field mouse—and must subsequently feed on the potential human host for an extended period of time (typically 24 to 72 hours) (Sood et al., 1997; Nadelman et al., 2001; des Vignes et al., 2001) for the patient to be at significant risk of infection. If the patient has never been in an endemic area for Lyme disease, the likelihood of infection is extremely small.

Once infection occurs, diagnosis of Lyme disease can be supported by appropriate laboratory observations. Laboratory confirmation of *B. burgdorferi* infection by serologic assays, culture and DNA amplification is comprehensively discussed in Chapters 9 and 10.

Establishing a cause and effect linkage between Lyme disease and a particular neurologic disorder may be the most challenging aspect. If the neurologic symptoms are within the well-defined range of disorders known to occur with nervous system Lyme, causality should be assumed and appropriate treatment instituted. If not, then more compelling evidence (e.g., specific abnormalities of cerebrospinal fluid if a central nervous system disorder is suspected) should be sought. Based on these simple principles, the American Academy of Neurology published straightforward guidelines for the diagnosis of nervous system Lyme disease (Halperin et al., 1996). Oschmann et al. have similarly proposed practical guidelines for the diagnosis of European neuroborreliosis (Oschmann et al., 1998), and slight modifications of these criteria have been useful during some studies.

CSF Abnormalities

Examination of the cerebrospinal fluid can be very important in the diagnosis of neuroborreliosis (Table 5.1). The circumstances under which a lumbar puncture is needed has been the subject of considerable discussion. Certainly when there is a significant risk of other disorders best diagnosed by CSF exam (e.g., other treatable CNS infections or a CNS malignancy), or in areas with high background rates of seropositivity, where blood serology has a low positive predictive value for neuroborreliosis, lumbar puncture (LP) is essential. In patients with parenchymal CNS involvement the information provided by CSF examination is essential. However, there are now numerous studies showing that Lyme meningitis and cranial neuritis are successfully treatable with oral doxycycline (at least with European strains); consequently many have suggested that in these patients, LP may not be necessary. Nevertheless, many experts do recommend an LP in all such patients; this question should be subjected to rigorous study.

Specific intrathecal antibody production to *B. burgdorferi sp.* is the most specific single finding in neuroborreliosis, although it may be absent in patients early in the course of the disease, and should not be expected to be present in patients who lack CNS involvement, such as those with ACA-associated neuropathy. Hansen and Lebech used a specific capture antibody index in their prospective study (OD-CSF/OD-serum) $\times$ (OD-CSF minus OD-serum). An index ≥ 0.3 for IgM or IgG was proposed as a cutoff value for definite intrathecal specific *B. burgdorferi sp.* antibody production (Hansen and Lebech, 1992). A similar approach has been used in US patients with neuroborreliosis. The somewhat different methods used (capture assay for some (Steere et al., 1990), pre-assay adjustment for immunoglobulin concentration in others (Halperin et al., 1989), leads to differing cutoff values. The perception is that the sensitivity of this technique may be lower in US patients, although some recent European studies also suggest a lower sensitivity (Ljøstad et al., 2007).

Although controversy remains regarding the proportion of patients with CNS Lyme disease who demonstrate this laboratory finding (Logigian et al., 1990; Halperin et al., 1991; Blanc et al., 2007; Ljøstad et al., 2007), at the very least it should be evident in patients with obvious CNS inflammatory disease. This means that if there is a vigorous immune-mediated

TABLE 5.1 CSF Findings in central nervous system *B. burgdorferi* infection

Measure	Sensitivity
Lymphocytic pleocytosis	Approaches 100%
Increased protein	Approaches 100%
Intrathecal antibody production (US)	
In presence of significant pleocytosis	90%
In absence of significant pleocytosis	50%
PCR	<10%
Culture	<10%
Immune complexes	Unknown

CNS process that is sufficiently active to result in an overall increase in intra-CNS antibody synthesis (increased IgG index, IgG synthesis rate, or oligoclonal bands), and this antibody production is due to a particular inciting organism, it is only reasonable to expect that antibody to that organism would be present in increased concentration.

As in any infection with central nervous system involvement, CSF is typically abnormal. Total CSF protein is usually elevated, due to increased blood–brain barrier permeability. In one study of 187 patients (Hansen and Lebech, 1992) total CSF protein varied between 0.2 and 12 g/L (mean 1.13). In another study of 330 neuroborreliosis patients with early or late neurological manifestations, CSF protein ranged from 0.13 to 10.7g/L (Oschmann et al., 1998). Higher values were often found in patients with progressive disease and long pretreatment durations. An elevated albumin ratio and IgG-index are commonly found. Oligoclonal bands were seen in 66% to 77% of European patients (Oschmann et al., 1998). In late neuroborreliosis intrathecal antibody production is even more intense. A CSF/blood glucose ratio $\leq$0.3 was found in 4% of the patients, lower values being associated with a progressive course of infection (Hansen and Lebech, 1992). Increased CSF lactate levels (>1.9 mmol/L) have been reported in 50% of patients with neuroborreliosis (Oschmann et al., 1998). Findings in US patients are qualitatively similar, though often less pronounced. CSF protein and cell counts may be somewhat lower, and intrathecal antibody production is more variable.

The cell count and CSF protein concentration decrease for two to six months or more following successful antibiotic treatment (Martin et al., 1993; Borg et al., 2005). In individuals with more longstanding neuroborreliosis, CSF normalizes more slowly (Kaiser, 1994), and the amount of intrathecally produced immunoglobulin does not necessarily decline during the initial period after treatment (Hammers Berggren et al., 1993). CSF IgG oligoclonal bands can still be demonstrated in one-third of patients 5 to 17 years after infection (Krüger et al., 1989). Other reported CSF biochemical markers of disease activity include elevated concentrations of astroglial protein GFAp (Dotevall et al., 1996), IL-2, IL-6, fibronectin (Weller et al., 1991), neopterin (Dotevall et al., 1990), and metalloproteinase with recent evidence that glia play a prominent role in this response (Ramesh et al., 2009).

Neuroimaging

Cranial computed tomography (CT) has generally been of limited utility in Lyme neuroborreliosis; magnetic resonance imaging (MRI) has been more informative. CT of 51 European patients with neuroborreliosis was abnormal in only three, all with chronic progressive encephalomyelitis. Multiple white matter lesions described as leukoencephalopathy were seen in these three (Hansen and Lebech, 1992). In other patients with European neuroborreliosis multiple sclerosis-like lesions have been described on MRI (Hansen, 1994). Three children with neurological Lyme disease had normal CT but abnormal MRI findings. Subcortical areas of ADEM-like enhanced signal intensities were reported, in spite of normal CT results. MRI in 16 of 21 patients with Lyme neuroborreliosis in North America demonstrated multifocal abnormalities primarily in the white and occasionally grey matter (Halperin et al., 1991). In one patient MRI demonstrated a focal inflammatory mass, with increased activity on PET imaging (Kalina et al., 2005). Isolated reports of angiographic changes compatible with cerebral vasculitis have also been published (Veenendaal-Hilbers et al., 1988), although whether these patients had a vasculitis caused by neuroborreliosis remains unclear (Halperin, 2008).

CLINICAL SPECTRUM OF NERVOUS SYSTEM LYME DISEASE

Virtually every known neurologic and psychiatric disorder has been attributed to Lyme disease at one time or another, much like in the early neurosyphilis literature. The challenge is to determine which ones are chance associations and which are caused by *Borrelia* infection. It is equally important to understand the pathophysiologic mechanisms responsible for the neurologic disorders that actually are caused by this infection.

Evolution of Clinical Symptoms

The neurological manifestations have been reviewed by many authors (Stiernstedt et al., 1988; Hansen, 1994; Garcia-Monco and Benach, 1995; Halperin, 1998, 2003b; Christen et al., 1993b). Systemic manifestations, such as headache and fever are common (Stiernstedt et al., 1988), and may occur simultaneous with, or within a few weeks following the onset of erythema migrans (EM). Both US and European reports have emphasized that most neurological abnormalities occur in the early dissemination phase of Lyme disease. The evolution of symptoms and signs in severe European neuroborreliosis has been thoroughly addressed in the prospective study by Hansen and Lebech (Hansen and Lebech, 1992). They found that the median latency between EM and sensory radiculitis was 19 days (range 5–90), the median time between sensory radiculitis and first paresis was 15 days (range 1–99), and last paresis was noted after further median time of 7 days (range 1–30). In another three series of patients with European neuroborreliosis median time between the appearance of EM and onset of radicular pain was reported to be 8 to 21 days (range 0–95 days) (Oschmann et al., 1998). In about four-fifths of the patients the EM had disappeared by the time of onset of neurological symptoms.

Meningitis and Intracranial Hypertension

The lymphocytic meningitis is generally similar to that in "aseptic" or viral meningitis, although compared to patients with viral meningitis, Lyme meningitis patients have a less acute onset and are more likely to have a cranial neuropathy or erythema migrans (Shah et al., 2005; Garro et al., 2009). At least in children, papilledema is more common. Typically patients have severe headaches, photophobia, and neck stiffness, but some may lack these typical symptoms and signs despite an obvious meningeal inflammatory reaction. Neck stiffness is reported in 45% of children (Christen and Hanefeld, 1993). Headache occurs in 18% to 64% of all patients with neuroborreliosis (Hansen and Lebech, 1992; Stiernstedt et al., 1988; Oschmann et al., 1998), but may be a less prominent symptom in adults. In contrast, some patients with severe headaches have normal CSF. CSF pleocytosis is a common but not invariable finding in patients with radiculitis or cranial neuritis, although it is often absent during the first few days after onset of symptoms (Steere, 1989).

Two closely related disorders deserve mention. Several reports have described normal pressure hydrocephalus (NPH) in patients with evidence of Lyme disease (Danek et al., 1996; Etienne et al., 2003). Although the number of cases described is small, since meningitis is one of the well-known predisposing factors for NPH, such an association is plausible. A larger number of reports has described the occurrence of pseudotumor cerebri in children with Lyme disease (Jacobson and Frens, 1989; Kan et al., 1998; Zemel, 2000). Since most of these patients have, at one time or another, evidenced a CSF pleocytosis, it is difficult to understand why this should be considered pseudotumor rather than intracranial hypertension associated with meningitis. Regardless, it is important to recognize that, particularly in children, the elevation in intracranial pressure can be significant and can lead to optic nerve compromise (Rothermel et al., 2001).

Cranial Nerve Palsy

Cranial neuritis is the most common focal finding, reported in 43% to 82% of European patients with Lyme neuroborreliosis (Stiernstedt et al., 1988), with an onset typically several weeks after EM has appeared, although in rare patients it occurs within the first week or two following initiation of antibiotic treatment. Facial nerve palsy is by far the most common cranial neuritis in Lyme disease. It was reported in 72% to 92% of patients with cranial nerve involvement in earlier studies (Pachner and Steere, 1985) but nowadays appears to be less frequent in adults, presumably due to earlier diagnosis and treatment. Facial palsy originally was found to be bilateral in as many as a third of cases (Pachner and Steere, 1985). Interestingly occasional patients with early facial (or other cranial) nerve involvement will have normal CSF. Clinical, electrophysiologic, and CSF findings all point to the facial nerve being involved in the periphery, not in the subarachnoid space (Halperin et al., 1990b; Halperin, 2003a). In some patients increased levels of astroglial and neuronal marker proteins in CSF, and accompanying focal brain abnormalities, do indicate simultaneous CNS involvement (Dotevall et al., 1999).

Less frequently the disease may affect the IIIrd (oculomotor) or VIth (abducens) nerve, causing diplopia, the Vth (trigeminal) nerve, causing facial numbness or pain, the VIIIth (vestibulo-acoustic) nerve, causing hearing loss, tinnitus, or vertigo, or the IXth or Xth (vagus and glossopharyngeal) nerves, causing hoarseness or dysphagia. Progressive sensorineural hearing loss has been reported in a few patients with *Borrelia* encephalomyelitis of long duration (Hansen and Lebech, 1992). Although there are numerous reports in the literature describing optic nerve involvement in patients with presumed Lyme disease, a careful review of these descriptions suggests that optic neuritis occurs quite rarely, if ever, as a result of Lyme disease (Sibony et al., 2005).

Radiculoneuritis

Painful radicular involvement is a typical and frequent symptom in early neuroborreliosis in Europe. The pain is often alarming and causes anxiety and restlessness. Pfister described the neuralgic radicular pain in neuroborreliosis as "severe, burning, tearing, migrating pain with characteristic exacerbations at night" (Pfister et al., 1993). Sensations of dysesthesia and hyperesthesia in the involved area are frequent. Slight contact as from the pressure of clothing may cause severe burning pain. The radicular pain may be located anywhere on the body and is almost always described as focal and asymmetric, and may migrate to adjacent dermatomes

Initially the cause of symptoms may be difficult to diagnose (Halperin et al., 1996), particularly in the 20% of patients in whom radicular pain is the only symptom (Pfister et al., 1993). The mismatch between the dramatic symptoms and the almost normal physical findings may be striking. In the Danish study that was performed in the years 1985 to 1990, when physicians were less cognizant of the manifestations of neuroborreliosis, 7% of the patients were initially suspected of being hysterical and some of them were seen by a psychiatrist before the diagnosis of *Borrelia* infection was made (Hansen and Lebech, 1992). The symptoms resemble zoster neuralgia or mechanical radiculopathies. Objective signs may not be prominent; sensory loss is only found in 30% of the patients (Pfister et al., 1993). Motor and reflex changes are similarly variable. This diagnosis should always be considered in a patient with appropriate symptoms, presenting in Spring through Autumn, who has been in an endemic area, particularly if there was no apparent mechanical precipitant. Nonsteroidal anti-inflammatory drugs do not usually control the neuralgic pain. Pain may transiently improve with steroids (Pfister et al., 1988), but steroids obviously do not treat the infection. Antibiotic treatment relieves the radicular pain within one to seven days, but dysesthesias may remain for many months, although the symptoms will be less pronounced (Hansen and Lebech, 1992).

Other Peripheral Nerve Involvement

Since the earliest descriptions of the classic triad, a wide range of other neuropathies has been linked to this infection (Halperin, 2003b). Mononeuropathies (damage to individual nerves, e.g., causing a radial or ulnar nerve palsy), plexopathies (lumbosacral or brachial), mononeuropathy multiplex (damaging multiple individual nerves), and distal "stocking glove" (actually a confluent mononeuropathy multiplex) neuropathies all occur. Paresis of limb or truncal muscles has been reported (Pfister et al., 1993; Hansen, 1994). In European patients with focal paresis or sensory impairment, the symptoms are most often located on the same side as the preceding tick bite or erythema migrans.

Although some patients may develop a fairly rapidly evolving polyneuropathy that clinically resembles the Guillain–Barré syndrome (Sterman et al., 1982), neurophysiologic testing rarely if ever indicates a demyelinating process (Muley and Parry, 2009), and CSF, if abnormal, usually demonstrates a pleocytosis rather than isolated protein elevation—that is, CSF and electrophysiologic abnormalities are the opposite of those seen classically in Guillain—Barré syndrome. Detailed neurophysiologic studies in large cohorts of patients with peripheral nervous system Lyme disease—including cranial neuropathies, radiculopathies, plexopathies, or diffuse neuropathies—indicate that all represent varying manifestations of a mononeuropathy multiplex (Halperin et al., 1990b). This pattern, with patchy, multifocal involvement of multiple individual nerves, is generally associated with a vasculopathy (e.g., diabetes) or vasculitis.

Limited neuropathologic observations indicate that peripheral nerve damage is axonal, with perivascular lymphoplasmocytic infiltrates (Meurers et al., 1990; Kristoferitsch, 1993; Camponovo and Meier, 1986; Halperin et al., 1987; Meier et al., 1989). No vessel wall necrosis has ever been demonstrated, so this is not a true vasculitis. Although abnormalities improve or resolve entirely with antimicrobial therapy, no studies have been able to demonstrate intact organisms in peripheral nerve, although one study demonstrated fragments of spirochetal DNA close to the sural nerve (Maimone et al., 1997).

Only rarely has a more diffuse peripheral neuropathy been reported as an isolated manifestation of early neuroborreliosis (without meningitis) (Oschmann et al., 1998). However, the neuropathy of patients with acrodermatitis chronica atrophicans (ACA) is well documented, occurring in 30% to 45% of cases (Asbrink and Hovmark, 1988). Sensory impairment is the most common finding, although peripheral paresis occurs. The symptoms predominately affect the extremity where ACA is found. Joint and skeletal symptoms secondary to the neurologic deficits have also been observed, analogous to the "Charcot joints" found in neurosyphilis (Asbrink and Hovmark, 1988) or in diabetic neuropathy.

An identical mononeuropathy multiplex has been observed in the only good animal model of neuroborreliosis—experimental infection in the rhesus macaque monkey (England et al., 1997). Clinically and electrophysiologically, virtually all infected monkeys develop a mononeuropathy multiplex. Neuropathologic examination of involved nerves demonstrates the same findings described in humans—vasocentric inflammation, patchy nerve damage, no primary demyelination, and no identifiable organisms. Despite extensive study in this animal model, the mechanism underlying peripheral nerve involvement remains elusive. However, it is now clear that regardless of the clinical presentation, all patients have a mononeuropathy multiplex that resolves with antimicrobial therapy. Although there has been considerable conjecture about the possibility of a role for molecular mimicry—including experimental evidence of interactions between specific anti-*B. burgdorferi* antibodies and neural tissue (Garcia-Monco et al., 1989, Sigal et al., 2001)—such a mechanism seems inconsistent with the clinical observation that nerve damage improves fairly rapidly following antimicrobial therapy. Nevertheless, recent evidence that *B. burgdorferi* lipoproteins might directly or indirectly induce astrocytic changes (Ramesh et al., 2003) may lead to some insights into the mechanisms underlying nervous system damage.

Encephalomyelitis

The term "encephalomyelitis," by definition, should be used only to describe patients with evident parenchymal inflammation in the spinal cord or brain. A tremendous amount of controversy in the neuroborreliosis literature can be directly attributed to a misuse of this term. In European neuroborreliosis many patients with radiculitis have spinal cord involvement at the affected level, leading to estimates that *Borrelia* myelitis occurs in up to 8% to 16% of affected patients (Stiernstedt et al., 1988; Martin et al., 1993; Hansen, 1994). Myelopathic findings typically include paraparesis, spinal (primarily sensory) ataxia, or neurogenic bladder (Stiernstedt et al., 1988).

The histopathological findings in human Lyme encephalomyelitis are extremely sparse. Perivascular infiltrates have been described and may disappear after treatment (Meurers et al., 1990). Glial nodules, increased numbers of astroglia, mild spongioform changes, granular ependymitis, and increased microglia have also been reported in a few biopsy specimens and autopsy reports (Miklossy et al., 1990; Reik, 1991). Single studies have described spirochetes in the brain. A spirochete "morphologically compatible with *B. burgdorferi*" was reported in one case report in a temporal lobe brain biopsy. Culture for *B. burgdorferi sp.* was negative, and confirmation with monoclonal antibodies or PCR was not performed (Pachner et al., 1989).

Just as in early reports from Europe (Ackermann et al., 1985), some US patients develop parenchymal CNS involvement (Halperin et al., 1989; Logigian et al., 1990). This, on rare occasion, may involve inflammation within the substance of the brain. The latter disorder, the only entity for which the term "encephalitis" should be used, probably occurs in less than 0.1% of patients with untreated Lyme disease, and the inflammation seems to affect white matter preferentially, sometimes leading to misdiagnosis as either a first episode of multiple sclerosis, or acute disseminated encephalomyelitis. In most instances it can be differentiated from these other two disorders by demonstrating the selective production of anti–*B. burgdorferi* antibodies in the CSF.

It is essential to differentiate between this brain infection, and the "toxic metabolic" encephalopathy seen in some patients with Lyme disease, comparable to that seen frequently in other patients with inflammatory systemic diseases—absent any CNS involvement. This disorder, which typically involves difficulties with concentration, memory, and other cognitive functions, has been well documented in patients with clear evidence of extra-neurologic involvement, with no evidence of nervous system infection, and has been clearly shown to resolve with antimicrobial therapy (Krupp et al., 1990; Halperin et al., 1990; Logigian et al., 1990). Termed "Lyme encephalopathy" this disorder is not typically a result of CNS infection, and no such diagnosis should be inferred in patients with findings limited to these isolated cognitive symptoms.

Late Neuroborreliosis

By analogy to syphilis, many refer to first-, second-, and third-stage neuroborreliosis. The term "third-stage Lyme neuroborreliosis" is typically used to describe an untreated *Borrelia* infection with neurological abnormalities that persist or are intermittent for more than six months. Although various time periods for stage III have been proposed by different authors, more than six months is the most widely used (Martin et al., 1993; Oschmann et al., 1998). It should be noted that other authors feel that since the pathophysiology of the disease does not change at six months, any time-based categorization is inherently arbitrary. All agree that late neurological abnormalities in Lyme borreliosis are typically a continuation of earlier manifestations. Focal brain or spinal cord damage can occur in later neuroborreliosis (Kaiser, 1994).

In a German study of neuroborreliosis patients evaluated between 1979 and 1994, late chronic progressive disease (duration of symptoms $\geq$ 6 months) was found in 9% of patients (Oschmann et al., 1998), while 4% of those with neuroborreliosis included between 1985 and 1990 in a Danish prospective study were characterized as third-stage neuroborreliosis (Hansen and Lebech, 1992). In these patients antibiotic therapy was effective in arresting the infection. However, as in any neurologic disorder, the more significant the nervous system damage that occurred prior to treatment, the greater the likelihood of post-treatment neurologic residua (Shadick et al., 1999).

It is essential to emphasize that there is no objective evidence of ongoing active spirochetal infection in humans after adequate antibiotic treatment for verified neuroborreliosis. Persistent live spirochetes in the CNS have never been demonstrated, and seem unlikely since there are no verified late relapses in neuroborreliosis (Krüger et al., 1989). Thus the term "chronic" neuroborreliosis is misleading and should be avoided (Feder et al., 2007). Remaining symptoms after antibiotic treatment for neuroborreliosis may be caused by an unrelated disorder or by permanent tissue damage after earlier Lyme borreliosis. Postinfectious autoimmune phenomena (Feder et al., 2007) have been postulated. Western blotting against extracts of brain tissue has demonstrated a variety of cross-reacting CSF antibodies, including antibodies to myelin basic protein and neurofilament protein (Kaiser, 1995). However, the absence of ongoing inflammatory changes following antibiotic treatment makes it unlikely that this is pathophysiologically significant. There is an obvious risk of overdiagnosis and overtreatment for postulated Lyme disease in these situations (Sigal, 1994; Klempner et al., 2001).

Some reports have attributed a variety of psychiatric disorders or other behavioral problems to CNS infection (Fallon et al., 1998). Although it is not uncommon for patients with depression, anxiety, or other behavioral problems to be more symptomatic when medically ill, it is inappropriate to conclude that the presence of such symptoms is indicative of CNS infection. First, in most instances these patients have had no evidence of CNS infection—CSF and MRI scans have been normal, as have been neurologic examinations. Second, it is not necessary to invoke such an explanation. Any event that leads to increased fatigue, malaise, or systemic symptoms can exacerbate psychiatric disease. Third, the few systematic studies that have addressed this issue indicate no higher incidence of psychiatric disease in patients with Lyme disease than in those with other comparable chronic inflammatory disorders (Krupp et al., 1989; Kaplan et al., 1992). Importantly, particularly in this era of Internet communication, many patients have acquired the impression that these symptoms reflect an underlying brain infection, and that this infection is incurable and causes irreparable brain damage that is consequently inevitably neurologically debilitating. This has resulted in widespread fear and misunderstanding about Lyme disease that has greatly amplified public anxiety about this infection. Since not one of these underlying assumptions is accurate, it is essential that this misunderstanding be corrected (Feder et al., 2007).

Unusual Features of Neuroborreliosis

Occasional reports attributing atypical neurological disorders—including cerebellitis, chorea, motor neuron disease (ALS-like), extrapyramidal findings (Oschmann et al., 1998), and myositis—to neuroborreliosis must be interpreted with caution. In each such report it is essential to determine whether the diagnostic criteria for neuroborreliosis were fulfilled and whether other co-existing disorders and alternative explanations for the clinical findings were adequately excluded.

Specific Features of Lyme Neuroborreliosis in Children

Neurological manifestations of pediatric borreliosis in Europe have been thoroughly reviewed by Christen (Christen and Hanefeld, 1993), and the pertinent pediatric data from both continents were recently reviewed by Sood (Sood, 2006). Clinical patterns may differ in children and adults. Tick bites in children were located in the head and neck area in 49% of cases (compared with 2% for adults) (Berglund et al., 1995). Peripheral facial palsy was the most common manifestation of neuroborreliosis in children, found in 55% of all cases (Christen and Hanefeld, 1993). In children, 33% to 64% of all cases of peripheral facial paresis have been attributed to *B. burgdorferi sp.* infections (Christen, 1993) reflecting how rarely facial nerve paresis occurs in children. In endemic areas bilateral facial palsy in children is almost pathognomonic for neuroborreliosis. Christen found that only a fourth of the children with facial palsy due to neuroborreliosis showed clinical signs of meningeal irritation despite the CSF pleocytosis (Christen et al., 1993). The typical neuralgic radicular pain in adult patients occurs infrequently in children with neuroborreliosis (Hansen and Lebech, 1992).

The dramatic symptom of facial palsy in children may be a reason for early diagnosis of Lyme disease in most cases. The lower frequency of positive antibody tests to *B. burgdorferi sp.* in children with neuroborreliosis may be due to shorter periods of clinical manifestations before evaluation, just as some adults presenting with facial palsy have not yet become seropositive (Jain et al., 1996; Halperin, 2003a). The outcome of neuroborreliosis in children is considered to be excellent with appropriate treatment (Thorstrand et al., 2002), and the rate of spontaneous remission seems to be high even without antibiotics (Christen et al., 1993b).

PATHOGENESIS

The precise mechanism of nervous system damage in neuroborreliosis is unknown; current knowledge was well summarized in a recent review (Rupprecht et al., 2008). Presence of spirochetes must play a primary role, as ongoing nervous system disease ends with antimicrobial therapy. Clinically, radicular pain and constitutional symptoms often improve rapidly after initiation of antibiotic treatment. Similarly the topographical association between the site of the tick bite (and the EM) and the location of focal neurological manifestations suggests a local interaction. In contrast, the occasional onset of facial palsy up to two weeks after the start of treatment suggests that other secondary mechanisms might be present.

There is experimental and clinical evidence that *B. burgdorferi sp.* invade the CNS early in the course of infection (Garcia Monco et al., 1990); spirochetes may disseminate directly through tissue or hematogenously. The number of spirochetes in the CNS appears to be remarkably small; however, they appear to elicit a quite vigorous inflammatory response (Pachner and Steiner, 2007). *Borrelia burgdorferi sp.* penetrate endothelial cells and induce an inflammatory response in the CNS, prominently around the vasculature. In vitro, spirochetes adhere to cells, upregulate cell-adhesion molecules and promote inflammatory reactions (Sellati et al., 1995). There is in vitro evidence of *Borrelia* spirochete attachment to astrocytes and oligodendrocytes, and spirochetes can induce injury to these cells (Garcia-Monco et al., 1989). *Borrelia burgdorferi sp.* may even adhere and induce toxicity to neurons (Thomas et al., 1994). However, *B. burgdorferi sp.* spirochetes have not been found in the brain parenchyma in animal studies (Garcia-Monco and Benach, 1997), and none of these other phenomena have ever been demonstrated in human disease or in animal models.

Infection-triggered B cell–mediated autoimmune mimicry has been suggested as a possible mechanism of injury in *B. burgdorferi sp.* infections. *Borrelia burgdorferi sp.* antigens have been shown to elicit a number of cross-reactive antibodies in the human host (summarized by Sigal in Sigal and Williams, 1997). Cross-reactive antibodies have been identified that recognize *B. burgdorferi sp.* epitopes and human axonal proteins. Others have reported serum auto-antibodies to cardiolipin, myelin basic protein, and gangliosides (GM1, GD1b, asialo GM1) in patients with neuroborreliosis (Aberer et al., 1989; Sigal, 1993; Garcia Monco et al., 1993; Kaiser, 1995). Such cross-reactive antibodies triggered by *B. burgdorferi sp.* might lead to injury to myelin in oligodendroglia and Schwann cells, axons, and neuronal soma. This is clinically reflected as neuropathy and white matter damage in patients with neuroborreliosis, although the neuropathies associated with this infection are not demyelinating, and antibodies have never been shown to be deposited in nerve or brain of affected patients or experimentally infected animals.

Other inflammatory mediators have been demonstrated in neuroborreliosis. Nitric oxide, produced by activated microglia as one of the means of killing *B. burgdorferi sp.*, has been proposed as an important mediator of neuronal and oligodendroglia cell damage in neuroborreliosis (Tatro et al., 1994). Cytokines may contribute. Increased levels of IL-1 and TNF-α have been reported in CSF of patients with neuroborreliosis, and elevated levels of neopterin and IL-6 in spinal fluid even correlated to the clinical findings (Dotevall et al., 1990; Weller et al., 1991; Nilsson et al., 1994). Recent evidence suggests production of CXCL13, a B cell chemoattractant, very early in infection, probably by brain microglia (Ramesh et al., 2009). *Borrelia burgdorferi sp.*–reactive T cells secreting interferon-γ have been reported in CSF of Lyme disease patients (Wang et al., 1995). Elevated CSF levels of neuroactive quinolonic acid, an excitotoxin known to be associated with immune stimulation, have also been reported in patients with neuroborreliosis (Halperin and Heyes, 1992).

TREATMENT

Historically one of the key considerations in choice of treatment has been whether the nervous system is involved. As has been detailed above, not every patient with altered behavior or systemic symptoms should be assumed to have nervous system infection. In brief, patients who have both Lyme disease and altered CNS function can be divided into three groups: (1) rare patients with patchy, multifocal brain (encephalitis), or spinal cord (myelitis) inflammation demonstrable on neurologic exam and MRI imaging, presumably analogous to the pathophysiologic process observed in peripheral nerve; (2) more commonly, patients with a benign self-limited inflammation of the meninges (meningitis), either in isolation or in combination with other peripheral or central nervous system manifestations; and (3) probably most commonly, patients with modest temporary memory and cognitive impairment, comparable to that observed in innumerable other systemic inflammatory diseases, with no underlying CNS infection, inflammation or other identifiable pathology.

For a variety of reasons the number of clinical trials limited to neuroborreliosis has been somewhat limited. Most treatment studies in the United States have accepted the assumption that nervous system involvement is fairly uncommon, and therefore have aggregated patients with arthritis, PNS disease, and CNS disease. Moreover the overwhelming fear prevalent among the patient population that the infection will lead to irreparable brain damage has limited the opportunity to study oral treatment regimens in individuals with meningitis or other neurologic disorders, despite extensive relevant European literature supporting such an approach (Halperin et al., 2007).

Although several European studies have demonstrated that oral doxycycline is highly effective in Lyme meningitis and cranial neuropathies (Dotevall and Hagberg, 1999; Karkkonen et al., 2001; Thorstrand et al., 2002), including a recent randomized, double blind controlled trial (Ljøstad et al., 2008), comparable studies have not been performed in the United States. A meta-analysis of multiple European studies indicates that absent parenchymal brain or spinal cord involvement, oral regimens (Halperin, 2003) are effective for neuroborreliosis, including meningitis, cranial neuropathies, and perhaps other PNS disorders (Halperin et al., 2007).

TABLE 5.2 Treatment recommendations

Disorder	Regimen
Acute neuroborreliosis (meningitis, radiculitis, cranial neuritis)	Ceftriaxone 2 grams/d for 14–21 days *or* cefotaxime 2 grams tid for 14–21 days, *or* penicillin 24 MU/d × 14–21 days *or POSSIBLY* po doxycycline 200–400 mg/d for 21–42 days
Encephalomyelitis	Ceftriaxone 2 grams/d for 28 days *or* cefotaxime 2 grams tid for 28 days, *or* penicillin 24 MU/d × 28 days
Chronic or recurrent neuroborreliosis (e.g., treatment failure after shorter courses of treatment)	Ceftriaxone 2 grams/day for 28 days *or* cefotaxime 2 grams tid for 28 days,

Source: Halperin et al. (2007).
Note: Tetracyclines such as doxycycline should not be used in pregnant women or in children age 8 or under.

However, meningitis and encephalomyelitis are still almost invariably treated with parenteral antimicrobials in the United States—typically ceftriaxone or cefotaxime. In contrast, a recent European Guideline recommends oral treatment for peripheral nervous system forms of neuroborreliosis, as well as for meningitis, reserving parenteral treatment for patients with parenchymal central nervous system involvement (Mygland et al., 2010). Duration of treatment has gradually increased over the years, although randomized clinical trials have never demonstrated that this is necessary. Current recommendations are summarized in Table 5.2. Treatment using these regimens is curative in over 90% of patients. Objective assessment of treatment response can be challenging. As in most neurologic diseases, cessation of the active disease process typically does not result in an immediate return to neurologic normalcy—recovery requires time, and may be incomplete. Even improvement in CSF measures of inflammation can lag significantly. Failure to recover completely should not be construed as evidence of persistent infection—the nervous system's ability to recover is, after all, limited.

This gives rise to one of the greatest therapeutic challenges—judging when treatment is sufficient. Measures of peripheral blood antibodies tend to decline only slowly after successful treatment, remaining positive for extended periods. Western blots tend to demonstrate antibodies to additional epitopes with prolonged and ongoing infection; presumably if infection is halted, blots should remain constant or demonstrate a slow decline in the number of bands. CSF serologic findings similarly are not overly helpful; persistence of apparent intrathecal antibody production has been demonstrated as much as 10 years after apparently successful treatment (Hammers Berggren et al., 1993). Somewhat more helpful in CNS disease, though, are measures of CSF protein concentration and pleocytosis, both of which generally improve following resolution of CNS infection. In the PNS, neurophysiologic testing can demonstrate objective improvement in nerve function. Ultimately decisions regarding adequacy of treatment depend on an aggregate assessment of these measures, as well as the patient's subjective impression of well-being. As demonstrated in a number of studies, many patients who have been given a diagnosis of Lyme disease can have persistently perceived subjective symptoms, but with no objective correlate, an observation that ultimately can make assessment of treatment response challenging (Shadick et al., 1999; Seltzer et al., 2000). Importantly, there have now been five randomized controlled trials showing additional antibiotic treatment in such individuals carries significant risk with minimal if any potential benefit (Klempner et al., 2001; Krupp et al., ; Fallon et al., 2007; Oksi et al., 2007).

PROGNOSIS AND OUTCOME

The prognosis after antibiotic treatment is generally excellent, although neurological symptoms in most patients do not resolve immediately with antimicrobial therapy. The pain disappears first, then the paresis starts to resolve. Patients may experience dysesthesias as well as systemic symptoms of fatigue and perceived cognitive difficulty for months after treatment. Sometimes symptoms resolve with fluctuations. Hansen found that 7% of patients had sensory complaints, and 2% suffered from residual radicular pain (Hansen and Lebech, 1992). Of the 95 patients with facial palsy, 15% were found to have slight and 3% severe post-treatment sequelae after unilateral palsy. Karlsson et al. found sequelae in 10% to 14% of patients with neuroborreliosis 12 months after treatment, mostly with residual facial palsy (Karlsson et al., 1994). Other studies have reported higher incidences of sequelae. One five-year follow-up study of neuroborreliosis patients found that 25% suffered from sequelae post-treatment, but only half of these had symptoms that affected their daily activity (Berglund et al., 2002). However, in the absence of information about the incidence of comparable symptoms in an uninfected control population, the significance of this is not at all clear. Treib et al. described that more than half of the patients with treated neuroborreliosis had self-reported symptoms of fatigue, headache, and concentration problems after a mean of 50 months (Treib et al., 1998). These symptoms, often referred to as "post-Lyme disease," do not respond to further antibiotic treatment if adequate treatment for neuroborreliosis has been given initially (Klempner et al., 2001; Feder et al., 2007; Fallon et al., 2007). Adequately treated neuroborreliosis in children seems to have an excellent prognosis (Christen et al., 1993; Thorstrand et al., 2002).

The duration of persistent symptoms in patients with neuroborreliosis if antibiotic treatment is not given has been estimated to be three to six months in most cases (Krüger et al., 1990), although in some patients continuing and progressive infection may occur (Bensch et al., 1987). In a long-term follow-up study of adult patients many years after untreated neuroborreliosis, Krüger et al. observed that 18% of the patients exhibited "mild to medium sequelae" up to 21 years after acute illness, while 32% had mild clinical sequelae (Krüger et al., 1989). Again, the significance of this observation is unclear in the absence of information about the incidence of such symptoms in uninfected control populations.

SUMMARY

The disease known as Lyme disease in the United States is actually quite similar to the disorders caused by *B. burgdorferi sensu lato* in Europe. Despite widely held beliefs that nervous system involvement is more common in European patients, the limited available epidemiologic data do not support this conclusion. Similarly the neurologic syndromes are rather comparable, with the same neurologic triad representing the predominant syndrome in both populations. Diagnosis requires a commonsense clinical approach, demonstrating objective evidence in support of both the neurologic diagnosis and the microbiological one. If the diagnosis is firm, several treatment regimens are available and highly effective.

REFERENCES

Aberer E, Brunner C, Suchanek G, Klade H, Barbour A, Stanek G, Lassmann H: Molecular mimicry and Lyme borreliosis. A shared antigenic determinant between *Borrelia burgdorferi* and human tissue. *Ann Neurol* 26:732–737; 1989.

Ackermann R, Gollmer E, Rehse KB: [Progressive *Borrelia* encephalomyelitis. Chronic manifestation of erythema chronicum migrans disease of the nervous system]. *Dtsch Med Wochenschr* 110:1039–1042; 1985.

Asbrink E, Hovmark A: Early and late cutaneous manifestations in *Ixodes*-borne borreliosis (erythema migrans borreliosis, Lyme borreliosis). *Ann N Y Acad Sci* 539:4–15; 1988.

Bannwarth A: Chronische lymphocytare meningitis, entzundliche polyneuritis und "rheumatismus." *Arch Psychiatr Nervenkr* 113:284–376; 1941.

Bensch J, Olcén P, Hagberg L: Destructive chronic *Borrelia* meningoencephalitis in a child untreated for 15 years. *Scand J Infect Dis* 19:697–700; 1987.

Berglund J, Eitrem R, Ornstein K, Lindberg A, Ringnér Å, Elmrud H, Carlsson M, Runehagen A, Svanborg C, Norrby R: An epidemiologic study of Lyme disease in southern Sweden. *N Engl J Med* 333:1319–1324; 1995.

Berglund J, Stjernber L, Ornstein K, Tykesson-Joelsson K, Walter H: 5-y Follow-up study of patients with neuroborreliosis. *Scand J Infect Dis* 34:421–425; 2002.

Blanc F, Jaulhac B, Fleury M, De Seze J, De Martino SJ, Remy V, Blaison G, Hansmann Y, Christmann D, Tranchant C: Relevance of the antibody index to diagnose Lyme neuroborreliosis among seropositive patients. *Neurology* 69:953–958; 2007.

Borg R, Dotevall L, Hagberg L, Maraspin V, Lotric-Furlan S, Cimperman J, Strle F: Intravenous ceftriaxone compared with oral doxycycline for the treatment of Lyme neuroborreliosis. *Scand Journal of Infect Dis* 37:449–454; 2005.

Camponovo F, Meier C: Neuropathy of vasculitic origin in a case of Garin-Bujadoux-Bannwarth syndrome with positive *Borrelia* antibody response. *J Neurol* 233:69–72; 1986.

CDC: Lyme disease. United States, 2003–2005. *MMWR Morb Mortal Wkly Rep* 56:573–576; 2007.

Christen HJ: Bacterial meningitis and Lyme neuroborreliosis in childhood. *Curr Opin Neurol Neurosurg* 6:403–409; 1993.

Christen HJ, Hanefeld F: [Lyme borreliosis in childhood]. *Monatsschr Kinderheilkd* 141:513–526; 1993.

Christen HJ, Hanefeld F, Eiffert H, Al E: Epidemiology and clinical manifestations of Lyme borreliosis in childhood. A prospective multicentre study with special regard to neuroborreliosis. *Acta Paediatr* 82(Suppl. 386): 1–76; 1993a.

Christen HJ, Hanefeld F, Eiffert H, Thomssen R: Epidemiology and clinical manifestations of Lyme borreliosis in childhood. A prospective multicentre study with special regard to neuroborreliosis. *Acta Paediatr* 82:1–75; 1993b.

Danek A, Uttner I, Yoursry T, Pfister HW: Lyme neuroborreliosis disguised as normal pressure hydrocephalus. *Neurology* 46:1743-L 1745; 1996.

Des Vignes F, Piesman J, Heffernan R, Schulze TL, Stafford KC, Fish D: Effect of tick removal on transmission of *Borrelia burgdorferi* and *Ehrlichia phagocytophila* by *Ixodes scapularis* nymphs. *J Infect Dis* 183:773–778; 2001.

Diza E, Papa A, Vezyri E, Tsounis S, Milonas I, Antoniadis A: *Borrelia valaisiana* in cerebrospinal fluid. *Emerg Infect Dis* 10:1692–1693; 2004.

Dotevall L, Fuchs D, Reibnegger G, Wachter H, Hagberg L: Cerebrospinal fluid and serum neopterin levels in patients with Lyme neuroborreliosis. *Infection* 18:210–214; 1990.

Dotevall L, Hagberg L: Successful oral doxycycline treatment of Lyme disease-associated facial palsy and meningitis. *Clin Infect Dis* 28:569–574; 1999.

Dotevall L, Rosengren LE, Hagberg L: Increased cerebrospinal fluid levels of glial fibrillary acidic protein (GFAp) in Lyme neuroborreliosis. *Infection* 24:125–129; 1996.

Dotevall L, Hagberg L, Karlsson JE, Rosengren LE: Astroglial and neuronal proteins in cerebrospinal fluid as markers of CNS involvement in Lyme neuroborreliosis. *Eur J Neurol* 6:169–178; 1999.

England JD, Bohm RP, Roberts ED, Philipp MT: Mononeuropathy multiplex in rhesus monkeys with chronic Lyme disease. *Ann Neurol* 41:375–384; 1997.

Etienne M, Carvalho P, Fauchais AL, Pestel-Caron M, Doucet J, Chassagne P: Lyme neuroborreliosis revealed as a normal pressure hydrocephalus. A cause of reversible dementia. *J Am Geriatr Soc* 51:579–580; 2003.

Fallon BA, Kochevar JM, Gaito A, Nields JA: The underdiagnosis of neuropsychiatric Lyme disease in children and adults. *Psychiatr Clin North Am* 21:693–703, viii; 1998.

Fallon BA, Keilp JG, Corbera KM, Petkova E, Britton CB, Dwyer E, Slavov I, Cheng J, Dobkin J, Nelson DR, Sackeim HA: A randomized, placebo-controlled trial of repeated IV antibiotic therapy for Lyme encephalopathy. *Neurology* [Epub ahead of print]; 2007.

Feder HM Jr, Johnson BJ, O'Connell S, Shapiro ED, Steere AC, Wormser GP: A critical appraisal of "chronic Lyme disease." *N Engl J Med* 357:1422–1430; 2007.

Fingerle V, Schulte-Spechtel UC, Ruzic-Sabljic E, Leonhard S, Hofmann H, Webere K, Pfisterc K, Strle F, Wilske B: Epidemiological aspects and molecular characterization of *Borrelia burgdorferi* s. l. from southern Germany with special respect to the new species *Borrelia spielmanii* sp. nov. *Int J Med Microbiol* 298:279–290; 2008.

Garcia-Monco JC, Benach JL: Lyme neuroborreliosis. *Ann Neurol* 37:691–702; 1995.

Garcia-Monco JC, Benach JL: Mechanisms of injury in Lyme neuroborreliosis. *Semin Neurol* 17:57–62; 1997.

Garcia-Monco JC, Fernandez-Villar B, Benach JL: Adherence of the Lyme disease spirochete to glial cells and cells of glial origin. *J Infect Dis* 160:497–506; 1989.

Garcia-Monco JC, Villar BF, Alen JC, Benach JL: *Borrelia burgdorferi* in the central nervous system. Experimental and clinical evidence for early invasion. *J Infect Dis* 161:1187–1193; 1990.

Garcia-Monco JC, Wheeler CM, Benach JL, Furie RA, Lukehart SA, Stanek G, Steere AC: Reactivity of neuroborreliosis patients (Lyme disease) to cardiolipin and gangliosides. *J Neurol Sci* 117:206–214; 1993.

Garin C, Bujadoux A: Paralysie par les tiques. *J Med Lyon* 71:765–767; 1922.

Garro AC, Rutman M, Simonsen K, Jaeger JL, Chapin K, Lockhart G: Prospective validation of a clinical prediction model for Lyme meningitis in children. *Pediatrics* 123:e829–e834; 2009.

Halperin J, Logigian E, Finkel M, Pearl R: Practice parameter for the diagnosis of patients with nervous system Lyme borreliosis (Lyme disease). *Neurology* 46:619–627; 1996.

Halperin JJ: Neuroborreliosis: central nervous system involvement. *Semin Neurol* 17:19–24; 1998.

Halperin JJ: Facial nerve palsy associated with Lyme disease. *Muscle Nerve* 28:516–517; 2003a.

Halperin JJ: Lyme disease and the peripheral nervous system. *Muscle Nerve* 28:133–143; 2003b.

Halperin JJ: Stroke in patients with Lyme Disease. *In* Caplan L (ed): *Uncommon Causes of Stroke*, 2nd ed. Cambridge, UK, Cambridge University Press; 2008.

Halperin JJ, Heyes MP: Neuroactive kynurenines in Lyme borreliosis. *Neurology* 42:43–50; 1992.

Halperin JJ, Volkman DJ, Wu P: Central nervous system abnormalities in Lyme neuroborreliosis. *Neurology* 41:1571–1582; 1991.

Halperin JJ, Little BW, Coyle PK, Dattwyler RJ: Lyme disease. A treatable cause of peripheral neuropathy. *Neurology* 37:1700–1706; 1987.

Halperin JJ, Luft BJ, Anand AK, Roque CT, Alvarez O, Volkman DJ, Dattwyler RJ: Lyme neuroborreliosis. Central nervous system manifestations. *Neurology* 39:753–759; 1989.

Halperin JJ, Krupp LB, Golightly MG, Volkman DJ: Lyme borreliosis-associated encephalopathy. *Neurology* 40:1340–1343; 1990a.

Halperin JJ, Luft BJ, Volkman DJ, Dattwyler RJ: Lyme neuroborreliosis. Peripheral nervous system manifestations. *Brain* 113:1207–1221; 1990b.

Halperin JJ, Shapiro ED, Logigian EL, Belman AL, Dotevall L, Wormser GP, Krupp LB, Gronseth G, Bever C: Practice parameter. Treatment of nervous system Lyme disease. *Neurology* 69:91–102; 2007.

Hammers-Berggren S, Hansen K, Lebech AM, Karlsson M: *Borrelia burgdorferi*-specific intrathecal antibody production in neuroborreliosis. A follow-up study. *Neurology* 43:169–175; 1993.

Hansen K: Lyme neuroborreliosis: improvements of the laboratory diagnosis and a survey of epidemiological and clinical features in Denmark 1985–1990. *Acta Neurol Scand Suppl* 151:1–44; 1994.

Hansen K, Lebech AM: The clinical and epidemiological profile of Lyme neuroborreliosis in Denmark 1985–1990. A prospective study of 187 patients with *Borrelia burgdorferi* specific intrathecal antibody production. *Brain* 115:399–423; 1992.

Hellerstrom S: Erythema migrans Afzelius with meningitis. *Acta Derm Venereol (Stockholm)* 31:227–234; 1951.

Jacobson DM, Frens DB: Pseudotumor cerebri syndrome associated with Lyme disease. *Am J Ophthalmol* 107:81–82; 1989.

Jain VK, Hilton E, Maytal J, Dorante G, Ilowite NT, Sood SK: Immunoglobulin M immunoblot for diagnosis of *Borrelia burgdorferi* infection in patients with acute facial palsy. *J Clin Microbiol* 34:2033–2035; 1996.

Kaiser R: Variable CSF findings in early and late Lyme neuroborreliosis: a follow-up study in 47 patients. *J Neurol* 242:26–36; 1994.

Kaiser R: Intrathecal immune response in patients with neuroborreliosis: specificity of antibodies for neuronal proteins. *J Neurol* 242:319–325; 1995.

Kalina P, Decker A, Kornel E, Halperin JJ: Lyme disease of the brainstem. *Neuroradiology* 47:903–907; 2005.

Kan L, Sood SK, Maytal J: 1998. Pseudotumor cerebri in Lyme disease: a case report and literature review. *Pediatr Neurol* 18:439–441; 1998.

Kaplan RF, Meadows ME, Vincent LC, Logigian EL, Steere AC: Memory impairment and depression in patients with Lyme encephalopathy. Comparison with fibromyalgia and nonpsychotically depressed patients. *Neurology* 42:1263–1267; 1992.

Karkkonen K, Stiernstedt SH, Karlsson M: Follow-up of patients treated with oral doxycycline for Lyme neuroborreliosis. *Scand J Infect Dis* 33:259–262; 2001.

Karlsson M, Hammers-Berggren S, Lindquist L, Stiernstedt G, Svenungsson B: Comparison of intravenous penicillin G and oral doxycycline for treatment of Lyme neuroborreliosis. *Neurology* 44:1203–1207; 1994.

Klempner M, Hu L, Evans J, Schmid C, Johnson G, Trevino R, Norton D, Levy L, Wall D, McCall J, Kosinski M, Weinstein A: Two controlled trials of antibiotic treatment in patients with persistent symptoms and a history of Lyme disease. *N Engl J Med* 345:85–92; 2001.

Kristoferitsch W: Chronic peripheral neuropathy. *In* Weber K, Burgdorfer W (eds): *Aspects of Lyme Borreliosis*. New York, Springer; 1993.

Krüger H, Kohlhepp W, Konig S: Follow-up of antibiotically treated and untreated neuroborreliosis. *Acta Neurol Scand* 82:59–67; 1990.

Krüger H, Reuss K, Pulz M, Rohrbach E, Pflughaupt KW, Martin R, Mertens HG: Meningoradiculitis and encephalomyelitis due to *Borrelia burgdorferi.* A follow-up study of 72 patients over 27 years. *J Neurology* 236:322–328; 1989.

Krupp LB, Larocca NG, Luft BJ, Halperin JJ: Comparison of neurologic and psychologic findings in patients with Lyme disease and chronic fatigue syndrome. *Neurology* 39:144; 1989.

Krupp LB, Fernquist S, Masur D, Halperin JJ: Cognitive impairment in Lyme disease. *Neurology* 40:304; 1990.

Krupp LB, Hyman LG, Grimson R, Coyle PK, Melville P, Ahnn S, Dattwyler R, Chandler B: Study and treatment of post Lyme disease (STOP-LD): A randomized double masked clinical trial. *Neurology* 60(12): 1923–1930; 2003.

Lebech A: Polymerase chain reaction in diagnosis of *Borrelia burgdorferi* infections and studies on taxonomic classification. *APMIS (suppl)*: 1–40; 2002.

Ljøstad U, Skarpaas T, Mygland A: Clinical usefulness of intrathecal antibody testing in acute Lyme neuroborreliosis. *Eur J Neurol* 14:873–876; 2007.

Ljøstad U, Skogvoll E, Eikeland R, Midgard R, Skarpaas T, Berg Å, Mygland Å: Oral doxycycline versus intravenous ceftriaxone for European Lyme neuroborreliosis: a multicentre, non-inferiority, double-blind, randomised trial. *Lancet Neurol* 7(8): 690–695; 2008.

Logigian EL, Kaplan RF, Steere AC: Chronic neurologic manifestations of Lyme disease. *N Engl J Med* 323:1438–1444; 1990.

Maimone D, Villanova M, Stanta G, Bonin S, Maladrini A, Guazzi GC, Annunziata P: Detection of *Borrelia burgdorferi* DNA and complement membrane attack complex deposits in the sural nerve of a patient with chronic polyneuropathy and tertiary Lyme disease. *Muscle Nerve* 20:969–975; 1997.

Martin R, Kohlhepp W, Mertens HG: Chronic central nervous system involvement. *In* Weber K, Burgdorfer W (eds): *Aspects of Lyme Borreliosis.* New York, Springer; 1993.

Meier C, Grahmann F, Engelhardt A, Dumas M: Peripheral nerve disorders in Lyme-Borreliosis. Nerve biopsy studies from eight cases. *Acta Neuropathol (Berl)* 79:271–278; 1989.

Meurers B, Kohlhepp W, Gold R, Rohrbach E, Mertens HG: Histopathologic findings in the central and peripheral nervous systems in neuroborreliosis. *Journal of Neurology* 237:113–116; 1990.

Miklossy J, Kuntzer T, Bogousslavsky J, Regli F, Janzer RC: Meningovascular form of neuroborreliosis: similarities between neuropathologic findings in a case of Lyme disease and those occurring in tertiary neurosyphilis. *Acta Neuropathogica* 80:568–572; 1990.

Muley SA, Parry GJ: Antibiotic responsive demyelinating neuropathy related to Lyme disease. *Neurology* 72:1786–1787; 2009.

Mygland A, Ljøstad U, Fingerle V, Rupprecht T, Schmutzhard E, Steiner I: EFNS guidelines on the diagnosis and management of European Lyme neuroborreliosis. *Eur J Neurol;* 17(1): 8–16; 2010.

Nadelman RB, Nowakowski J, Fish D, Falco RC, Freeman K, McKenna D, Welch P, Marcus R, Aguero-Rosenfeld ME, Dennis DT, Wormser GP: Prophylaxis with single-dose doxycycline for the prevention of Lyme disease after an *Ixodes scapularis* tick bite. *N Engl J Med* 345:79–84; 2001.

Nilsson I, Alves M, Nässberger L: Response of soluble IL-2 receptor, Interleukin-2 and Interleukin-6 in patients with positive and negative *Borrelia burgdorferi* serology. *Infection* 22:316–320; 1994.

Oksi J, Nikoskelainen J, Hiekkanen H, Lauhio A, Peltomaa M, Pitkäranta A, Nyman D., Granlund H, Carlsson SA, Seppälä I, Valtonen V, Viljanen M: Duration of antibiotic treatment in disseminated Lyme borreliosis. A double-blind, randomized, placebo-controlled, multicenter clinical study. *Eur J Clin Microbiol Infect Dis* 26; 2007 (Epub in advance of publication).

Ornstein K, Berglund J, Bergstrom S, Norrby R, Barbour A: Three major Lyme *Borrelia* genospecies (*Borrelia burgdorferi* sensu stricto, *B. afzelii* and *B. garinii*) identified by PCR in cerebrospinal fluid from patients with neuroborreliosis in Sweden. *Scand J Infect Dis* 34:341–346; 2002.

Oschmann P, Dorndorf W, Horing C, Schäfer C, Wellensiek HJ, Pflughaupt KW: Stages and syndromes of neuroborreliosis. *Neurol* 836:1–11; 1998.

Pachner AR, Steere AC: Neurological findings of Lyme disease. *Yale J Biol Med* 57:481–483; 1984.

Pachner AR, Steere AC: The triad of neurologic manifestations of Lyme disease. *Neurology* 35:47–53; 1985.

Pachner AR, Steiner I: Lyme neuroborreliosis: infection, immunity, and inflammation. *Lancet Neurol* 6:544–552; 2007.

Pachner AR, Duray P, Steere AC: 1989. Central nervous system manifestations of Lyme disease. *Arch Neurol* 46:790–795; 1989.

Pfister HW, Einhaupl KM, Franz P, Garner C: Corticosteroids for radicular pain in Bannwarth's syndrome. A double blind, randomized, placebo controlled trial. *Ann NY Acad Sci* 539:485–487; 1988.

Pfister HW, Preac MV, Wilske B, Rieder G, Forderreuther S, Schmidt S, Kapfhammer HP: Catatonic syndrome in acute severe encephalitis due to *Borrelia burgdorferi* infection. *Neurology* 43:433–435; 1993.

Ramesh G, Alvarez AL, Roberts ED, Dennis VA, Lasater BL, Alvarez X, Philipp MT: Pathogenesis of Lyme neuroborreliosis: *Borrelia burgdorferi* lipoproteins induce both proliferation and apoptosis in rhesus monkey astrocytes. *Eur J Immunol* 33:2539–2550; 2003.

Ramesh G, Borda JT, Gill A, Ribka EP, Morici LA, Mottram P, Martin DS, Jacobs MB, Didier PJ, Philipp MT: 2009. Possible role of glial cells in the onset and progression of Lyme neuroborreliosis. *J Neuroinflammation* 6:23; 2009.

Reik L: *Lyme Disease and the Nervous System*. New York, Thieme Medical Publishers, 1991.

Reik L, Steere AC, Bartenhagen NH, Shope RE, Malawista SE: Neurologic abnormalities of Lyme disease. *Medicine* 58:281–294; 1979.

Rothermel H, Hedges T.R. III, Steere AC: Optic neuropathy in children with Lyme disease. *Pediatrics* 108:477–481; 2001.

Rupprecht TA, Koedel U, Fingerle V, Pfister HW: The pathogenesis of Lyme neuroborreliosis. From infection to inflammation. *Mol Med* 14:205–212; 2008.

Schaltenbrand G: Chronische aseptische Meningitis. *Nervenarzt* 20:433–442; 1949.

Schaltenbrand G: [Radiculomyelomeningitis after tick bite]. *Munch Med Wochenschr* 104:829–834; 1962.

Sellati T, Burns M, Ficazzola M, Furie M: *Borrelia burgdorferi* upregulates expression of adhesion molecules on endothelial cells and promotes transendothelial migration of neutrophils in vitro. I. *Infect Immun* 63:4439–4447; 1995.

Seltzer E, Gerber M, Cartter M, Freudigman K, Shapiro E: Long-term outcomes of persons with Lyme disease. *JAMA* 283:609–616; 2000.

Shadick NA, Phillips CB, Sangha O, Logigian EL, Kaplan RF, Wright EA, Fossel AH, Fossel K, Berardi V, Lew RA, Liang MH: Musculoskeletal and neurologic outcomes in patients with previously treated Lyme disease. *Ann Intern Med* 131:919–926; 1999.

Shah SS, Zaoutis TE, Turnquist J, Hodinka RL, Coffin SE: Early differentiation of Lyme from enteroviral meningitis. *Pediatr Infect Dis J* 24:542–545; 2005.

Sibony P, Halperin J, Coyle P, Patel K: Reactive Lyme serology in patients with optic neuritis and papilledema. *J Neuro-Ophthal* 25:71–82; 2005.

Sigal LH: Cross-reactivity between *Borrelia burgdorferi* flagellin and a human axonal 64,000 molecular weight protein. *J Infect Dis* 167:1372–1378; 1993.

Sigal LH: Persisting complaints attributed to chronic Lyme disease: possible mechanisms and implications for management. *Am J Med* 96:365–374; 1994.

Sigal LH, Williams S: A monoclonal antibody to *Borrelia burgdorferi* flagellin modifies neuroblastoma cell neuritogenesis in vitro. A possible role for autoimmunity in the neuropathy of Lyme disease. *Infect Immun* 65:1722–1728; 1997.

Sigal LH, Williams S, Soltys B, Gupta R: H9724, a monoclonal antibody to *Borrelia burgdorferi*'s flagellin, binds to heat shock protein 60 (HSP60) within live neuroblastoma cells. A potential role for HSP60 in peptide hormone signaling and in an autoimmune pathogenesis of the neuropathy of Lyme disease. *Cell Mol Neurobiol* 21:477–495; 2001.

Smith RP Jr., Muzaffar SB, Lavers J, Lacombe EH, Cahill BK, Lubelczyk CB, Kinsler A, Mathers AJ, Rand PW: *Borrelia garinii* in seabird ticks (*Ixodes uriae*), Atlantic Coast, North America. *Emerg Infect Dis* 12:1909–1912; 2006.

Sood SK, Salzman MB, Johnson BJ, Happ CM, Feig K, Carmody L, Rubin LG, Hilton E, Piesman J: Duration of tick attachment as a predictor of the risk of Lyme disease in an area in which Lyme disease is endemic. *J Inf Dis* 175:996–999; 1997.

Sood SK: What we have learned about Lyme borreliosis from studies in children. *Wien Klin Wochenschr* 118:638–642; 2006.

Steere AC: Lyme disease. *N Engl J Med* 321:586–596; 1989.

Steere AC, Malawista SE, Hardin JA, Ruddy S, Askenase W, Andiman WA: Erythema chronicum migrans and Lyme arthritis. The enlarging clinical spectrum. *Ann Intern Med* 86:685–698; 1977.

Steere AC, Berardi VP, Weeks KE, Logigian EL, Ackermann R: Evaluation of the intrathecal antibody response to *Borrelia burgdorferi* as a diagnostic test for Lyme neuroborreliosis. *J Infect Dis* 161:1203–1209; 1990.

Sterman AB, Nelson S, Barclay P: Demyelinating neuropathy accompanying Lyme disease. *Neurology* 32:1302–1305; 1982.

Stiernstedt G, Gustafsson R, Karlsson M, Svenungsson B, Skoldenberg B: Clinical manifestations and diagnosis of neuroborreliosis. *Ann NY Acad Sci* 539:46–55; 1988.

Tatro JB, Romero LI, Beasley D, Steere AC, Reichlin S: *Borrelia burgdorferi* and *Escherichia coli* lipopolysaccharides induce nitric oxide and interleukin-6 production in cultured rat brain cells. *J Infect Dis* 169:1014–1022; 1994.

Thomas DD, Cadavid D, Barbour AG: Differential association of *Borrelia* species with cultured neural cells. *J Infect Dis* 169:445–448; 1994.

Thorstrand C, Belfrage E, Bennet R, Malmborg P, Eriksson M: Successful treatment of neuroborreliosis with ten day regimens. *Pediatr Infect Dis J* 21:1142–1145; 2002.

Treib J, Fernandez A, Haass A, Grauer MT, Holzer G, Woessner R: Clinical and serologic follow-up in patients with neuroborreliosis [see comments]. *Neurology* 51:1489–1491; 1998.

Van Dam AP, Kuiper H, Vos K, Al E: Different genospecies of *Borrelia burgdorferi* are associated with distinct clinical manifestations of Lyme borreliosis. *Clin Infec Dis* 17:708–717; 1993.

Veenendaal-Hilbers JA, Perquin WV, Hoogland PH, Doornbos L: Basal meningovasculitis and occlusion of the basilar artery in two cases of *Borrelia burgdorferi* infection. *Neurology* 38:1317–1319; 1988.

Wang W, Fredrikson S, Sun J, Link H: Lyme neuroborreliosis: evidence for persistent up-regulation of *Borrelia burgdorferi*-reactive cells secreting interferon-gamma. *Scand J Immunol* 42:694–700; 1995.

Weber K, Pfister HW: History of Lyme borreliosis in Europe. *In* Weber K, Burgdorfer W (eds): *Aspects of Lyme Borreliosis.* New York, Springer, 1993.

Weller M, Stevens A, Sommer N, Wietholter H, Dichgans J: Cerebrospinal fluid interleukins, immunoglobulins, and fibronectin in neuroborreliosis. *Arch Neurol* 48:837–841; 1991.

Zemel L: Lyme disease and pseudotumor. *Mayo Clin Proc* 75:315; 2000.

6

LYME ARTHRITIS

Frank Dressler, Patricia I. Irigoyen, Norman T. Ilowite,
and Hans-Iko Huppertz

The first description of Lyme arthritis was in 1977 (Steere et al., 1977) when a cluster of 39 children and 12 adults in and around Old Lyme, Connecticut, who were initially thought to have juvenile or adult rheumatoid arthritis, was studied. Subsequently it became clear that this arthritis was caused by the spirochete *Borrelia burgdorferi* (Burgdorfer et al., 1982, Steere et al., 1983) and that arthritis was one of many possible manifestations of the illness now known as Lyme borreliosis or Lyme disease (Steere, 2001; Stanek and Strle, 2003; Huppertz and Dressler, 2010). In retrospect the oldest published instance was probably the description of several patients with "rheumatism" accompanying lymphocytic meningitis and inflammatory polyneuritis in Germany in 1941 (Bannwarth, 1941).

EPIDEMIOLOGY

Lyme disease has been conclusively demonstrated to occur only in the temperate zones of the Northern Hemisphere (Steere, 2001; Stanek and Strle, 2003). In Europe, the disease occurs most commonly in central Europe but is endemic between southern Sweden and the northern Mediterranean and between Portugal and Russia. Data from the Slovenian National Registry document annual incidences of Lyme disease of 176 to 223 per 100,000 between 2003 and 2007 (Ministry of Health of the Republic of Slovenia, 2008).

Lyme Borreliosis in Europe and North America: Epidemiology and Clinical Practice, First Edition.
Edited by Sunil K. Sood.

A study in southern Sweden found an incidence of 69 per 100,000; Lyme arthritis was present in 7% of all cases (Berglund et al., 1995). In a population-based study in Würzburg, Germany, the incidence was 111 per 100,000, with higher rates in children younger than 16 years and an overall occurrence of Lyme arthritis in 5% of all patients (Huppertz et al., 1999). In a community-based Connecticut cohort study of 201 consecutive children with newly diagnosed Lyme disease, 13 (6%) had arthritis and 5% had facial palsy (Gerber et al., 1996). In Europe Lyme arthritis and neuroborreliosis have been reported with similar frequency. On both continents cases have been reported in all ages, but a bimodal age distribution is seen, with peaks in school-age children and adults between 40 and 74 years of age (Gerber et al., 1996; Huppertz et al., 1999a; CDC, 2007).

Compared with adults, children more frequently had manifestations other than isolated erythema migrans in the Würzburg study (Huppertz et al., 1999). Peak incidence of disease occurred in July (29%) and fewer than 8% of cases occurred between December and March. Early onset of cutaneous disease and neural involvement are closely related to tick activity in the spring to autumn months, but there is no seasonal pattern to late manifestations such as Lyme arthritis (Huppertz et al., 1995b; Huppertz et al., 1999a; Steere, 2001; Stanek and Strle, 2003). There is no sex predilection. Although Lyme disease may affect several members of the same family, genetic factors appear to have no influence on its occurrence.

MICROBIOLOGY

Lyme disease is caused by infection with one of several species of *B. burgdorferi* sensu lato. *Borrelia burgdorferi* sensu lato has been subdivided into several species, of which only *B. burgdorferi* sensu stricto has been found to cause human disease in North America. In addition *B. garinii* and *B. afzelii* have been identified regularly in patients in Europe, including cases with Lyme arthritis (Steere, 2001; Stanek and Strle, 2003). Recently the first case of Lyme arthritis due to infection with *B. spielmanii* was presented at the 2010 International Lyme Borreliosis Conference in Ljubljana, Slovenia.

PATHOPHYSIOLOGY

Induction of the host immune response by *B. burgdorferi* is intrinsic to the development of Lyme arthritis. Immune cells first encounter the organism at the site of the tick bite, stimulating an innate immune response in macrophages and dendritic cells, and an adaptive response in T cells, resulting in the production of cytokines. Despite these local responses, *B. burgdorferi* is in some patients able to disseminate to many sites including synovial tissue, further stimulating strong innate and adaptive pro-inflammatory responses required for host defense, but also involved in initiation or perpetuation of joint inflammation (Steere and Glickstein, 2004).

In order to survive in varied hosts, *B. burgdorferi* has developed an extensive set of outer surface lipoproteins that allow it to evade immune destruction. The spirochetes use the mechanism of sequential variation of outer surface proteins to attempt to evade the host immune response. As the exposed antigenic structure of the spirochete is in constant flux, the humoral system must continuously mount new responses. This allows for the persistence of the organism despite a strong antibody response and results in prolonged inflammation in the host. The pathologic changes of arthritis appear to be due largely to this host inflammatory response (Steere and Glickstein, 2004).

Differential expression of the outer surface proteins also contributes to the clinical expression of Lyme disease. Certain plasmid encoded outer surface proteins, referred to as OspA to OspF, are differentially expressed as the spirochete's environment changes. For example, *B. burgdorferi* expresses OspA and OspB in the mid-gut of the tick, but OspC is preferentially expressed after transfer to a mammalian host (Steere, 2001). Only a few OspC genotypes are associated with disseminated disease in humans (Steere and Glickstein, 2004). Another example is the increased expression of OspA in the human in the context of an inflammatory environment, as revealed by the almost universal presence of OspA antibodies in North American patients with Lyme arthritis (Kalish et al., 1993).

The outer surface proteins also play a role in pathogenesis via their binding capacities. Best understood is the organism's ability to bind different proteoglycans, complex molecules of glycosaminoglycan (GAG) side chains covalently bound to a protein core. A vital part of connective tissue and endothelial lining, proteoglycans are ubiquitous adhesion substrates for spirochetes. Of note, all known binding substrates for the spirochete are present in synovium, perhaps also explaining tropism of the organism to the joint (Coburn et al., 2002). The organism's decorin binding proteins (DBP) are associated with the pathogenesis of Lyme arthritis (Coburn et al., 2005; Cabello et al., 2007). Decorin is a proteoglycan found associated with collagen, and DBP promote alignment with collagen fibers, probably explaining the presence of the spirochete in the heart, nervous system, and synovial space.

The role of DBP in clinical manifestations is substantiated by the evidence of attenuated arthritis in decorin-deficient mice. Other proteoglycan binding proteins are involved in recognition of glycosaminoglycan (GAG) chains of cell-associated and extracellular matrix proteoglycans. Specifically, *B. burgdorferi* binds to heparin sulfate proteoglycans on the surface of mammalian cells. As heparin sulfate GAGs are increased with inflammation, binding sites would become more available to the spirochete during an inflammatory response. This may set up a vicious cycle in which these adhesion pathways allow *B. burgdorferi* to cause persistent infection.

Synovial Immune Response

Outer surface lipoproteins of *B. burgdorferi* bind to CD14 and toll-like receptors on macrophages. In disseminated infection this initial stimulus results in T and B cell activation in the lymph nodes, with subsequent antibody production (Steere, 2001). Disseminated spirochetes settle in the synovial space, prompting accumulation of joint fluid along with a neutrophilic infiltrate. There is a concentration of *B. burgdorferi* specific TH1 inflammatory responses in the synovial space, causing further inflammation and pannus formation (Steere, 2001). A *B. burgdorferi*–specific CD8 cytotoxic T cell response has been found in patients with Lyme arthritis (Busch et al., 1996). Interestingly these cells were found only after the disappearance of arthritis. *Borrelia burgdorferi* also stimulates synovial γ/δ T cells in patients with Lyme arthritis, leading to high and long expression of Fas ligand associated with cytolytic activity (Glatzel et al., 2002; Roessner et al., 2003). The persistent synovial inflammation stimulates more spirochete binding by revealing more adhesion sites. This may account for the persistence of infection, if untreated, over months or years.

Based on mouse models it has recently been suspected that there is an additional role for TH17 lymphocytes based on data that show a role for Interleukin 17 in Lyme arthritis

(Nardelli et al., 2008). This still needs to be confirmed in further animal studies and then in humans.

Molecular Mimicry and Induction of Autoimmunity

Steere and Glickstein propose four main hypotheses for the mechanism of antibiotic-treatment resistant (antibiotic-refractory) Lyme arthritis: persistent infection, retained spirochetal antigens, and infection-induced autoimmunity resulting from either epitope mimicry or bystander activation (Steere and Glickstein, 2004). One or more of these processes may play a role in resistant disease.

Although it is possible that live spirochetes might be protected from antibiotics and survive in the joint, such as intracellularly in Type 1 or 2 synovial cells, by antigenic drift, or by some immunodeficiency of the host, there is little data to support that this occurs in humans (Fikrig et al., 1995; Girschick et al., 1996; Franz et al., 2001). After appropriate treatment, PCR results for *B. burgdorferi* DNA become negative in the synovial fluid as well as in synovial tissue samples of patients who underwent synovectomy. Mouse models support this reasoning: no live spirochetes were found in mice six months after completion of treatment (Steere, 2001). Also patients with antibiotic-refractory Lyme arthritis who are treated with immunosuppressive therapies, such as those used in reactive or rheumatoid arthritis, do not have exacerbation of symptoms or re-emergence of positive PCR results. In addition studies looking for retained spirochete antigens found no persistent *B. burgdorferi* proteins using immunohistochemical techniques. Similarly, although retained spirochetal antigens (in the absence of live organisms) might be able to perpetuate synovial inflammation, this has only been demonstrated in a rat model and not in human disease (Gondolf et al., 1994). Instead, antibiotic-refractory Lyme arthritis appears to be a sterile inflammatory arthritis due to infection-induced autoimmunity either from T cell epitope mimicry or from nonspecific bystander activation of a T cell response to a self-epitope that is not related to the spirochetal protein.

Certain aspects of the immune environment appear to predispose patients to treatment-resistant Lyme arthritis. For example, the HLA-DR4 allele of the MHC molecule is associated with development of antibiotic-refractory Lyme arthritis. This finding has been refined to show that most patients with antibiotic-refractory Lyme arthritis have HLA-DRB1*0401, 0101, or 0404 alleles (Steere, 2001). These are the same MHC alleles that confer increased risk for rheumatoid arthritis. These findings are more significant as it has been shown that the HLA type does not confer risk for infection with *B. burgdorferi* overall but merely to the outcome. More recently a DR4-positive mouse model has been established (Iliopoulou et al., 2008; Iliopoulou et al., 2009). The HLA associations have not been confirmed in European patients, perhaps also because of the greater species diversity there. Another immune parameter that correlates with treatment resistance is cellular and humoral responses to the OspA outer surface lipoprotein (Kalish et al., 1993; Kamradt et al., 1996; Shin et al., 2007). T cell lines from patients with antibiotic-refractory Lyme arthritis preferentially recognized OspA, which is different from patients with antibiotic-responsive arthritis (Kamradt et al., 1996). In particular, reactivity to one OspA epitope was observed in treatment-resistant patients. The epitope of OspA presented by the HLA-DRB1*0401 molecule resides between amino acids 165–173, as predicted by a computer algorithm and confirmed using transgenic mice lacking MHC class II molecules (Gross et al., 1998), as well as in studies of antibiotic-refractory arthritis (Chen et al., 1999). Sequences of this epitope are

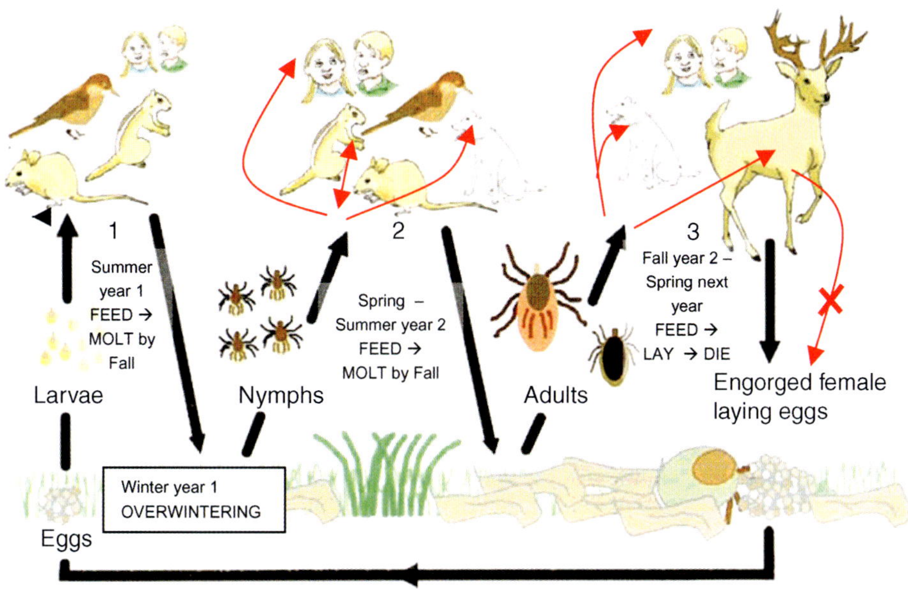

Figure 1.5 Life cycle of the blacklegged tick or "deer" tick, *Ixodes scapularis*. 1, 2, 3 = Feeding on new host. During feeding, infection is transmitted as shown by direction of red arrow. X = transmission blocked. Source: Modified from Kirby Stafford.

(a)

(b)

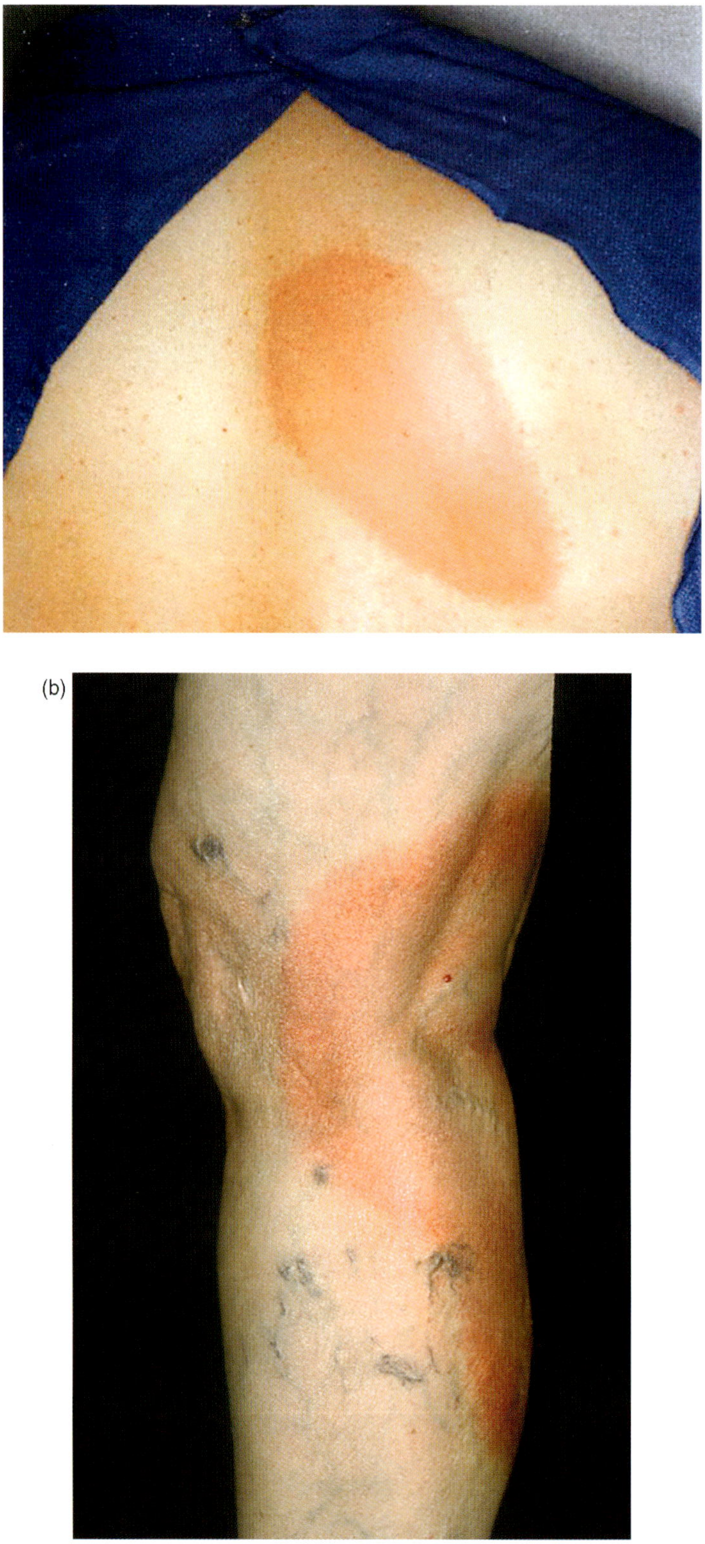

Figure 3.1 Solitary erythema migrans: (a) Plaque-like (United States—VKS), (b) large macular lesion (Europe—RRM).

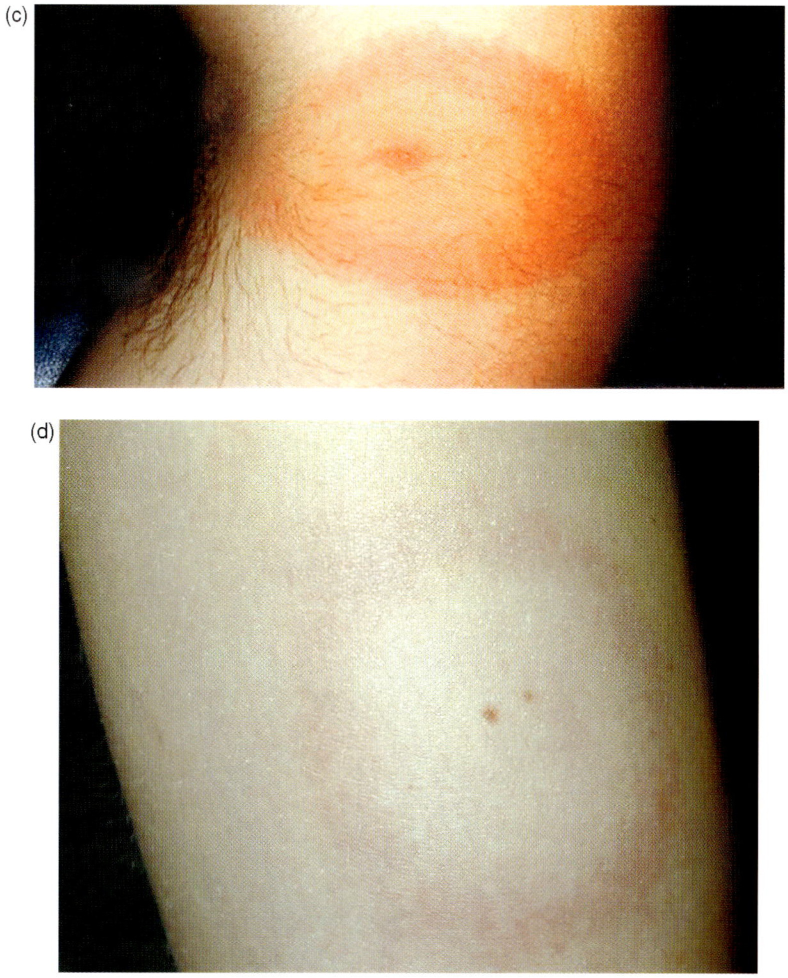

Figure 3.1 Solitary erythema migrans: (c) Dark annular (United States—VKS), (d) faint annular (Europe—RRM).

(a)

(b)

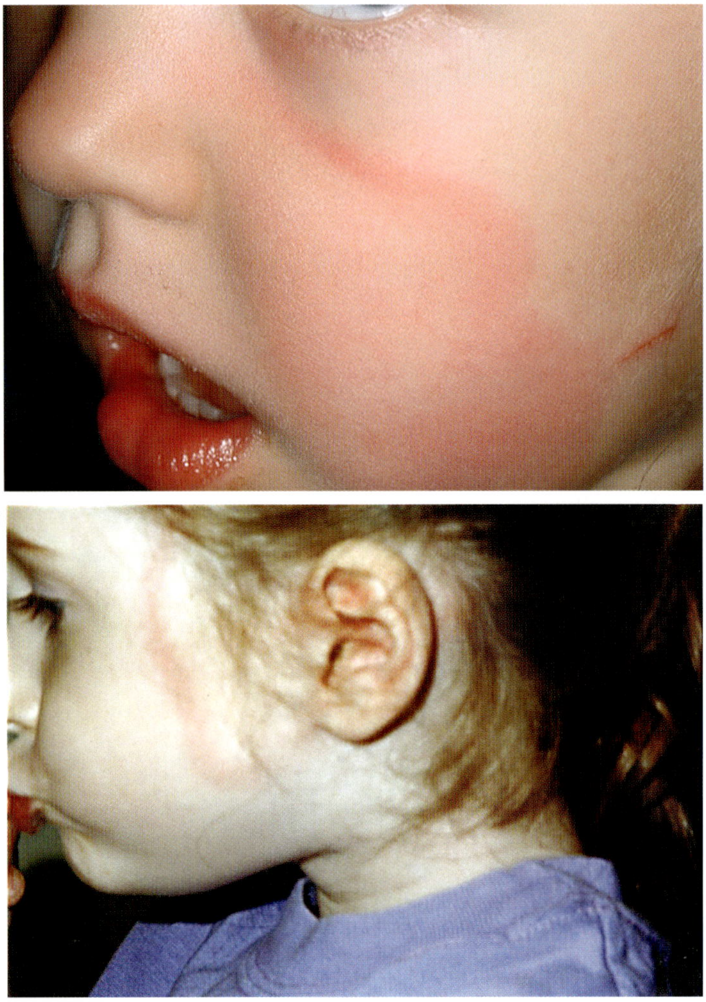

Figure 3.2 Erythema migrans on the head/face of a child: (a) On the face of a two-year-old girl (Europe—RRM); (b) scalp lesion only partially visible on the face (United States—VKS).

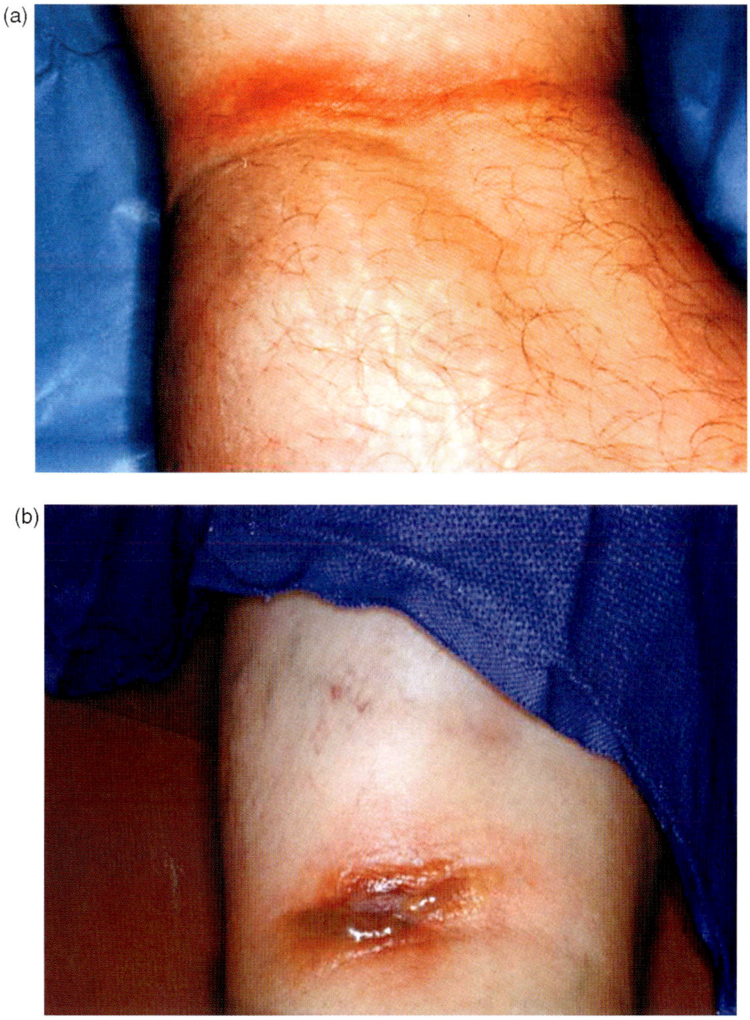

Figure 3.3 Atypical EM (United States—VKS): (a) Linear, (b) bullous.

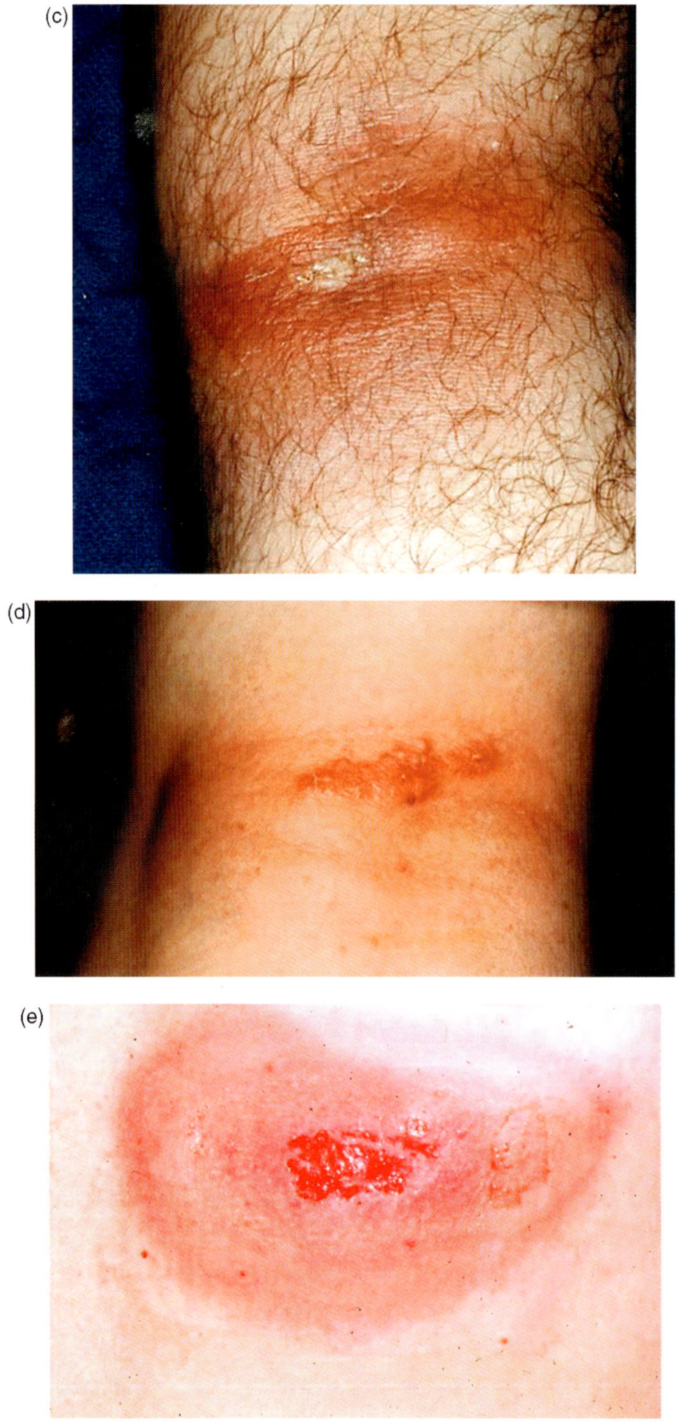

Figure 3.3 Atypical EM (United States—VKS): (c) Pustular, (d) vesicular, (e) ulcerated.

(a) (b)

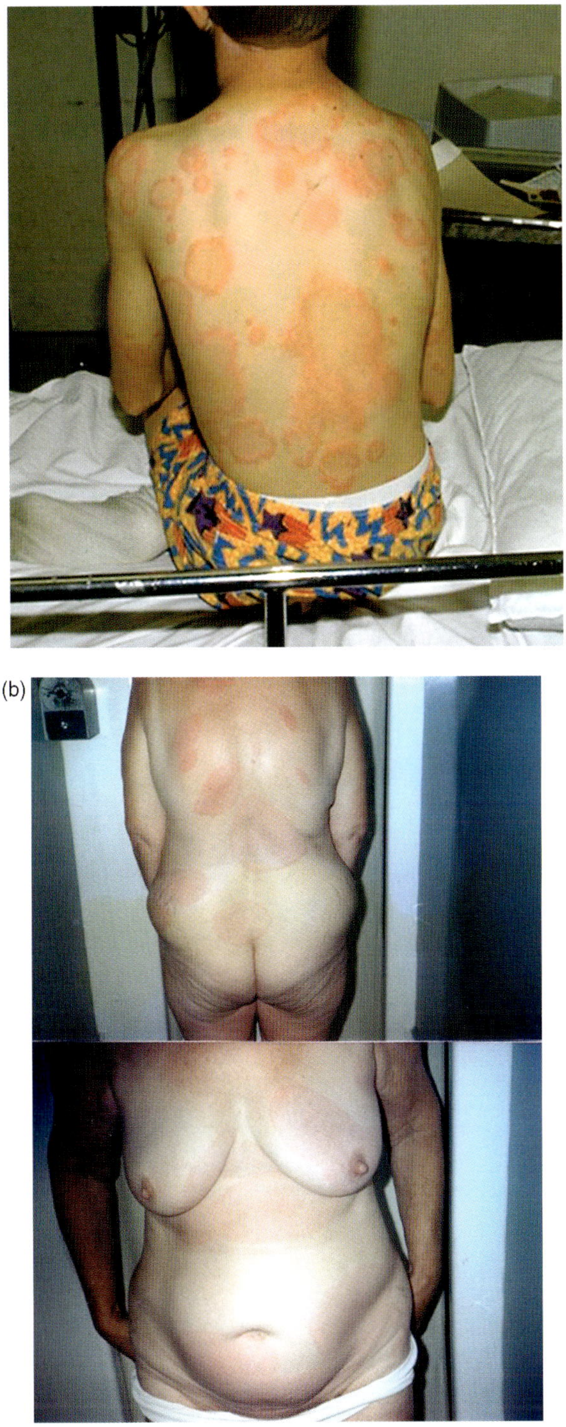

Figure 3.4 Disseminated erythema migrans: (a) Child (United States—Lorry Rubin), (b) adult (United States—VKS).

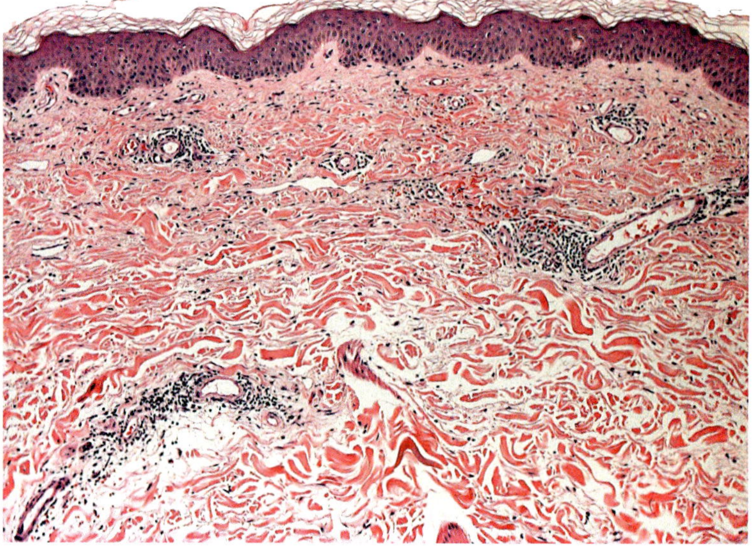

Figure 3.5 Histopathology of erythema migrans (hematoxylin/eosin, ×40) (RRM).

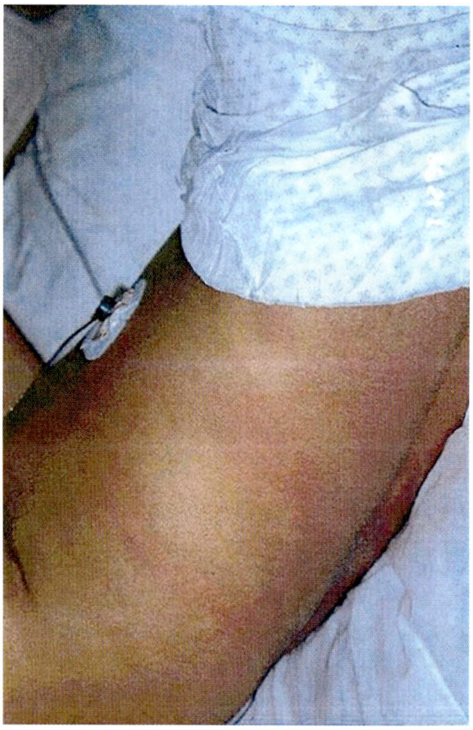

Figure 4.1 (b) Erythema migrans rash of patient with *B. burgdorferi* RFLP type 2 isolated on blood culture. Source: Haddad FA, Nadelman RB: Lyme disease and the heart. *Front Biosci* 8: s769–s782; 2003.

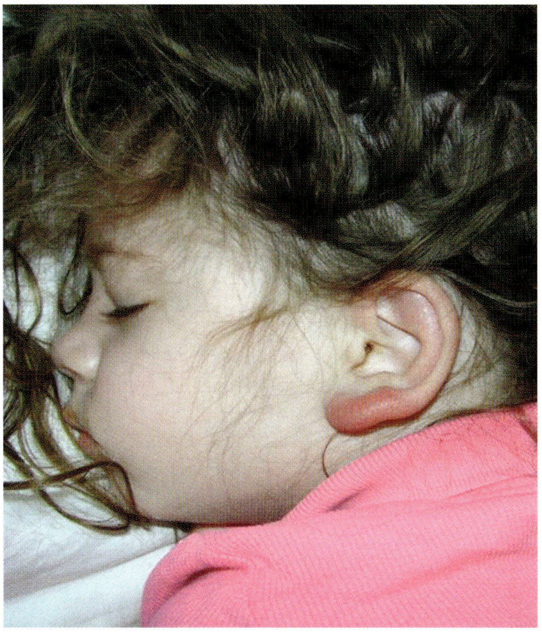

Figure 7.1 Borrelial lymphocytoma. Five-year-old girl from southern California who, while visiting Norway in August 2006, had a tick removed from her left ear lobe. (*See text for full caption.*)

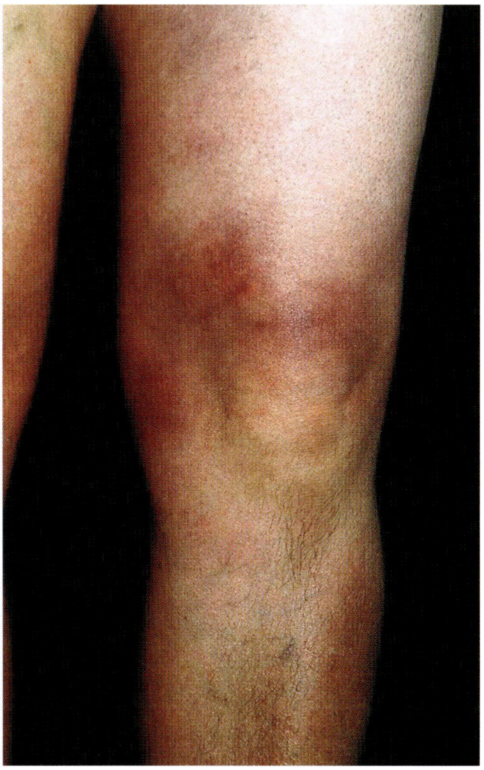

Figure 7.2 Acrodermatitis chronica atrophicans. Example of the acute stage (disease duration <3 months) around the knee of a 50-year-old male patient.

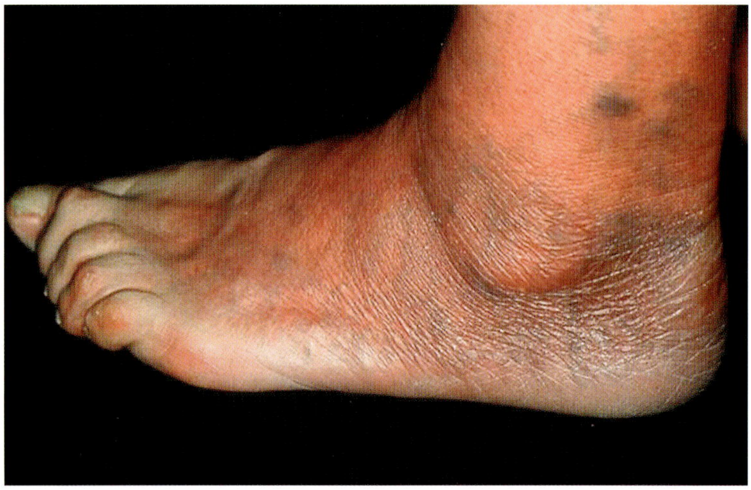

Figure 7.3 Acrodermatitis chronica atrophicans. Example of a subacute stage (3–6 months disease duration) on the ankle. Note co-existence of inflammatory erythema and swelling, and atrophy of the skin.

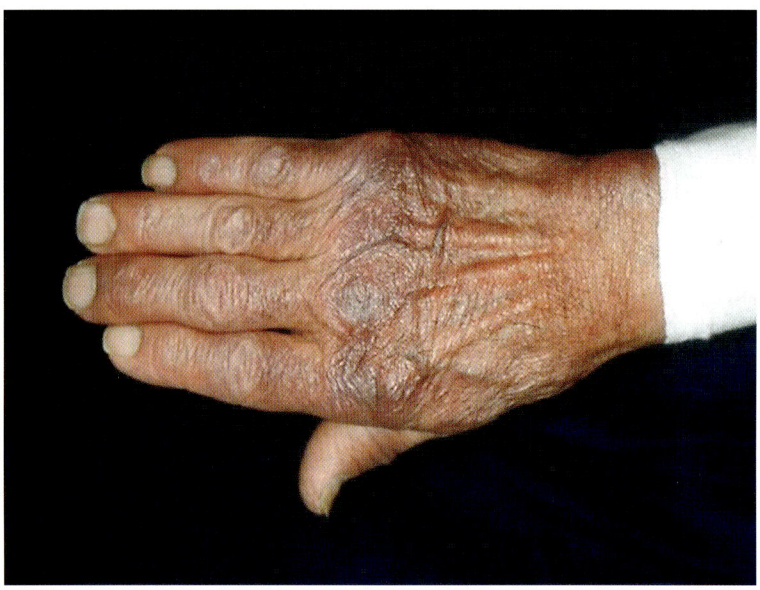

Figure 7.4 Acrodermatitis chronica atrophicans. Example of a chronic stage of ACA (>6 months disease duration) on the hand of 75-year-old male patient. Note the significant atrophy of skin overlying the knuckles and the bluish-red discoloration and prominent appearance of blood vessels.

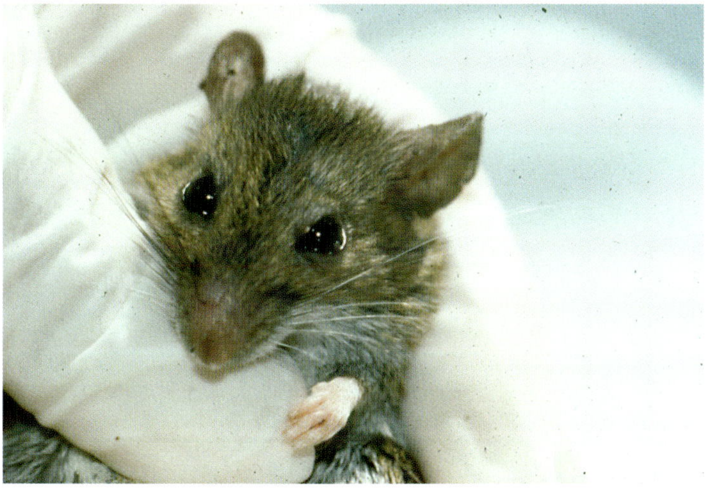

Figure 12.1 *Peromyscus leucopus* with ticks attached (arrow). Source: Kirby Stafford.

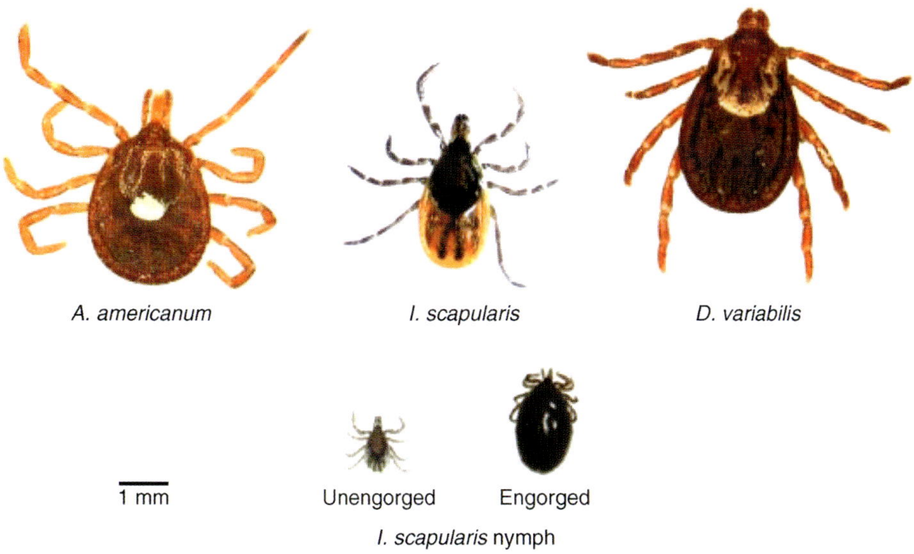

Figure 12.2 Adult female *Amblyomma americanum* (Lone Star Tick), adult Female, and nymphal *Ixodes scapularis* (Deer Ticks), and adult female *Dermacentor variabilis* (Dog Tick). Source: Hayes E and Piesman, J: *N Engl J Med* 348:2424–2430; 2003. Reproduced with permission.

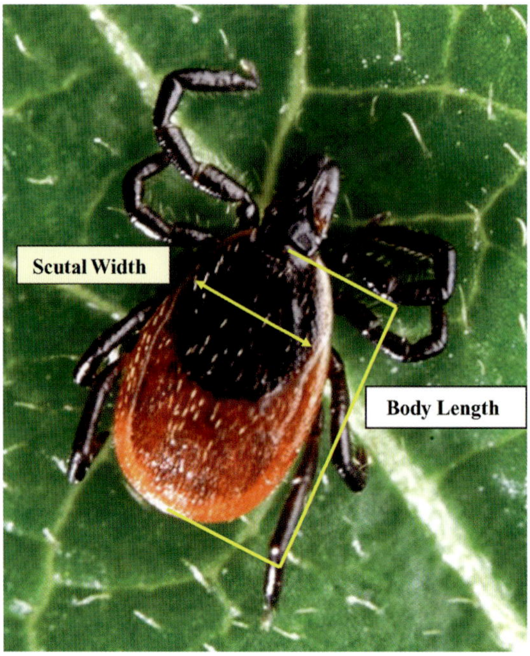

Figure 12.3 Measurements for scutal index with ocular micrometer. For calculation method refer to Falco RC et al., *Am J Epidemiol* 143:187–192; 1996. Source: USDA. Image adapted from http://commons.wikimedia.org/wiki/Image:Adult_deer_tick.jpg/Adult_deer_tick.jpg.

(a)

(b)

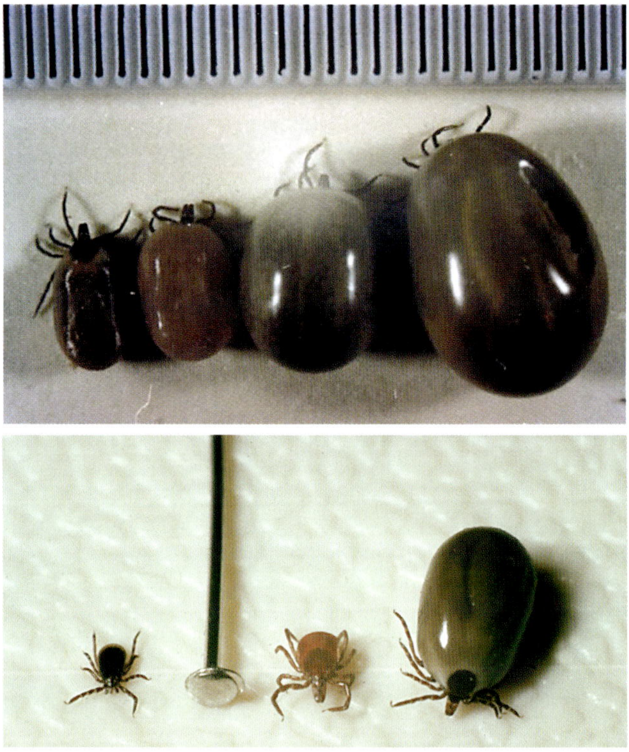

Figure 12.4 (a) Engorgement of *Ixodes* tick. Source: Jeremy Gray, University of Dublin. (b) Flat (unfed) and engorged *Ixodes scapularis* ticks. Source: Pfizer.

different in *B. garinii* and *B. afzelii*, the main European strains, which may explain the decreased frequency of antibiotic-refractory Lyme arthritis in Europe (Steere et al., 2001).

One hypothesis for explaining the significance of the strength of OspA T cell responses in antibiotic-refractory patients is molecular mimicry. This theory suggests that the reactive OspA epitope, recognized by the HLA alleles that confer risk, is cross-reactive to a self-peptide. A proposed self-antigen is human LFA-1, an adhesion molecule expressed by lymphoid and myeloid lineage cells. The light chain (hLFA-1$\alpha_{L332-340}$) of LFA-1 has partial homology to $OspA_{165-173}$ and is also predicted to bind HLA-DRB1*0401, but the LFA-1 peptide only weakly competed with binding to $OspA_{165-173}$ -reactive T cells in treatment-resistant Lyme arthritis (Steere et al., 2003). Moreover, the specificity of these responses was questioned (Kalish et al., 2003).

Alternatively, or additionally, pro-inflammatory responses in joints might cause persistent synovial inflammation due to failure to adequately regulate innate or adaptive immune responses. Genetically determined differences in the regulation of many pro-inflammatory cytokines, including TNF and IL-1, could conceivably influence this persistent inflammation in the joint. High levels of inflammatory chemokines and cytokines have been found in synovial fluid and tissue from patients with antibiotic-resistant Lyme arthritis throughout the course of their illnesses (Shin et al., 2007). Although defects in number or function of regulatory cells might contribute to self-perpetuated inflammation, there are no data to support this in Lyme arthritis. In summary, antibiotic-refractory Lyme arthritis appears to be due to infection-induced autoimmunity, and not to resistant protected live organisms or retained spirochetal antigens. Successful treatment regimens of patients with antibiotic-refractory or chronic arthritis are largely based on this hypothesis, adding further support to its validity. Recently two membrane glycolipids of *B. burgdorferi* have been shown to elicit strong IgG responses in patients with Lyme arthritis (Jones et al., 2009). These antibodies were long-lasting, and correlated with lack of re-infection, suggesting the possibility of membrane glycolipids as vaccine candidates.

PATHOLOGY

The synovitis of Lyme arthritis resembles that of rheumatoid arthritis, with villous hypertrophy, synovial cell hyperplasia, and infiltration of lymphocytes and plasma cells (Johnston et al., 1985). Lymphoid follicles and endarteritis may also be present. In one study, spirochetes were detected in 2 of 17 synovia, mainly in a perivascular distribution (Johnston et al., 1985). Other studies using special silver stains have also identified *B. burgdorferi* in synovium or synovial fluid (Snydman et al., 1986; De Koning et al., 1987). Myositis may in part account for the myalgia and fatigue that occur in this disease, and DNA from *B. burgdorferi* has been demonstrated in the muscle of such patients (Frey et al., 1998).

CLINICAL PRESENTATION

Lyme arthritis appears to be slightly more common in North America than in Europe. (Steere et al., 1987; Bianchi et al., 1990; Valesova and Trnavsky, 1990; Herzer, 1991; Huppertz and Karch, 1991; Hammers-Berggren et al., 1992; Huppertz et al., 1995b; Gerber et al., 1998; Sigal, 1998a; Steere, 2001; Huppertz and Dressler, 2010; Stanek and Strle, 2003). Myalgia, myositis, and enthesitis are not a common finding, although *B. burgdorferi* have been found by polymerase chain reaction in rare patients with enthesitis or nodular fasciitis (Reimers et al., 1993; Häupl et al., 1993; Schnarr et al., 2002). Arthralgia and myalgia start as early as days to weeks after infection, sometimes together with erythema migrans or flu-like symptoms. However, arthritis appears typically months to years after infection (Steere et al., 1987).

In a Connecticut series of 55 patients with untreated Lyme disease, 51% of patients went on to develop frank arthritis on average six months after initial presentation. (Steere et al., 1987). In half of these patients, migratory arthralgia preceded the development of arthritis. The typical pattern of arthritis was asymmetric monoarticular or oligoarticular arthritis in large joints, most commonly involving the knees. Effusions were quite large in several patients, and three had ruptured Baker's cysts. In patients with knee arthritis, the swelling was frequently disproportional to the pain. In contrast to septic arthritis, Lyme arthritis is not commonly associated with a hot, erythematous, extremely painful joint, or with high fever. In a recent study of acute monarthritis, fever was a negative predictor for Lyme versus septic arthritis and knee involvement was a positive predictor (Thompson et al., 2009).

Polyarthritis was less common than oligoarthritis (Huppertz et al., 1995b). Symmetric rheumatoid arthritis-like polyarthritis but also asymmetrical and proximal interphalangeal joint involvement were sometimes noted. Enthesitis, inflammation of the tendon insertion into bone, was found in a subset of patients. The temporomandibular joints were frequently involved (Steere et al., 1987).

Lyme arthritis, like other inflammatory arthritides, was associated with morning stiffness lasting 15 minutes to 2 hours (Steere et al., 1987). Morning stiffness was most prominent in patients with hand involvement. Subcutaneous nodules, while rare, were also seen. Overall, Lyme arthritis was associated with fatigue, normal or mildly elevated ESR values, and markedly elevated IgG antibodies to *Borrelia* antigens. Synovial fluid showed a moderate leukocytosis with a neutrophilic preponderance.

The natural history of Lyme arthritis is one of a remitting and relapsing course. Among the initial series of untreated patients, most had up to 12 recurrent episodes of arthritis, the frequency of these episodes tapering off with time (Steere et al., 1987). Eleven percent of patients developed persistent chronic arthritis for greater than one year. Chronic arthritis usually involved the knee, but chronic arthritis of the hip and the shoulder were also seen. Eight patients went on to develop radiographic abnormalities associated with chronic inflammatory arthritis.

Lyme arthritis is indistinguishable from other arthritides on plain radiographs. However, MRI can help differentiate between Lyme arthritis and septic arthritis. In particular, muscle edema and regional lymphadenopathy were more common in children with Lyme arthritis (Ecklund et al., 2005). Subcutaneous edema on MRI imaging was more suggestive of septic arthritis. In pediatric patients presenting with acute, painful monarthritis, the absence of subcutaneous edema gave an estimated probability of Lyme disease as 99%, with $<1\%$ probability of septic arthritis (Ecklund et al., 2005).

In summary, while classically a monarthritis or oligoarthritis involving the knee, the natural history of Lyme arthritis can resemble most other inflammatory arthritides. Lyme arthritis should be considered within the differential diagnosis of any arthritic condition, including long-standing disease. In Europe an expert group has recently provided clinical definitions for manifestations of Lyme borreliosis including Lyme arthritis (Stanek et al., 2011).

Pediatric Lyme Arthritis

The largest series of pediatric patients with Lyme arthritis were reported from the northeastern United States and Germany: 90 patients from Connecticut (Gerber et al., 1998), 106 from New England (Tory et al., 2010), and 109 from Germany (Huppertz and Michels, 1996), 62 of whom have been described in detail (Huppertz et al., 1995b). Two-thirds of all children presented with monarthritis of one knee. Both knees or other large joints were affected in other patients (Huppertz et al., 1995b; Huppertz and Michels, 1996; Gerber et al., 1998). Polyarticular involvement of small joints was rare. At onset the arthritis was usually episodic and relatively painless. Swelling lasted only a few days and disappeared spontaneously. Among the109 German children with Lyme arthritis, 70 had monarthritis, 32 oligoarthritis, and 7 polyarthritis (Huppertz and Michels, 1996). The pattern of oligoarticular involvement differed from that found in patients with early-onset oligoarticular JIA/JRA. Patients with Lyme arthritis had symmetrical, unilateral, or predominantly unilateral arthritis, but never showed an oblique pattern of joint involvement, defined as no joint involvement that was also present contralaterally (e.g., right knee and left ankle involved, but left knee and right ankle not involved in that patient) (Huppertz and Michels, 1996). Symptomatic ocular involvement with keratitis, anterior or intermediate uveitis, occurred in 3 of 84 children with Lyme arthritis in Germany (Huppertz et al., 1999b). In a recent review of 99 children age 2 to 18 years with Lyme arthritis in the northeastern United States, Tory et al. found that 76 (77%) had antibiotic-responsive arthritis following 2 courses of 28 days of oral or intravenous antibiotics (Tory et al., 2010). Of the 23 patients with antibiotic-refractory arthritis, defined as persistence of arthritis more than three months after initiation of the first antibiotic regimen, 6 children received further antibiotics and remission followed in 3. The other 17 patients were treated with nonsteroidal anti-inflammatory drugs ($n = 11$) or intraarticular steroids ($n = 6$). Six patients were lost to follow-up prior to remission of their arthritis, and five eventually went onto treatment with disease-modifying antirheumatic drugs. Importantly none of the patients went on to develop chronic debilitating arthritis or permanent joint deformities, and the overall prognosis was excellent.

APPROACH TO DIAGNOSIS

Clinical characteristics of patients with arthritis that suggest a diagnosis of Lyme arthritis include residence in or travel to an endemic area, a preceding tick bite, the presence of episodic oligoarthritis involving the knee joint, and the absence of arthralgias preceding the onset of arthritis. Specific criteria have been combined to form a clinical diagnostic score that would confirm or exclude Lyme arthritis in two thirds of pediatric patients with arthritis (Huppertz et al., 1998) (Table 6.1). This score has not been validated in adults. For a diagnosis of Lyme arthritis, joint swelling and effusion, or painful limitation of motion in the absence of trauma must be observed by a physician. Arthralgias or reports by the patient alone that the joint was swollen are not objective signs of arthritis in this context. The clinical presentation of Lyme arthritis may be indistinguishable from that of other rheumatic diseases with arthritis, and laboratory tests are necessary in all patients with arthritis living in or having traveled to an endemic area.

Lyme arthritis occurred in a woman following autologous chondrocyte transplantation (Marlovits et al., 2004). The authors speculated that *B. burgdorferi* was asymptomatically

TABLE 6.1 Diagnosis of Lyme arthritis in children and adolescents using a clinical score

Criterion	Score
Episodic arthritis	+ 4
Arthralgia before onset of arthritis	– 3
Age at onset of arthritis	+ 0.3 × age in years
Initial arthritis in knee joint	+ 2
History of tick bite	+ 2
Number of joints involved	– 0.4 × number of large joints affected
If a criterion is found in the patient, its indicated value is added to (or subtracted from) the total score. If it is not found, the item is scored "0." Values of 6 or greater indicate the presence of Lyme arthritis. Values of 2.5 or below exclude the diagnosis.	
Example: A 10-year-old boy without prior arthralgia or history of a tick bite developed arthritis in a knee. The arthritis resolved after 10 days but recurred after a 3-months interval.	
Episodic arthritis present	+ 4
No initial arthralgias	+ 0
Age at onset × 0.3	+ 3
Initial arthritis in knee	+ 2
No history of tick bite	+ 0
One large joint affected	– 0.4
Total	8.6
This patient's serum contained IgG antibodies to *B. burgdorferi* by enzyme immunoassay and immunoblot. He was treated with ceftriaxone for 2 weeks. Arthritis disappeared during therapy and has not recurred in the subsequent 2 years.	

Source: Adapted from Huppertz HI, Bentas W, Haubitz I, et al: Diagnosis of pediatric Lyme arthritis using a clinical score. *Eur J Pediatr* 157: 304; 1998, table 3.

present in the patient's joint prior to the transplant procedure. Myositis has only rarely been demonstrated in adults (Reimers et al., 1992), and myalgia alone has been reported in children (Cristofaro et al., 1987). A dermatomyositis-like picture was described in an adult patient (Hoffmann et al., 1995). *Borrelia burgdorferi* was isolated from a child with subacute multifocal osteomyelitis (Oksi et al., 1994). Fibromyalgia may follow Lyme borreliosis and does not respond to antibiotic therapy (Sigal and Patella, 1992).

COURSE OF THE DISEASE AND PROGNOSIS

The overall prognosis of Lyme arthritis is excellent. Whereas the natural history of Lyme arthritis is typically relapsing and remitting, appropriate and timely antibiotic therapy cures the majority of patients. Even in antibiotic-refractory patients, erosive disease is rare, and the disease tends to remit spontaneously, albeit over the course of several years.

Of 90 children with Lyme arthritis treated with appropriate antibiotics, 4 had ongoing musculoskeletal complaints 7 years later (Gerber et al., 1998). Of 51 German children with Lyme arthritis examined 1 year after initiation of antibiotic treatment, 8 patients had chronic arthritis defined as lasting longer than 3 months and 4 had persistent arthralgias in joints previously affected by arthritis (Bentas et al., 2000). Chronic arthritis occurred mostly as monarthritis of one knee (6 of 8 patients), and the remaining 2 patients had one finger joint or both knees, elbows, and wrists affected. Risk factors for a prolonged course of disease were female gender, age above 10 years, and intra-articular steroids prior to antibiotic treatment (Bentas et al., 2000). The reason for a higher incidence of chronic arthritis in this and another German study is unclear (Huppertz et al., 1995b). It can be speculated that some patients were infected with *B. afzelii* and *B. garinii*, but whether this accounts for the different outcome from North American children is unknown (Sood and Ilowite, 2000). Also recruitment of the children from multiple centers could have skewed the population toward more severe disease. In another study of 94 children arthritis resolved more than 6 months after antibiotic treatment in 39% and more than 12 months in 13% of patients (Brescia et al., 2009). Chronic arthritis despite adequate antibiotic treatment was also reported in 2 Belgian children (Hendrickx et al., 2004). In rare cases flares of arthritis in a previously affected joint were observed several years after antibiotic treatment and the initial disappearance of arthritis. Onset of new joint involvement following successfully treated Lyme disease is frequently due to development of another disease entity, such as rheumatoid arthritis.

Erosion of cartilage is particularly rare in children (Huppertz et al., 1995b; Hendrickx et al., 2004). Arthralgias in joints previously affected by arthritis may persist for several months but usually do not restrict the physical or educational performance of adolescents. Late neurologic complications occurred in untreated children with Lyme arthritis (Szer et al., 1991) but have not been found after appropriate treatment (Adams et al., 1994). However, transient neurocognitive abnormalities have been described (Bloom et al., 1998). Late development of keratitis has occurred in both treated and untreated children (Szer et al., 1991; Huppertz et al., 1999b).

Szer and colleagues (Szer et al., 1991) studied 46 American children with Lyme arthritis with onset of disease between 1976 and 1979 and who did not receive any antibiotics during the first 4 years of disease. All except one patient had arthralgias during the early phase, with a median time from onset to development of arthritis of 3 months (range 2 to 24 months). The number of children with recurrent episodes declined each year. Older children tended to have arthritis of longer duration. At the end of the study 12 children (31%) still had occasional brief episodes of arthralgia. One child had marked fatigue, and 2 developed keratitis. All 46 children had persistently positive IgG antibody responses. IgM responses were more frequent and IgG titers higher in children with recurrent symptoms than in those who became asymptomatic.

In Europe the frequency of chronic arthritis in adults has ranged from 2 of 16 (13%) Italian (Bianchi et al., 1990) to 10 of 65 (15%) German (Herzer, 1991) to 7 of 37 (19%) Czechoslovakian patients (Valesova and Trnavsky, 1990). Erosions were described in 2 of 65 German patients (Herzer, 1991).

The poor prognosis of Lyme arthritis that is observed in some American adults has been associated with the presence of antibodies to OspA and of the DRB1*0401 and 0101 alleles (Johnston et al., 1985). The risk of treatment failure increased with increasing age and when intra-articular steroids were given before antibiotics (Dattwyler et al., 1988; Bentas et al., 2000).

Antibiotic-Refractory Lyme Arthritis

Lyme arthritis that fails to respond adequately to antibiotic therapy is herein referred to as antibiotic-refractory Lyme arthritis, and has also been termed antibiotic–treatment-resistant and antibiotic-resistant by other authors. The term antibiotic-resistant Lyme arthritis does not imply that the spirochetes have developed antibiotic resistance. Moreover the nonresponse of the disease manifestation to repeated courses of antibiotics is probably due to the mechanisms that are discussed in the Pathophysiology section of this chapter. The incidence of clinically apparent antibiotic-refractory Lyme arthritis is about 10%. Twenty-three percent of pediatric patients in a recent retrospective review met the author's definition of antibiotic-refractory Lyme arthritis, but this was likely a reflection of a referral bias of refractory cases to a large tertiary care center (Tory et al., 2010). Diagnosis of antibiotic-refractory Lyme arthritis requires persistent objective findings of arthritis, such as joint effusion, following appropriate courses of antibiotic therapy (see Figure 6.2). Antibiotic-refractory Lyme arthritis usually occurs in the joint or joints initially affected, most commonly the knee.

Post–Lyme Disease Syndrome

Post–Lyme disease syndrome refers to patients who continue to have subjective complaints for more than a year following definitive identification and appropriate treatment for Lyme disease (Wormser et al., 2006). Commonly patients present with fatigue, diffuse body aches, and subtle neurocognitive symptoms. Controlled studies have found no persistent spirochetal infection nor any role for antibiotics in this condition (Feder et al., 2007).

At this time there are no diagnostic criteria to differentiate post–Lyme disease syndrome from similar syndromes such as chronic fatigue syndrome or fibromyalgia. There are no standardized therapies for these patients, although improving sleep habits may be helpful, and careful evaluation for other underlying medical conditions is essential.

LABORATORY EXAMINATION

The erythrocyte sedimentation rate is elevated in about one-half of patients, especially during the early phase of Lyme arthritis. The mean synovial fluid white blood cell count ranges from less than 1000 to over 50,000/mm,^{3} with a predominance of neutrophils in samples with high cell numbers (Huppertz et al., 1995b).

Laboratory methods to confirm infection with *B. burgdorferi* are reviewed in Chapters 9 and 10. Direct tests, such as culture or polymerase chain reaction (PCR) to detect borrelial DNA sequences, and indirect tests, such as serology may be used. A summary of laboratory testing in Lyme arthritis is presented in Table 6.2. Serological tests are the most frequently used and universally available. A screening test, commonly an ELISA, should be combined with a more specific serologic test such as Western blot. Examples of typical Western blot results in patients with Lyme arthritis are shown in Figure 6.1. Although the laboratory evaluation of North American patients with Lyme disease has been standardized (CDC, 1995; Tugwell et al., 1997), these recommendations cannot be used in European patients. Some of the common problems with standardization of test procedures for the diagnosis of Lyme disease have been reviewed (Sigal, 1998b). "Seronegative" Lyme

TABLE 6.2 Laboratory diagnosis of Lyme arthritis

Method	Assessment
Culture of *B. burgdorferi*	Requires weeks; rarely successful
Histochemistry using silver stain or monoclonal antibodies	Rarely successful in synovial tissue
Polymerase chain reaction for borrelial DNA	Efficiency varies widely: Urine 5–85% Synovium (6–90%) (Higher in membrane than in fluid)
Enzyme immunoassay or immunofluorescence assay	High sensitivity, low specificity
Immunoblot	Confirmatory test with high specificity
Lymphocyte-proliferation assay with borrelial antigens	Sensitivity and specificity <80% Limited availability

Note: All diagnostic tests bear the risk of false-negative or false-positive results. No test is of value in a patient with low pre-test probability of having Lyme arthritis.
Source: Adapted from Huppertz HI: Lyme arthritis. *In* Wahn U, Seger R, Wahn V (eds): *Paediatrische Allergologie and Immunologie*. Munich, Urban and Fischer, 1999, pp. 598–602.

arthritis has been described (Dressler et al., 1991; Zoschke et al., 1991; Huppertz et al., 1996; Holl-Wieden et al., 2007), but it occurs so rarely that vigorous attempts must be undertaken by centers with special experience with Lyme arthritis to exclude other diagnoses. In these cases the cellular immune response induced by *B. burgdorferi* can be tested (Dressler et al., 1991; Zoschke et al., 1991; Huppertz et al., 1996; Rutkowski et al., 1997). However, lymphoproliferative assays are not well standardized and have high rates of false-positive and false-negative results (Dressler et al., 1991; Zoschke et al., 1991; Huppertz et al., 1996).

Synovial fluid analysis is of limited help in diagnosing Lyme arthritis, since the white blood cell count and types of cells vary greatly (Huppertz et al., 1995a). However, synovial fluid examinations help to exclude septic arthritis and other infection-associated arthritides, provide material for PCR, and confirm the presence of inflammation. A positive PCR result from an experienced laboratory indicates persistent infection, while a negative result does not exclude Lyme arthritis. Positive results by PCR have been obtained more commonly in synovial tissue than in synovial fluid, particularly in antibiotic-refractory patients (Jaulhac et al., 1996; Priem et al., 1998).

TREATMENT

Antibiotic Regimens

Recommendations for the treatment of Lyme disease were developed by the Infectious Diseases Society of America (IDSA) and depend on disease manifestation (Wormser et al., 2006). A summary of antibiotic treatment recommendations for Lyme arthritis is presented in Table 6.3. In patients with erythema migrans or neuroborreliosis, there were insignificant differences between the efficacy of penicillins, cephalosporins, and doxycycline, while macrolide antibiotics were inferior to other antibiotics. It is not known whether

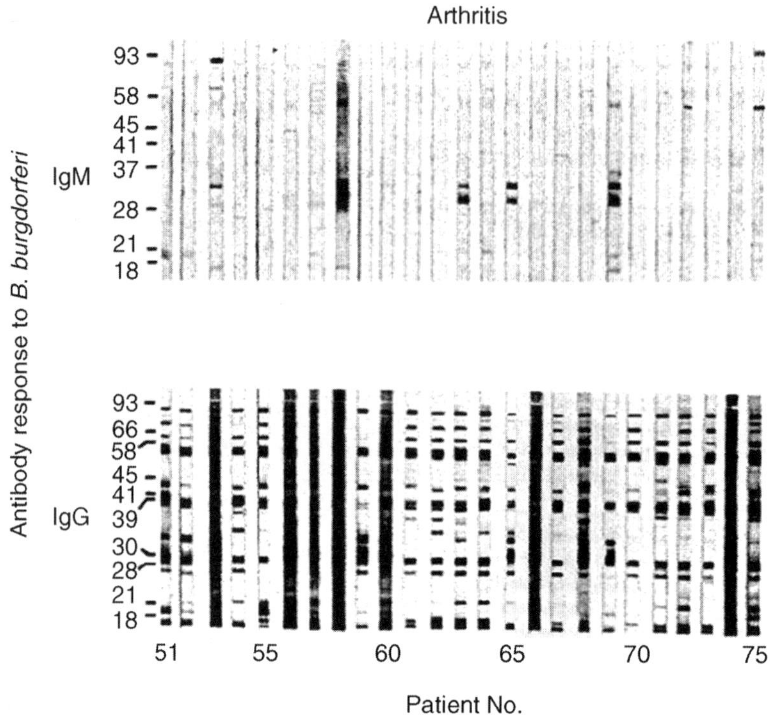

Figure 6.1 Western blots of immunoglobulin M (IgM) and IgG antibody responses of 25 American patients with Lyme arthritis to a sonicated whole-cell lysate of *Borrelia burgdorferi sensu stricto* strain G39/40. Molecular weight (in kilodaltons) is indicated on the left side. Characteristic of Lyme arthritis, strong IgG responses against many antigens are demonstrated. In North America, criteria for a positive IgG blot are the detection of least five of the following 10 bands: 18 kD, 21 kD OspC, 28 kD, 30 kD, 39 kD BmpA, 41 kD flagellin, 45 kD, 58 kD, 66 kD, and 93 kD. All patients met these criteria. A minority of patients also have IgM responses to a smaller number of antigens. Molecular weights may vary depending on the strain used for testing. Source: Adapted from Dressler F, Whalen JA, Reinhardt BN, et al: Western blotting in the serodiagnosis of Lyme disease. *J Infect Dis* 167: 392; 1993. By permission of the publisher, the University of Chicago.

TABLE 6.3 Current recommendations for treatment of Lyme arthritis

Manifestation	Drugs[a]	Dose[a]	Duration
Lyme arthritis	Ceftriaxone	50–100 mg/kg/d in 1 dose	2–4 wk
	Cefotaxime	50–150 mg/kg/d in 3 doses	2–4 wk
	Amoxicillin	50 mg/kg/d in 3–4 doses	4 wk
	Doxycycline	4 mg/kg/d in 2 doses	4 wk
	Cefuroxime axetil	30 mg/kg/d in 2 doses	4 wk

Note: Large, well-designed controlled clinical trials upon which to base recommendations specifically for Lyme arthritis are lacking. All listed drugs have been effective in such studies of erythema migrans or neuroborreliosis.
[a]Ceftriaxone and cefotaxime IV; amoxicillin, doxycycline and cefuroxime axetil orally. Maximum daily doses of amoxicillin = 1.5 g; doxycycline = 200 mg; cefuroxime axetil = 1 g; ceftriaxone = 2 g; cefotaxime = 6 g. Doxycycline should not be administered to patients <9 yr of age.

these results are applicable to patients with Lyme arthritis, in whom a variety of antibiotics have been used, including parenteral penicillin G, oral penicillins, amoxicillin with or without probenecid, ceftriaxone, cefotaxime, cefuroxime, erythromycin, roxithromycin (plus cotrimoxazole), azithromycin, tetracycline, and doxycycline (Steere et al., 1994; Huppertz et al., 1995b). Oral antibiotic therapy for 4 weeks has been recommended as first-line treatment by the IDSA; however, there has never been a controlled trial of oral versus intravenous antibiotic therapy in Lyme arthritis.

An approach to treatment is shown in Figure 6.2. Ceftriaxone 50 mg/kg/day can be used intravenously as a single daily 20-minute infusion for 14 days, and treatment can be provided as an outpatient. Patients with Lyme arthritis have also been treated successfully with oral antibiotics, including amoxicillin or doxycycline, for 4 weeks. This approach to treatment is more convenient for the patient and more cost-effective than intravenous

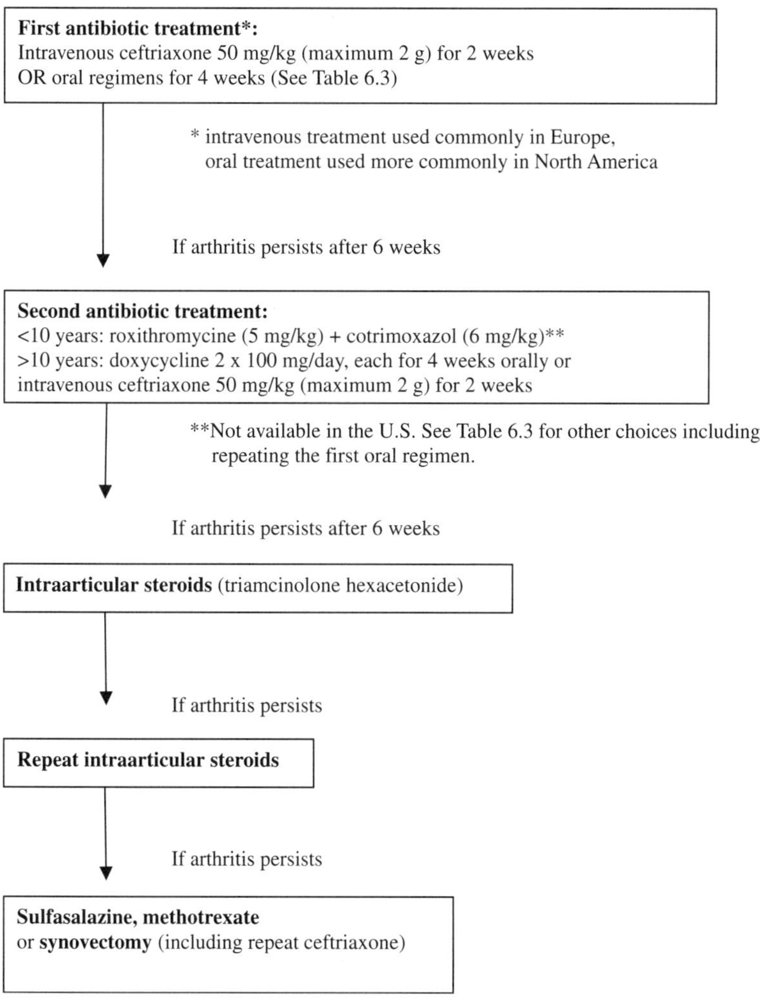

Figure 6.2 Sequential treatment of Lyme arthritis. Source: Adapted from Huppertz HI: Lyme arthritis. *In* Wahn U, Seger R, Wahn V (eds): *Paediatrische Allergologie und Immunologie.* Munich, Urban and Fischer, 1999, pp. 598–602.

regimens, but should not be used in patients with Baker cysts, nervous system, or cardiac involvement (Eckman et al., 1997). Children under the age of 9 years who are allergic to penicillin, amoxicillin, or cephalosporins, should receive macrolide antibiotics, although these drugs are less effective than beta-lactam antibiotics (Hansen et al., 1992; Luft et al., 1996). This disadvantage may be overcome by a combination of roxithromycin and cotrimoxazole (Gasser et al., 1995). Lyme arthritis during pregnancy needs to be treated with antibiotics that do not pose a risk to the fetus, such as amoxicillin, intravenous penicillin G, or cephalosporins.

At least two courses of sufficient duration and well-documented compliance are required before one assumes failure of antibiotic therapy. In fact the failure of treatment with appropriate antibiotics should lead to reevaluation of the diagnosis of Lyme arthritis. There is no evidence that treatment extending beyond one month is of any additional benefit. The success of antibiotic treatment must be determined clinically because serologic results remain positive for a long time after resolution of all manifestations (Rose et al., 1996; Hilton et al., 1997).

Symptomatic Treatment of Lyme Arthritis

For symptomatic relief, NSAIDs (most commonly naproxen or ibuprofen) are quite effective. For children, we recommend anti-inflammatory doses of naproxen 15 to 20 mg/kg divided in 2 doses for 4 to 6 weeks, or until resolution of symptoms. Ibuprofen can also be used at doses of 40 mg/kg/day divided in 4 doses. In patients with history of gastritis or peptic ulcer disease, selective Cox 2 inhibitors may be preferable. Physiotherapy should be used to maintain joint mobility in a similar manner as in other arthritides.

Treatment of Antibiotic-Refractory Arthritis

Patients who continue to have persistent arthritis following two courses of appropriate doses and duration of antibiotics are considered to have antibiotic-refractory Lyme arthritis. Therapy in such patients has been reviewed (Steere and Angelis, 2006). Following confirmation of disease eradication by synovial fluid PCR, intra-articular corticosteroids can be recommended. If arthritis still persists, second-line antirheumatic medications such as hydroxychloroquine, methotrexate, or sulfasalazine or arthroscopic synovectomy (Schoen et al., 1991) should be considered. Onset of new joint symptoms or other evidence of systemic inflammatory disease must prompt full evaluation for other autoimmune disorders.

PREVENTION

Prompt antibiotic treatment of the early manifestations of Lyme disease almost always prevents late manifestations such as arthritis. Two human vaccines were developed with recombinant fragments of OspA of *B. burgdorferi* sensu stricto. These vaccines were found to be safe. After three injections vaccine efficacy in adults was 76% to 92% (Steere et al., 1998; Sigal et al., 1998). One of these vaccines was also safe and efficacious in children (Feder et al., 1999), and recommendations for the use of the vaccine were published

(CDC, 1999). However, neither vaccine was intended for use in Europe or Asia due to the greater strain variation. Economic reasons led to withdrawal of the single licensed vaccine from the American market. New vaccines are under development. Principal considerations regarding the prevention of Lyme borreliosis are described in Chapter 12.

REFERENCES

Adams WV, Rose CD, Eppes SC, Klein JD: Cognitive effects of Lyme disease in children. *Pediatrics* 94:185–189; 1994.

Bannwarth A: Chronische lymphocytäre Meningitis, entzündliche Polyneuritis und "Rheumatismus." *Arch Psychiatr Nervenkr* 113:284–376; 1941.

Bentas W, Karch H, Huppertz HI: Lyme arthritis in children and adolescents. Outcome 12 months after initiation of antibiotic therapy. *J Rheumatol* 27:2025–2030; 2000.

Berglund J, Eitrem R, Ornstein K, Lindberg A, Ringer A, Elmrud H, Carlsson M, Runehagen A, Svanborg C, Norrby R: An epidemiologic study of Lyme disease in southern Sweden. *N Engl J Med* 333:1319–1327; 1995.

Bianchi G, Rovetta G, Monteforte P, Fumarola D, Trevisan G, Crovato F, Cimmino MA: Articular involvement in European patients with Lyme disease. A report of 32 Italian patients. *Br J Rheumatol* 29:178–180; 1990.

Bloom BJ, Wyckoff PM, Meissner HC, Steere AC: Neurocognitive abnormalities in children after classic manifestations of Lyme disease. *Pediatr Infect Dis J* 17:189–196; 1998.

Brescia AC, Rose CD, Fawcett PT: Prolonged synovitis in pediatric Lyme arthritis cannot be predicted by clinical or laboratory parameters. *Clin Rheumatol* 28:591–593; 2009.

Burgdorfer W, Barbour AG, Hayes SF, Benach JL, Grunwaldt E, Davis JP: Lyme disease. A tick-borne spirochetosis? *Science* 216:1317–1319; 1982.

Busch DH, Jassoy C, Brinckmann U, Girschick H, Huppertz HI: Detection of *Borrelia burgdorferi*-specific CD8 + cytotoxic T cells in patients with Lyme arthritis. *J Immunol* 157:3534–3541; 1996.

Cabello FC, Godfrey HP, Newman SA: Hidden in plain sight. *Borrelia burgdorferi* and the extracellular matrix. *Trends Microbiol* 15:350–354; 2007.

CDC: Recommendations for test performance and interpretation from the Second National Conference on Serologic Diagnosis of Lyme Disease. *MMWR Morb Mortal Wkly Rep* 44:590–591; 1995.

CDC: Recommendations for the use of Lyme disease vaccine. Recommendations of the Advisory Committee on Immunization Practices (ACIP). *MMWR Recomm Rep* 48:1–17, 21–25; 1999.

CDC: Lyme disease. United States, 2003–2005. *MMWR Morb Mortal Wkly Rep* 56:573–576; 2007.

Chen J, Field JA, Glickstein L, Molloy PJ, Huber BT, Steere AC: Association of antibiotic treatment-resistant Lyme arthritis with T cell responses to dominant epitopes of outer surface protein A of *Borrelia burgdorferi*. *Arthritis Rheum* 42:1813–1822; 1999.

Coburn J, Medrano M, Cugini C: *Borrelia burgdorferi* and its tropisms for adhesion molecules in the joint. *Curr Opin Rheumatol* 14:394–398; 2002.

Coburn J, Fischer JR, Leong JM: Solving a sticky problem: new genetic approaches to host cell adhesion by the Lyme disease spirochete. *Mol Microbiol* 57:1182–1195; 2005.

Cristofaro RL, Appel MH, Gelb RI, Williams CL: Musculoskeletal manifestations of Lyme disease in children. *J Pediatr Orthop* 7:527–530; 1987.

Dattwyler RJ, Halperin JJ, Volkman DJ, Luft BJ: Treatment of late Lyme borreliosis. Randomised comparison of ceftriaxone and penicillin. *Lancet* 1:1191–1194; 1988.

De Koning J, Bosma RB, Hoogkamp-Korstanje JA: Demonstration of spirochaetes in patients with Lyme disease with a modified silver stain. *J Med Microbiol* 23:261–267; 1987.

Dressler F, Yoshinari NH, Steere AC: The T-cell proliferative assay in the diagnosis of Lyme disease. *Ann Intern Med* 115:533–539; 1991.

Eckman MH, Steere AC, Kalish RA, Pauker SG: Cost effectiveness of oral as compared with intravenous antibiotic therapy for patients with early Lyme disease or Lyme arthritis. *N Engl J Med* 337:357–363; 1997.

Ecklund K, Vargas, S., Zurakowski D, Sundel RP: MRI features of Lyme arthritis in children. *AJR Am J Roentgenol* 184:1904–1909; 2005.

Feder HM Jr, Beran J, Van Hoecke C, Abraham B, De Clercq N, Buscarino C, Parenti, D L: Immunogenicity of a recombinant *Borrelia burgdorferi* outer surface protein A vaccine against Lyme disease in children. *J Pediatr* 135:575–579; 1999.

Feder HM Jr, Johnson BJ, O'Connell S, Shapiro ED, Steere AC, Wormser GP, Agger WA, Artsob H, Auwaerter P, Dumler JS, Bakken JS, Bockenstedt LK, Green J, Dattwyler RJ, Munoz J, Nadelman RB, Schwartz I, Draper, T., McSweegan E, Halperin JJ, Klempner MS, Krause PJ, Mead P, Morshed M, Porwancher R, Radolf JD, Smith RP Jr, Sood S, Weinstein A, Wong SJ, Zemel L: A critical appraisal of "chronic Lyme disease". *N Engl J Med* 357:1422–1430; 2007.

Fikrig E, Liu B, Fu LL, Das S, Smallwood JI, Flavell RA, Persing DH, Schoen RT, Barthold SW, Malawista SE: An ospA frame shift, identified from DNA in Lyme arthritis synovial fluid, results in an outer surface protein A that does not bind protective antibodies. *J Immunol* 155:5700–5704; 1995.

Franz JK, Fritze O, Rittig M, Keysser G, Priem S, Zacher J, Burmester GR, Krause A: Insights from a novel three-dimensional in vitro model of lyme arthritis. Standardized analysis of cellular and molecular interactions between *Borrelia burgdorferi* and synovial explants and fibroblasts. *Arthritis Rheum* 44:151–162; 2001.

Frey M, Jaulhac B, Piemont Y, Marcellin L, Boohs PM, Vautravers P, Jesel M, Kuntz, J.L, Monteil H, Sibila J: Detection of *Borrelia burgdorferi* DNA in muscle of patients with chronic myalgia related to Lyme disease. *Am J Med* 104:591–594; 1998.

Gasser R, Wendelin I, Reisinger E, Bergloff J, Feigl B, Schafhalter I, Eber B, Grisold M, Klein W: Roxithromycin in the treatment of Lyme disease–update and perspectives. *Infection* 23(suppl 1): S39–S43; 1995.

Gerber MA, Shapiro ED, Burke GS, Parcells VJ, Bell GL:, Lyme disease in children in southeastern Connecticut Pediatric Lyme Disease Study Group. *N Engl J Med* 335:1270–1274; 1996.

Gerber MA, Zemel LS, Shapiro ED: Lyme arthritis in children. Clinical epidemiology and long-term outcomes. *Pediatrics* 102:905–908; 1998.

Girschick HJ, Huppertz HI, Russmann H, Krenn V, Karch H: Intracellular persistence of *Borrelia burgdorferi* in human synovial cells. *Rheumatol Int* 16:125–132; 1996.

Glatzel A, Entschladen F, Zollner TM, Kraiczy P, Brade V, Kaufmann R, Janssen O, Lengl-Janssen B, Wesch D, Kabelitz D: The responsiveness of human V delta 1 gamma delta T cells to *Borrelia burgdorferi* is largely restricted to synovial-fluid cells from patients with Lyme arthritis. *J Infect Dis* 186:1043–1046; 2002.

Gondolf KB, Mihatsch M, Curschellas E, Dunn JJ, Batsford SR: Induction of experimental allergic arthritis with outer surface proteins of *Borrelia burgdorferi*. *Arthritis Rheum* 37:1070–1077; 1994.

Gross DM, Forsthuber T, Tary-Lehmann M, Etling C, Ito K, Nagy ZA, Field JA, Steere AC, Huber BT: Identification of LFA-1 as a candidate autoantigen in treatment-resistant Lyme arthritis. *Science* 281:703–706; 1998.

Hammers-Berggren S, Andersson U, Stiernstedt G: *Borrelia* arthritis in Swedish children: Clinical manifestations in 10 children. *Acta Paediatr* 81:921–924; 1992.

Hansen K, Hovmark A, Lebech AM, Lebech K, Olsson I, Halkier-Sorensen L, Olsson E, Asbrink E: Roxithromycin in Lyme borreliosis: Discrepant results of an in vitro and in vivo animal susceptibility study and a clinical trial in patients with erythema migrans. *Acta Derm Venereol* 72:297–300; 1992.

Häupl T, Hahn G, Rittig M, Krause A, Schoerner C, Schonherr U, Kalden JR, Burmester GR: Persistence of *Borrelia burgdorferi* in ligamentous tissue from a patient with chronic Lyme borreliosis. *Arthritis Rheum* 36:1621–1626; 1993.

Hendrickx G, De Boeck H, Goossens A, Demanet C, Vandenplas Y: Persistent synovitis in children with Lyme arthritis: two unusual cases. An immunogenetic approach. *Eur J Pediatr* 163:646–650; 2004.

Herzer P: Joint manifestations of Lyme borreliosis in Europe. *Scand J Infect Dis* 77(suppl): 55–63; 1991.

Hilton E, Tramontano A, Devoti J, Sood SK: Temporal study of immunoglobin M seroreactivity to *Borrelia burgdorferi* in patients treated for Lyme borreliosis. *J Clin Microbiol* 35:774–776; 1997.

Hoffmann JC, Stichtenoth DO, Zeidler H, Follmann M, Brandis A, Stanek G, Wollenhaupt J: Lyme disease in a 74-year-old forest owner with symptoms of dermatomyositis. *Arthritis Rheum* 38:1157–1160; 1995.

Holl-Wieden A, Suerbaum S, Girschick HJ: Seronegative Lyme arthritis. *Rheumatol Int* 27:1091–1093; 2007.

Huppertz HI, Karch H: Die Lyme-Arthritis im Kindesalter: Monarthritis des Kniegelenks, klinisch nicht unterscheidbar von Monarthritiden unbekannter Ursache. *Monatsschr Kinderheilkd* 139:759–764; 1991.

Huppertz HI, Michels H: Pattern of joint involvement in children with Lyme arthritis. *Br J Rheumatol* 35:1016–1018; 1996.

Huppertz HI, Dressler F: Lyme disease. *In* Cassidy JT, Petty RE, Laxer RM, Lindsley CB (eds): *Textbook of Pediatric Rheumatology*, 6th ed. Philadelphia, Elsevier Saunders; 2010, pp. 579–590.

Huppertz HI, Karch H, Heesemann J: Diagnostic value of synovial fluid analysis in children with reactive arthritis. *Rheumatol Int* 15:167–170; 1995a.

Huppertz HI, Karch H, Suschke HJ, Doring E, Ganser G, Thon A, Bentas W: Lyme arthritis in European children and adolescents. The Pediatric Rheumatology Collaborative Group. *Arthritis Rheum* 38:361–368; 1995b.

Huppertz HI, Mosbauer S, Busch DH, Karch H: Lymphoproliferative responses to *Borrelia burgdorferi* in the diagnosis of Lyme arthritis in children and adolescents. *Eur J Pediatr* 155:297–302; 1996.

Huppertz HI, Bentas W, Haubitz I, Girschick HJ, Ganser G, Thon A, Suschke HJ, Schauer-Petrowskaja C, Minden K, Schuchmann L: Diagnosis of paediatric Lyme arthritis using a clinical score. *Eur J Pediatr* 157:304–308; 1998.

Huppertz HI, Bohme M, Standaert SM, Karch H, Plotkin SA: Incidence of Lyme borreliosis in the Wurzburg region of Germany. *Eur J Clin Microbiol Infect Dis* 18:697–703; 1999a.

Huppertz HI, Munchmeier D, Lieb W: Ocular manifestations in children and adolescents with Lyme arthritis. *Br J Ophthalmol* 83:1149–1152; 1999b.

Iliopoulou BP, Alroy J, Huber BT: Persistent arthritis in *Borrelia burgdorferi*-infected HLA-DR4-positive CD28-negative mice post-antibiotic treatment. *Arthritis Rheum* 58:3892–3901; 2008.

Iliopoulou BP, Guerau-De-Arellano M, Huber BT: HLA-DR alleles determine responsiveness to *Borrelia burgdorferi* antigens in a mouse model of self-perpetuating arthritis. *Arthritis Rheum* 60:3831–3840; 2009.

Jaulhac B, Chary-Valckenaere I, Sibilia J, Javier RM, Piemont Y, Kuntz JL, Monteil H, Pourel J: Detection of *Borrelia burgdorferi* by DNA amplification in synovial tissue samples from patients with Lyme arthritis. *Arthritis Rheum* 39:736–745; 1996.

Johnston YE, Duray PH, Steere AC, Kashgarian M, Buza J, Malawista SE, Askenase PW: Lyme arthritis. Spirochetes found in synovial microangiopathic lesions. *Am J Pathol* 118:26–34; 1985.

Jones KL, Seward RJ, Ben-Menachem G, Glickstein LJ, Costello CE, Steere AC: Strong IgG antibody responses to *Borrelia burgdorferi* glycolipids in patients with Lyme arthritis, a late manifestation of the infection. *Clin Immunol* 132:93–102; 2009.

Kalish RA, Leong JM, Steere AC: Association of treatment-resistant chronic Lyme arthritis with HLA-DR4 and antibody reactivity to OspA and OspB of *Borrelia burgdorferi. Infect Immun* 61:2774–2779; 1993.

Kalish RS, Wood JA, Golde W, Bernard R, Davis LE, Grimson RC, Coyle PK, Luft BJ: Human T lymphocyte response to *Borrelia burgdorferi* infection. No correlation between human leukocyte function antigen type 1 peptide response and clinical status. *J Infect Dis* 187:102–108; 2003.

Kamradt T, Lengl-Janssen B, Strauss AF, Bansal G, Steere AC: Dominant recognition of a *Borrelia burgdorferi* outer surface protein A peptide by T helper cells in patients with treatment-resistant Lyme arthritis. *Infect Immun* 64:1284–1289; 1996.

Luft BJ, Dattwyler RJ, Johnson RC, Luger SW, Bosler EM, Rahn DW, Masters EJ, Grunwaldt E, Gadgil SD: Azithromycin compared with amoxicillin in the treatment of erythema migrans. A double-blind, randomized, controlled trial. *Ann Intern Med* 124:785–791; 1996.

Marlovits S, Khanakah G, Striessnig G, Vecsei V, Stanek G: Emergence of lyme arthritis after autologous chondrocyte transplantation. *Arthritis Rheum* 50:259–264; 2004.

Ministry of Health of the Republic of Slovenia: *Epidemiological report on communicable diseases in Slovenia.* Ljubljana. Institute of Public Health of the Republic of Slovenia; 2008.

Nardelli DT, Callister SM, Schell RF: Lyme arthritis: current concepts and a change in paradigm. *Clin Vaccine Immunol* 15:21–34; 2008.

Oksi J, Mertsola J, Reunanen M, Marjamaki M, Viljanen MK: Subacute multiple-site osteomyelitis caused by *Borrelia burgdorferi. Clin Infect Dis* 19:891–896; 1994.

Priem S, Burmester GR, Kambradt T, Wolbart K, Rittig MG, Krause A: Detection of *Borrelia burgdorferi* by polymerase chain reaction in synovial membrane, but not in synovial fluid from patients with persisting Lyme arthritis after antibiotic therapy. *Ann Rheum Dis* 57:118–121; 1998.

Reimers CD, Neubert U, Kristoferitsch W, Pfluger KH, Mayr WR: *Borrelia burgdorferi* infection in Europe. An HLA-related disease? *Infection* 20:197–200; 1992.

Reimers CD, De Koning J, Neubert U, Preac-Mursic V, Koster JG, Muller-Felber W, Pongratz DE, Duray PH: *Borrelia burgdorferi* myositis: report of eight patients. *J Neurol* 240:278–283; 1993.

Roessner K, Wolfe J, Shi C, Sigal LH, Huber S, Budd RC: High expression of Fas ligand by synovial fluid-derived gamma delta T cells in Lyme arthritis. *J Immunol* 170:2702–2710; 2003.

Rose CD, Fawcett PT, Gibney KM, Doughty RA: Residual serologic reactivity in children with resolved Lyme arthritis. *J Rheumatol* 23:367–369; 1996.

Rutkowski S, Busch DH, Huppertz HI: Lymphocyte proliferation assay in response to *Borrelia burgdorferi* in patients with Lyme arthritis: Analysis of lymphocyte subsets. *Rheumatol Int* 17:151–158; 1997.

Schnarr S, Wahl A, Jurgens-Saathoff B, Mengel M, Kreipe HH, Zeidler H: Nodular fasciitis, erythema migrans, and oligoarthritis. Manifestations of Lyme borreliosis caused by *Borrelia afzelii. Scand J Rheumatol* 31:184–186; 2002.

Schoen RT, Aversa JM, Rahn DW, Steere AC: Treatment of refractory chronic Lyme arthritis with arthroscopic synovectomy. *Arthritis Rheum* 34:1056–1060; 1991.

Shin JJ, Glickstein LJ, Steere AC: High levels of inflammatory chemokines and cytokines in joint fluid and synovial tissue throughout the course of antibiotic-refractory lyme arthritis. *Arthritis Rheum* 56:1325–1335; 2007.

Sigal LH: Musculoskeletal manifestations of Lyme arthritis. *Rheum Dis Clin North Am* 24:323–351; 1998a.

Sigal LH: Pitfalls in the diagnosis and management of Lyme disease. *Arthritis Rheum* 41:195–204; 1998b.

Sigal LH, Patella SJ: Lyme arthritis as the incorrect diagnosis in pediatric and adolescent fibromyalgia. *Pediatrics* 90:523–528; 1992.

Sigal LH, Zahradnik JM, Lavin P, Patella SJ, Bryant G, Haselby R, Hilton E, Kunkel M, Adler-Klein D, Doherty T, Evans J, Molloy PJ, Seidner AL, Sabetta JR, Simon HJ, Klempner MS, Mays J, Marks D, Malawista SE: A vaccine consisting of recombinant *Borrelia burgdorferi* outer-surface protein A to prevent Lyme disease. Recombinant Outer-Surface Protein A Lyme Disease Vaccine Study Consortium. *N Engl J Med* 339:216–222; 1998.

Snydman DR, Schenkein DP, Berardi VP, Lastavica CC, Pariser KM: *Borrelia burgdorferi* in joint fluid in chronic Lyme arthritis. *Ann Intern Med* 104:798–800; 1986.

Sood SK, Ilowite NT: Lyme arthritis in children. Is chronic arthritis a common complication? *J Rheumatol* 27:1836–1838; 2000.

Stanek G, Strle F: Lyme borreliosis. *Lancet* 362:1639–1647; 2003.

Stanek G, Fingerle V, Hunfeld KP, Jaulhac B, Kaiser R, Krause A, Kristoferitsch W, O'Connell S, Ornstein K, Strle F, Gray J: Lyme borreliosis. Clinical case definitions for diagnosis and management in Europe. *Clin Microbiol Infect;* 17(1):69–79; 2011.

Steere AC: Lyme disease. *N Engl J Med* 345:115–125; 2001.

Steere AC, Angelis SM: Therapy for Lyme arthritis. Strategies for the treatment of antibiotic-refractory arthritis. *Arthritis Rheum* 54:3079–3086; 2006.

Steere AC, Glickstein L: Elucidation of Lyme arthritis. *Nat Rev Immunol* 4:143–152; 2004.

Steere AC, Malawista SE, Snydman DR, Shope RE, Andiman WA, Ross MR, Steele FM: Lyme arthritis. An epidemic of oligoarticular arthritis in children and adults in three connecticut communities. *Arthritis Rheum* 20:7–17; 1977.

Steere AC, Grodzicki RL, Kornblatt AN, Craft JE, Barbour AG, Burgdorfer W, Schmid GP, Johnson E, Malawista SE: The spirochetal etiology of Lyme disease. *N Engl J Med* 308:733–740; 1983.

Steere AC, Schoen RT, Taylor E: The clinical evolution of Lyme arthritis. *Ann Intern Med* 107:725–731; 1987.

Steere AC, Levin RE, Molloy PJ, Kalish RA, Abraham J.H. III, Liu NY, Schmid CH: Treatment of Lyme arthritis. *Arthritis Rheum* 37:878–888; 1994.

Steere AC, Sikand VK, Meurice F, Parenti DL, Fikrig E, Schoen RT, Nowakowski J, Schmid CH, Laukamp S, Buscarino C, Krause DS: Vaccination against Lyme disease with recombinant *Borrelia burgdorferi* outer-surface lipoprotein A with adjuvant. Lyme Disease Vaccine Study Group. *N Engl J Med* 339:209–215; 1998.

Steere AC, Gross D, Meyer AL, Huber BT: Autoimmune mechanisms in antibiotic treatment-resistant lyme arthritis. *J Autoimmun* 16:263–268; 2001.

Steere AC, Falk B, Drouin EE, Baxter-Lowe LA, Hammer J, Nepom GT: Binding of outer surface protein A and human lymphocyte function-associated antigen 1 peptides to HLA-DR molecules associated with antibiotic treatment-resistant Lyme arthritis. *Arthritis Rheum* 48:534–540; 2003.

Szer IS, Taylor E, Steere AC: The long-term course of Lyme arthritis in children. *N Engl J Med* 325:159–163; 1991.

Thompson A, Mannix R, Bachur R: Acute pediatric monoarticular arthritis. Distinguishing lyme arthritis from other etiologies. *Pediatrics* 123:959–965; 2009.

Tory HO, Zurakowski D, Sundel RP: Outcomes of children treated for Lyme arthritis: Results of a large pediatric cohort. *J Rheumatol* 37:1049–1055; 2010.

Tugwell P, Dennis DT, Weinstein A, Wells G, Shea B, Nichol G, Hayward R, Lightfoot R, Baker P, Steere AC: Laboratory evaluation in the diagnosis of Lyme disease. *Ann Intern Med* 127:1109–1123; 1997.

Valesova M, Trnavsky K: Joint manifestations of Lyme borreliosis in Czechoslovakian patients. *Z Rheumatol* 49:192–196; 1990.

Wormser GP, Dattwyler RJ, Shapiro ED, Halperin JJ, Steere AC, Klempner MS, Krause PJ, Bakken JS, Strle F, Stanek G, Bockenstedt L, Fish D, Dumler JS, Nadelman RB: The clinical assessment, treatment, and prevention of lyme disease, human granulocytic anaplasmosis, and babesiosis. Clinical practice guidelines by the Infectious Diseases Society of America. *Clin Infect Dis* 43:1089–1134; 2006.

Zoschke DC, Skemp AA, Defosse DL: Lymphoproliferative responses to *Borrelia burgdorferi* in Lyme disease. *Ann Intern Med* 114:285–289; 1991.

7

BORRELIAL LYMPHOCYTOMA AND ACRODERMATITIS CHRONICA ATROPHICANS

Mark B. Salzman and Robert R. Müllegger

INTRODUCTION AND ETIOLOGY

The skin is the most frequently affected tissue in Lyme borreliosis. There are three distinct skin manifestations: erythema migrans (EM), borrelial lymphocytoma (BL), and acrodermatitis chronica atrophicans (ACA). Together these are sometimes referred to as dermatoborrelioses. EM, the hallmark of early Lyme borreliosis, is the only common skin manifestation and is discussed elsewhere. BL and ACA occur in Europe, and it is extremely rare for them to be encountered in North America.

In Europe there are three genospecies of *Borrelia burgdorferi* sensu lato that have been clearly established to be pathogenic and have been associated with Lyme borreliosis: *B. afzelii*, *B. garinii,* and *B. burgdorferi* sensu stricto (Picken et al., 1998). *Borrelia burgdorferi* sensu stricto causes borreliosis both in North America and in Europe, but *B. afzelii* and *B. garinii* occur only in Europe and parts of Asia (Strle et al., 1997). Although the vast majority of ACA and many of the BLs are caused by *B. afzelii*, *B. burgdorferi* sensu

Lyme Borreliosis in Europe and North America: Epidemiology and Clinical Practice, First Edition. Edited by Sunil K. Sood

stricto has been detected in skin lesions of patients with BL and ACA (Picken et al., 1997b; Maraspin et al., 2002). Among 85 adult patients in Slovenia with BL, 11/46 (23.9%) were confirmed by culture. Eight of the nine typed strains were *B. afzelii* and one was *B. bissettii* (Maraspin et al., 2002). Among 22 isolates from 21 patients with ACA from Slovenia who had skin biopsies for culture, 17 were *B. afzelii,* 4 were *B. garinii*, and one was *B. burgdorferi* sensu stricto (Picken et al., 1998).

In contrast, in a study of 25 skin biopsies from mainly German patients, the two BL isolates were both identified as *B. garinii* species, and all six of the ACA isolates were grouped into *B. afzelii* species (Busch et al., 1996). Additional studies from central Europe and unpublished observations of one of the authors (RM) in Austria indicate that ACA skin lesions there are exclusively caused by *B. afzelii* (Wienecke et al., 1994; Lunemann et al., 2001). Ohlenbusch et al., using PCR in patients from Germany, compared genospecies from 7 patients with ACA, 11 with EM, and 17 with cerebrospinal fluid (CSF) specimens (Ohlenbusch et al., 1996). They also typed isolates from 47 infected ticks in the same region. Sixty-six percent of the infected ticks harbored *B. garinii*, 28% *B. afzelii*, and 6% *B. burgdorferi* sensu stricto. However, all 7 of the ACA lesions yielded *B. afzelii*. Among the 11 EM lesions, 5 (46%) were caused by *B. garinii,* 4 (29%) by *B. afzelii*, and 2 (18%) by *B. burgdorferi* sensu stricto. Among the 17 CSF specimens, 65% were *B. garinii,* 29% were *B. afzelii*, and 6% were *B. burgdorferi* sensu stricto. Thus the genospecies from CSF specimens and EM lesions mirrored the prevalence of infection in the tick population, but only *B. afzelii* was associated with persistent ACA lesions. Similarly Fingerle et al. found that the most common *B. burgdorferi* sensu lato species in 475 ticks from southern Germany was *B. garinii* (34%), whereas *B. afzelii*, which was present in only 25% of tick samples, was the dominant subtype in the skin (67%) (Fingerle et al., 2008). Again, *B. garinii* was detected most often in CSF. Lenormand et al. (Lenormand et al., 2009) reported that among 9 patients (8 adults and 1 child) from France with BL between 1994 and 2007, three were caused by *B. afzelii*, one by *B. garinii*, and one by *B. burgdorferi* sensu stricto, using PCR evidence. Only *B. garinii* was also identified by culture. The patient with the *B. burgdorferi* sensu stricto had negative serology. In a study from Mexico (Gordillo-Perez et al., 2007), two patients with BL were reported, with *B. burgdorferi* sensu stricto identified by PCR in one of the cases. In a study from Austria (Müllegger et al., 2007), 8 of 9 BL cases were *B. afzelii* by PCR and one was *B. burgdorferi* sensu stricto. Among 19 ACA cases, 15 were *B. afzelii*, 2 *B. burgdorferi* sensu stricto, and 2 mixed *B. afzelii*/*B. burgdorferi* sensu stricto.

We can conclude from all these studies that *B. afzelii* is the etiology of the vast majority, if not the only etiology, of ACA lesions, whereas at least two genospecies (*B. afzelii* and *B. garinii*) cause BL. Although *B. afzelii* accounted for 8 of 9 isolates from the BL lesions in Slovenia and 8 of 9 isolates from BL lesions in Austria, this may just represent the prevalence of *B. afzelii* in the tick population in those regions. Whether *B. burgdorferi* sensu stricto can be the etiology of either ACA or BL is unclear given the rare reports of its identification in either lesion. Even if it can, the very uncommon occurrence would explain the near absence of these lesions in North America. Discordance between the prevalence of different genospecies of *B. burgdorferi* sensu lato in ticks and the lesional skin of patients, particularly the predominance of *B. afzelii* in ACA, point to the importance of host factors in the outcome of *Borrelia* infection.

BORRELIAL LYMPHOCYTOMA

History

Spiegler in 1894 and Fendt in 1900 first described a lesion that became known as pseudolymphoma of Spiegler and Fendt (Spiegler, 1894; Fendt, 1900). In 1921, Kaufmann-Wolf described scrotal nodules in children, which were termed lymphocytoma cutis (Kaufmann-Wolf, 1921). It became known as lymphadenosis benigna cutis after its description by Bäfverstadt in 1943 (Bäfverstedt, 1943). It was also called lymphadenosis benigna cutis solitaria. Four decades later in 1983, one year after Willy Burgdorfer discovered *B. burgdorferi*, spirochetes were demonstrated in silver stain sections of skin biopsies from lymphadenosis benigna cutis and ACA (Frithz and Lagerholm, 1983). In 1986, *B. burgdorferi* was isolated from a lymphadenosis benigna cutis skin biopsy (Hovmark et al., 1986). Within a few years of this association of the lesion with borreliosis, it became known as BL instead of lymphadenosis benigna cutis.

Incidence

BL is an uncommon manifestation of Lyme borreliosis and occurs more commonly in children than in adults. In a study of 1471 cases of Lyme borreliosis over a one-year period in Sweden (Berglund et al., 1995), 7% of children (16 cases) and 2% of adults (25 cases) had lymphocytoma. In contrast, 77% of all patients had EM. Similarly, in an Austrian series of more than 1000 patients with dermatoborrelioses, 5% had BL, two-thirds of whom were children (Müllegger, 2001). In Bulgaria, among 1257 patients with Lyme borreliosis, only 0.3% had either BL or ACA (Christova and Komitova, 2004).

Clinical Manifestations

BL presents clinically as a solitary erythematous plaque or nodule that typically is bluish-red in color and usually presents on the ear (lobe) or breast (Figure 7.1). The lesion ranges in size from 1 to 5 centimeters (Müllegger, 2004). In general, there are no local symptoms. BL may arise in the vicinity of a previous or concurrent EM lesion (Müllegger, 2004). Although its clinical presentation is very characteristic, in particular at the sites mentioned above, it may be misdiagnosed as cellulitis or perichondritis. Other differential diagnoses include cutaneous lymphomas or other malignancies, keloids, lupus erythematosus, sarcoidosis, arthropod bite or foreign body granuloma, granulomatous contact metal dermatitis to earrings, and granuloma annulare. Breast lesions in adults may cause concern about a possible malignancy.

In a study of 8 children from Germany, the lymphocytoma developed between 1 and 6 months after the tick bite, and the correct diagnosis was made a mean of 1.8 months after its appearance with a range of 1 week to 3 months (Pohl-Koppe et al., 1998). Although it is often considered an early disseminated stage infection, it is frequently present at the site of a tick bite and may develop at the site of a previous EM lesion (Müllegger, 2004). Therefore it may represent a localized infection with a longer incubation period and longer course than EM, and one that eventually resolves spontaneously. When present at

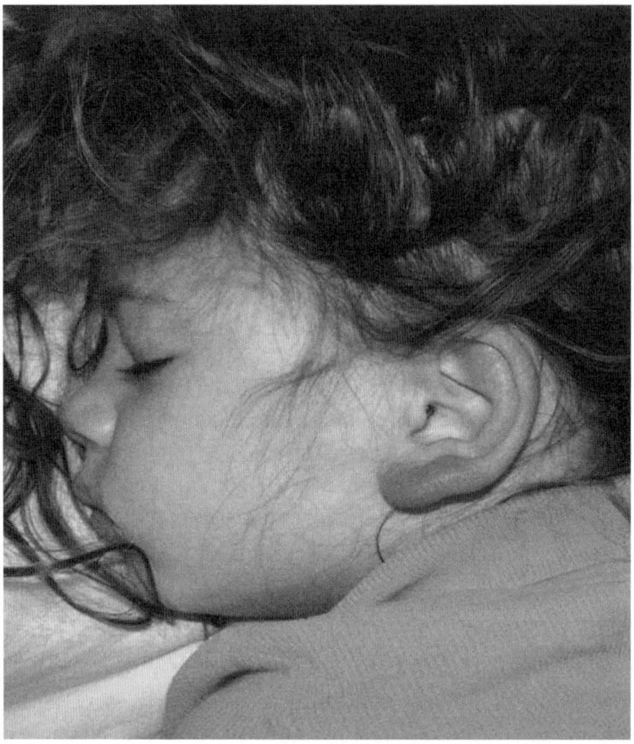

Figure 7.1 Borrelial lymphocytoma. Five-year-old girl from southern California who, while visiting Norway in August 2006, had a tick removed from her left ear lobe. Two months later she had a painful red bump at the site of the tick bite which increased in size over the next several months. Two-tier serology for *B. burgdorferi* infection was positive in the United States and the lesion slowly resolved after a 30-day course of amoxicillin. (*See insert for color representation*).

a site where there was no known tick bite, it may represent either early disseminated or localized infection, as a tick-bite history is commonly negative in BL patients (Müllegger, 2004).

The ear lobe and the breast areola are the most common sites, with the ear lobe more common in children and the breast more common in adults. (Pohl-Koppe et al., 1998, Maraspin et al., 2002) Pohl-Koppe et al reported on 8 children and reviewed the literature on 25 additional pediatric cases and found that 23 of the 33 cases (70%) involved the earlobe or conchae with 7 of the 33 cases (21%) involving the breast (Pohl-Koppe et al., 1998). The children with breast involvement were older with a median age of 12 years. One of those patients had both ears and one areola involved. One patient had the left ear affected at the same time as an EM lesion on the left cheek. Atypical locations included the scrotum, nose, forearm, and temple. It was unclear if patients who had more than one lesion had more than one tick bite causing disease or had dissemination from a single tick bite. Among the 25 reviewed patients, 11 (44%) had a preceding EM lesion and one patient had multifocal EM at the same time as the lymphocytoma. Other occasional accompanying manifestations of Lyme borreliosis in children include seventh-nerve palsy, arthritis, and carditis (Asbrink et al., 1989).

Maraspin et al. reported on 85 adult patients from Slovenia with involvement of the breast areola in 68 (80%), the earlobe in 8 (9.4%) and other locations in nine (10.6%) (Maraspin et al., 2002). An EM lesion was present in 67 (78.8%). Six (7.1%) had multiple EM, one had meningitis, one meningoradiculitis and arthritis, one radiculoarthritis and arthritis, one seventh-nerve palsy and meningitis, and two arthritis. Thus, overall, 6 (7.1%) had extracutaneous disease. In addition one patient also had ACA. A problem with the descriptions of preceding or concomitant EM lesions is that they often lack direct proof of the etiologic agent. Austrian experience suggests that BL occurs as an independent lesion in the majority of cases.

Diagnosis

The diagnosis of BL should be confirmed by serological testing, biopsy, or both. A biopsy is unnecessary if the lesion is typical, for example, on the earlobe of a child who has positive serology or a concomitant EM lesion. Since the incubation period from the time of tick bite to the presentation of the lymphocytoma can range from 1 to 6 months (Pohl-Koppe et al., 1998; Maraspin et al., 2002; Müllegger, 2004), a patient with a shorter incubation period may present with negative serology. Serum IgG and/or IgM antibody titers are positive in at least two-thirds of pediatric and adult patients (Asbrink et al., 1989; Strle et al., 1992; Pohl-Koppe et al., 1998; Colli et al., 2004).

A biopsy is indicated if the lesions are other than on the earlobe, especially with lesions on the breast where malignancy is in the differential diagnosis. Histologically the lesion consists of a dense lymphocytic infiltration of the cutis and subcutis that is polyclonal with a predominance of B lymphocytes, usually with germinal centers (Colli et al., 2004). Isolation of the borrelial species can be attempted in select laboratories to confirm the diagnosis in equivocal cases (see Chapter 9). Because there is monoclonality in a small percentage of patients, the histopathologic picture may resemble cutaneous lymphoma, and sensitivity of direct detection methods (culture, PCR) is low. A careful correlation of all available diagnostic modalities is needed to make the correct diagnosis (Colli et al., 2004).

Treatment

Practice guidelines from the Infectious Diseases Society of America state that patients with BL should be treated with the same regimens that are recommended for EM (Wormser et al., 2006). Amoxicillin, cefuroxime, or doxycycline for 14 to 21 days are recommended. Macrolides such as azithromycin, clarithromycin, or erythromycin are inferior and should be reserved for patients who cannot tolerate first-line medications. Parenteral ceftriaxone should be reserved for treatment failures or when there are neurological manifestations or advanced atrioventricular heart block. Amoxicillin, cefuroxime, and doxycycline are first-line antibiotics in Europe as well, but there is a trend for 3 to 4 week treatment duration because of the subacute nature of the lesion (Müllegger, 2004). It should be noted that recommendations on both continents are based on small and uncontrolled studies.

Maraspin et al. treated 85 adults with doxycycline, azithromycin, amoxicillin, cefuroxime, phenoxymethylpenicillin (which is no longer recommended), or ceftriaxone (Maraspin et al., 2002). The median time to complete disappearance of the lymphocytoma was 28 days with a range of 7 to 270 days. Disappearance took longer in the patients who had the skin lesion for a prolonged duration prior to treatment. Treatment failure occurred in 11 (12.9%), who then underwent retreatment. Untreated lesions eventually resolve spontaneously in several months to beyond one year. Serologic follow-up is not necessary after treatment. Among patients who were treated, 25% to 50% remained seropositive two months later (Müllegger and Glatz, 2009).

ACRODERMATITIS CHRONICA ATROPHICANS

History

Acrodermatitis chronica atrophicans (ACA), also known as Pick–Herxheimer disease, was first described by Buchwald in Germany in 1883 (Buchwald, 1883) and then by Pick in 1894 (Pick, 1895). Herxheimer and Hartmann in 1902 described 12 cases and reviewed 14 other published cases (Herxheimer and Hartmann, 1902). They proposed the name ACA for a skin condition that started with an inflammatory stage on the extremities and had a year-long course. They also described the later stages as looking atrophic and like cigarette paper. In 1921 a case was described that started with severe left elbow pain that was followed about 6 months later by ACA (Jessner, 1921). This was probably the first association of arthritis and ACA. In 1946 Svarts described penicillin treatment of two patients with ACA of 5 to 6 years duration (Svarts, 1946). The effect of penicillin was remarkable, and an infection was postulated as the etiology. Hauser in 1955 observed that cases of ACA followed the distribution of sheep ticks, with most patients being from rural areas and very few cases in the cities (Hauser, 1955).

Asbrink et al. in 1984 recovered spirochetes from a skin lesion of a patient with ACA and concluded that it was probably the etiologic agent of ACA (Asbrink et al., 1984). The authors also stated that their findings were consistent with the hypothesis that the same spirochete caused both EM and ACA with ACA being a late manifestation.

Incidence

The incidence of ACA varies throughout Europe. Among 1471 patients with Lyme borreliosis in Sweden over a one-year period in 1992 to 1993, there were 47 cases (3.2%) of ACA (Berglund et al., 1995). In Bulgaria only 0.3% of patients had either BL or ACA (Christova and Komitova, 2004). In Norway, all manifestations of Lyme borreliosis except EM are reportable. During 1995 to 2004, 5% of 1506 cases were ACA (Nygard et al., 2005). However, since EM is the most common manifestation, this percentage would be much lower if cases of EM were included. The extrapolated incidence from 15 years of experience in Austria is 4 per 100,000 persons per year (Müllegger, 2004).

ACA is rarely seen in North America. In a retrospective study from the Mayo Clinic in Rochester, Minnesota, 6 patients between 1912 and 1961 were identified in the dermatology files with the diagnosis of ACA. All 5 patients from whom biological data were available were European immigrants (DiCaudo et al., 1994). Other presumed cases of ACA in the United States were reported from California, New York, and eastern Pennsylvania (Lavoie et al., 1986; Kaufman et al., 1989; Edwards et al., 1992; Smetanick et al., 2010).

Clinical Manifestations

ACA is a late manifestation of Lyme borreliosis. It is more common in women, and most patients are older than 40 years but cases in children have been described (Nadal et al., 1988; Zalaudek et al., 2005). It develops months to years after a tick bite. In 9 of 50 (18%) Swedish patients, there was a history of EM on the same extremity 0.5 to 8 years earlier (Asbrink et al., 1986). It is most often located on the extensor surfaces of the hands, feet, or other distal extremity. It starts with localized swelling, which may be painful, often with a slightly bluish-red discoloration that is usually unilateral but can be bilateral (Figure 7.2). Sometimes the erythema can be mild and swelling may dominate the clinical picture, and the patient may be misdiagnosed with venous stasis or lymphedema. The lesion slowly enlarges and may spread to additional extremities over months to years or even decades. Initially the lesions may develop slowly and insidiously with waxing and waning of the erythema and swelling (Figure 7.3). Atrophy develops as the edema subsides gradually over many years. The skin may become violaceous, thin, wrinkled, and translucent and has been described as cigarette paper-like. The veins may appear prominent as the result of the

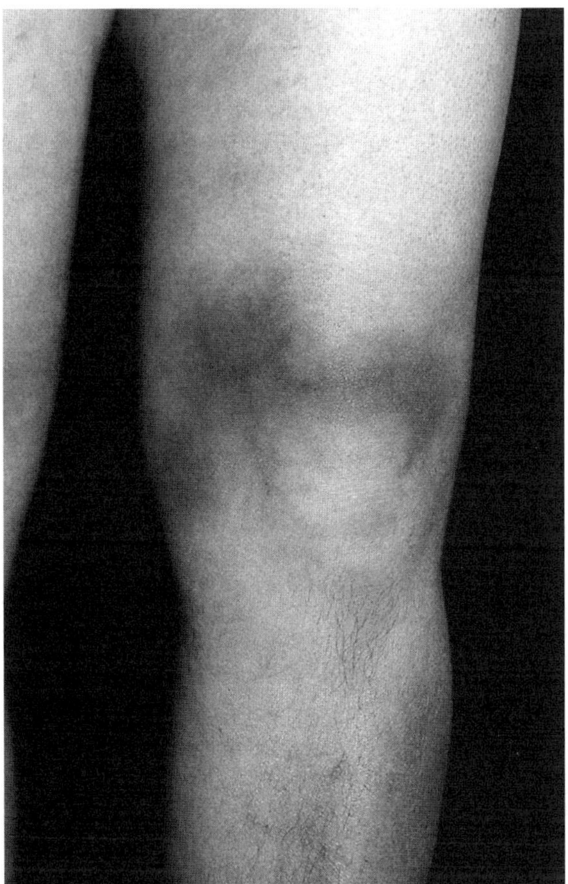

Figure 7.2 Acrodermatitis chronica atrophicans. Example of the acute stage (disease duration <3 months) around the knee of a 50-year-old male patient. (*See insert for color representation*).

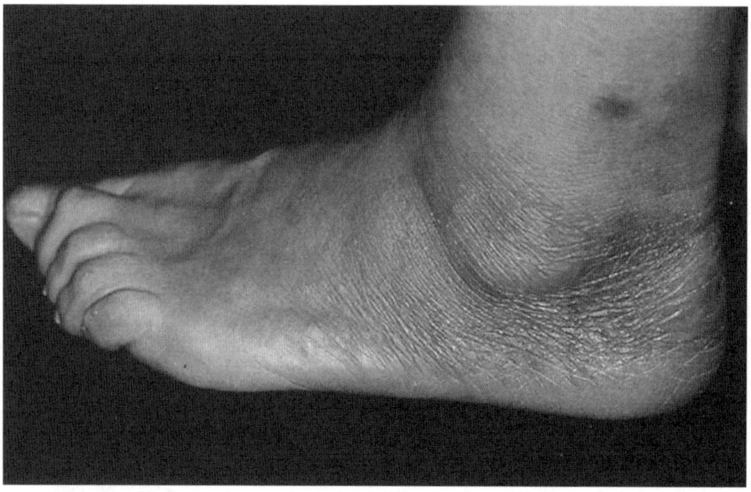

Figure 7.3 Acrodermatitis chronica atrophicans. Example of a subacute stage (3–6 months disease duration) on the ankle. Note co-existence of inflammatory erythema and swelling, and atrophy of the skin. (*See insert for color representation*).

translucency of the atrophic skin and patients may be misdiagnosed with phlebitis or venous insufficiency (Asbrink, 1991) (Figure 7.4).

Fibrotic nodules may develop, often over the elbows and knees or fibrotic bands over the extensor surfaces of the distal arms or legs and may be confused with rheumatic nodules (Asbrink, 1993). Sclerotic lesions resembling scleroderma develop in 10% to 20% of

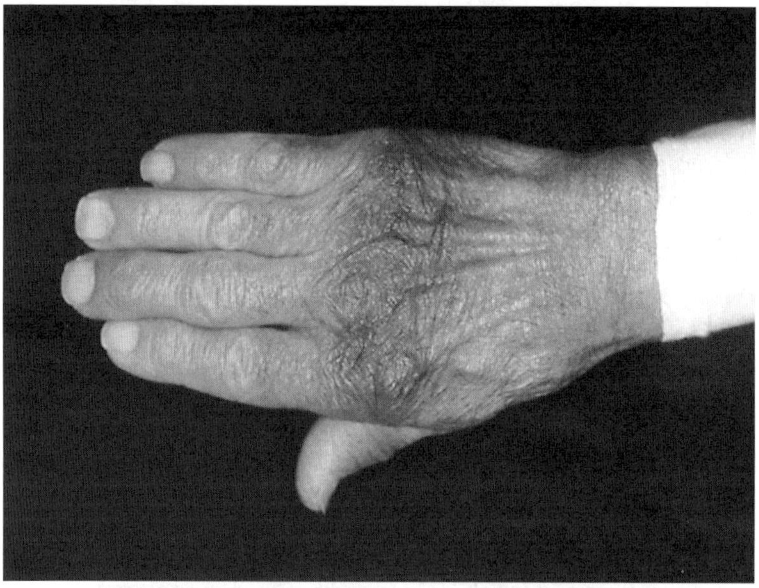

Figure 7.4 Acrodermatitis chronica atrophicans. Example of a chronic stage of ACA (>6 months disease duration) on the hand of a 75-year-old male patient. Note the significant atrophy of skin overlying the knuckles and the bluish-red discoloration and prominent appearance of blood vessels. (*See insert for color representation*).

patients (Asbrink, 1991; Müllegger, 2004). Minor trauma to the skin heals slowly. Pain and/or paresthesia may be present. The pain may be exaggerated and muscle weakness and cramps can occur. The pain is sometimes severe and usually intermittent. These signs and symptoms may be mistaken for dermatomyositis (Asbrink, 1991).

A peripheral neuropathy of mild to moderate severity develops in about 60% of patients (Kindstrand et al., 1997). This is usually sensory, but a motor neuropathy can occur and usually follows the distribution of the cutaneous ACA lesions. Neuropathy sometimes occurs on limbs without visible signs of ACA. Sural nerve biopsies have revealed axonal degeneration with perivascular infiltration with lymphocytes and plasma cells and obliteration of the epineural vasa nervorum (Asbrink, 1993). It has been postulated that this vasculitis of epineural vessels causes ischemic nerve damage. However, since the neuropathy usually follows the distribution of cutaneous ACA lesions, the damage is more likely due to the borrelial infection and an accompanying inflammatory response (Kindstrand et al., 2000).

Musculoskeletal pain with involvement of the bones and joints can occur, especially with long-standing disease. This is especially true of the bony prominences overlying the ACA lesions such as the knuckles, olecranon, and malleoli (Asbrink, 1993). Knee arthritis has been found to precede the lesion or occur simultaneously in about 20% of ACA patients (Asbrink, 1991). Other manifestations include subluxations of the small joints of the hands and feet, olecranon bursitis, epicondylitis, Achilles tendonitis, and periosteal bone thickening usually underlying the ACA lesions (Müllegger, 2004). Nonspecific symptoms such as headache, myalgia, fatigue, weight loss, and neuropsychiatric symptoms have been described (Müllegger, 2004).

Pediatric cases of ACA are extremely rare (Nadal et al., 1988). A 15-year-old girl from Austria with bluish-red skin changes that initially occurred over her left knee with moderate swelling was misdiagnosed as venous insufficiency for 6 years. Over the 6 years her disease spread down to the pretibial region and later involved both elbows. Eventually there was marked atrophy that did not fully resolve with 6 weeks of oral doxycycline (Zalaudek et al., 2005). Another case report involved an 11-year-old girl from Germany who had ACA involving all 4 limbs for 2 years that eventually involved her trunk (Brzonova et al., 2002). She had a history of a tick bite without erythema migrans 5 years previous to presentation. After a 4 week course of intravenous ceftriaxone, slow improvement occurred and eventually her skin normalized. Clinicians should keep ACA in the differential diagnosis of suggestive skin changes in children because delayed initiation of therapy may lead to irreversible skin changes.

Diagnosis

As the clinical appearance of ACA is not distinctive, the diagnosis should always be supported by serology, and confirmed by histopathology given the possibility of false-positive serology (Asbrink et al., 1986). The diagnosis should be considered in a patient with an acral bluish-red discoloration or swelling with or without atrophy of the skin especially in an older woman from northern, central, or eastern Europe (Asbrink, 1991). Patients are always seropositive (IgG antibodies); a negative serology rules out the diagnosis of ACA (Asbrink et al., 1986). It is therefore difficult to reconcile case reports of seronegative ACA with DNA detection by PCR (Berger et al., 2003).

If a biopsy is taken, a pronounced patchy or band-like lymphohistiocytic infiltration of the dermis is present with a variable admixture of plasma cells (Asbrink et al., 1986, Colli et al., 2004). The subcutaneous fat is frequently involved with this inflammatory cell infiltration. The density of the cell infiltrates, including the number of plasma cells, is related to the stage of disease. In the acute phase of the disease, the infiltrate is intense but decreases later in the course (Colli et al., 2004). During this chronic stage, atrophy of the epidermis (thinning and loss of rete redges) and dermis (reduction of collagen and elastic fibers) are typically found. The presence of telangiectases, both blood vessels and lymphatics, may be a prominent feature (Brehmer-Andersson, 1993). In addition vacuoles resembling fat cells have been observed in the dermis, often close to the epidermis, in a number of cases. In atypical or difficult cases, isolation of *Borrelia* or detection of *Borrelia*-specific DNA by PCR from skin lesions can be attempted, but the sensitivity is low (Asbrink et al., 1984; Rijpkema et al., 1997; Picken et al., 1997a) (see Chapter 9).

Treatment

No prospective randomized trials of therapy for ACA have been conducted. Practice guidelines from the Infectious Diseases Society of America recommend a 21-day course of doxycycline, amoxicillin, or cefuroxime (Wormser et al., 2006). As with EM, macrolides such as azithromycin are inferior and should be reserved for patients who are unable to take first-line medications. In Europe the same antibiotics are recommended as first-line treatment, but minocycline, ceftriaxone, cefotaxime, and oral or parenteral penicillin have also been used with success, and the duration of therapy is emphasized over the route of administration (Müllegger, 2004). Parenteral therapy has not been shown to be superior to oral therapy, but a 4-week course may be superior to 2 weeks. For example, Aberer et al. compared 14 patients treated with ceftriaxone for 15 days with 32 patients treated orally with penicillin or doxycycline for 20 to 30 days (Aberer et al., 1996). Four of the 14 (29%) treated with the ceftriaxone showed an incomplete response after 6 to 12 months. Also patients treated for 30 days needed re-treatment less often than patients treated for 20 days. Therefore some authors recommend a minimum of 4 weeks of antibiotics for ACA (Müllegger, 2004). The prognosis of ACA is good if treatment is given during the acute inflammatory stage, but there is usually only a partial response to treatment in the chronic atrophic phase. This factor needs to be controlled for in any comparative treatment trial.

Serologic follow-up of ACA patients after antibiotic therapy shows a decline in anti-*Borrelia* titers over years, although the vast majority of patients remain positive. The persistence of antibody titers is generally independent of clinical outcome after therapy and unrelated to the duration or type of antibiotic treatment (Müllegger and Glatz, 2009).

Borrelia burgdorferi AND SCLEROSING SKIN CONDITIONS

In addition to its proven role in EM, BL, and ACA, it has been speculated that *B. burgdorferi* can cause circumscribed scleroderma (CS) and lichen sclerosus et atrophicus (LSA), two sclerosing, sometimes overlapping skin diseases of unknown origin. Following initial suggestive serologic, immunohistochemical, and culture studies in the 1980s (Aberer et al., 1987), conflicting data have been reported. Indirect evidence for the involvement of *B. burgdorferi* in the etiopathogenesis of CS comes from Austria and Switzerland, where one-third to one-half of patients are seropositive (Buechner et al., 1995). In contrast, serologic investigations in most other European countries, the United States, and Japan yielded negative results (Hoesly et al., 1987; Raguin et al., 1992; Akimoto et al., 1996). Rarely, *Borrelia* have been isolated on culture from CS and LSA lesions in central Europe (Aberer et al., 1987; Weber et al., 1988; Breier et al., 1999; Breier et al., 2001). In Europe and Japan, *Borrelia*-specific DNA was amplified by PCR from the skin of 25 of a total of 165 (15%) CS patients, and 21 (40%) of 52 LSA patients (Fujiwara et al., 1997; Goodlad et al., 2002). In contrast, PCR for *Borrelia* sp. was always negative in US patients (Fan et al., 1995; Fujiwara et al., 1997; Colome-Grimmer et al., 1997). The studies with negative PCR results were more rigorous in that they investigated larger numbers of patients and applied more than one primer set. In other reports the association has been alleged based on diagnostic methods that are far less specific such as immunohistology, focus-floating microscopy, silver staining, or lymphoproliferative response assays (Buechner et al., 1995; Eisendle et al., 2007). In case reports, *B. burgdorferi* infection has been implicated in the causation of two additional sclerosing disorders, progressive facial hemiatrophy and eosinophilic fasciitis (Shulman syndrome), based on silver staining, immunohistology, or PCR (Stern et al., 1992; Granter et al., 1994). However, consistently negative serologic results were obtained in a recent case series of 12 patients with facial hemiatrophy (Sommer et al., 2006).

The preponderance of evidence suggests that *B. burgdorferi* has the potential to induce CS or LSA in a subgroup of patients, particularly in central Europe, but not in North America (Weide et al., 2000). This may be due to the prevalence of distinct *B. burgdorferi* subtypes in that geographic region. Because anecdotal experience suggests that some of these patients benefit from antibiotics effective against *B. burgdorferi*, they should be considered as a therapeutic option in those areas.

REFERENCES

Aberer E, Breier F, Stanek G, Schmidt B: Success and failure in the treatment of acrodermatitis chronica atrophicans. *Infection* 24:85–87; 1996.

Aberer E, Stanek G, Ertl M, Neumann R: Evidence for spirochetal origin of circumscribed scleroderma (morphea). *Acta Derm Venereol* 67:225–231; 1987.

Akimoto S, Ishikawa O, Miyachi Y: The absence of antibodies against *Borrelia burgdorferi* in the sera of Japanese patients with localized scleroderma. *J Rheumatol* 23:573–574; 1996.

Asbrink E: Cutaneous manifestations of Lyme borreliosis. Clinical definitions and differential diagnoses. *Scand J Infect Dis Suppl* 77:44–50; 1991.

Asbrink E: Acrodermatitis chronica atrophicans. *Clin Dermatol* 11:369–375; 1993.

Asbrink E, Hovmark A, Hederstedt B: The spirochetal etiology of acrodermatitis chronica atrophicans Herxheimer. *Acta Derm Venereol* 64:506–512; 1984.

Asbrink E, Hovmark A, Olsson I: Clinical manifestations of acrodermatitis chronica atrophicans in 50 Swedish patients. *Zentralbl Bakteriol Mikrobiol Hyg [A]* 263:253–261; 1986.

Asbrink E, Hovmark A, Olsson I: Lymphadenosis benigna cutis solitaria: *Borrelia* lyphocytoma in Sweden. *Aentralbl Bakteriol Mikrobiol Hyg A* 18(suppl):156–163; 1989.

Bäfverstedt B: Uber Lymphadenosis benigna cutis. *Acta derm Venereol (Stockh)* 24:1–202; 1943.

Berger TG, Schoerner C, Schell H, Simon M, Schuler G, Rollinghoff M, Gessner A: Two unusual cases of diffuse acrodermatitis chronica atrophicans seronegative for Lyme borreliosis. *Eur J Clin Microbiol Infect Dis* 22:392–395; 2003.

Berglund J, Eitrem R, Ornstein K, Lindberg A, Ringer A, Elmrud H, Carlsson M, Runehagen A, Svanborg C, Norrby R: An epidemiologic study of Lyme disease in southern Sweden. *N Engl J Med* 333:1319–1327; 1995.

Brehmer-Andersson E: Histopathologic patterns of acrodermatitis chronica atrophicans. *Clin Dermatol* 11:385–392; 1993.

Breier FH, Aberer E, Stanek G, Khanakaha G, Schlick A, Tappeiner G: Isolation of *Borrelia afzelii* from circumscribed scleroderma. *Br J Dermatol* 140:925–930; 1999.

Breier FH, Khanakah G, Stanek G, Kunz G, Aberer E, Schmidt B, Tappeiner G: Isolation and polymerase chain reaction typing of *Borrelia afzelii* from a skin lesion in a seronegative patient with generalized ulcerating bullous lichen sclerosus et atrophicus. *Br J Dermatol* 144:387–392; 2001.

Brzonova I, Wollenberg A, Prinz JC: Acrodermatitis chronica atrophicans affecting all four limbs in an 11-year-old girl. *Br J Dermatol* 147:375–378; 2002.

Buchwald A: Ein Fall von diffuser idiopathischer Haut-Artophie. *Arch Derm Syphilol* 10:553–556; 1883.

Buechner SA, Lautenschlager S, Itin P, Bircher A, Erb P: Lymphoproliferative responses to *Borrelia burgdorferi* in patients with erythema migrans, acrodermatitis chronica atrophicans, lymphadenosis benigna cutis, and morphea. *Arch Dermatol* 131:673–677; 1995.

Busch U, Hizo-Teufel C, Bohmer R, Fingerle V, Rossler D, Wilske B, Preac-Mursic V: *Borrelia burgdorferi* sensu lato strains isolated from cutaneous Lyme borreliosis biopsies differentiated by pulsed-field gel electrophoresis. *Scand J Infect Dis* 28:583–589; 1996.

Christova I, Komitova R: Clinical and epidemiological features of Lyme borreliosis in Bulgaria. *Wien Klin Wochenschr* 116:42–46; 2004.

Colli C, Leinweber B, Müllegger R, Chott A, Kerl H, Cerroni L: *Borrelia burgdorferi*-associated lymphocytoma cutis: clinicopathologic, immunophenotypic, and molecular study of 106 cases. *J Cutan Pathol* 31:232–240; 2004.

Colome-Grimmer MI, Payne DA, Tyring SK, Sanchez RL: *Borrelia burgdorferi* DNA and *Borrelia hermsii* DNA are not associated with morphea or lichen sclerosus et atrophicus in the southwestern United States. *Arch Dermatol* 133:1174; 1997.

Dicaudo DJ, Su WP, Marshall WF, Malawista SE, Barthold S, Persing DH: Acrodermatitis chronica atrophicans in the United States. Clinical and histopathologic features of six cases. *Cutis* 54:81–84; 1994.

Edwards L, Hoshaw RA, Burgdorf WH: Acrodermatitis chronica atrophicans. *Arch Dermatol* 128:858–860; 1992.

Eisendle K, Grabner T, Zelger B: Morphoea. A manifestation of infection with *Borrelia* species? *Br J Dermatol* 157:1189–1198; 2007.

Fan W, Leonardi CL, Penneys NS: Absence of *Borrelia burgdorferi* in patients with localized scleroderma (morphea). *J Am Acad Dermatol* 33:682–684; 1995.

Fendt H: Beiträge zur Kenntnis der sogenannten sarcoiden Geschwülste der Haut. *Archiv für Dermatologie und Syphilis* 53:213–242; 1900.

Fingerle V, Schulte-Spechtel UC, Ruzic-Sabljic E, Leonhard S, Hofmann H, Weber K, Pfister K, Strle F, Wilske B: Epidemiological aspects and molecular characterization of *Borrelia burgdorferi* s.l. from southern Germany with special respect to the new species *Borrelia spielmanii* sp. nov. *Int J Med Microbiol* 298:279–290; 2008.

Frithz A, Lagerholm B: Acrodermatitis chronica atrophicans, erythema chronicum migrans and lymphadenosis benigna cutis. Spirochetal diseases? *Acta Derm Venereol* 63:432–436; 1983.

Fujiwara H, Fujiwara K, Hashimoto K, Mehregan AH, Schaumburg-Lever G, Lange R, Schempp C, Gollnick H: Detection of *Borrelia burgdorferi* DNA (*B garinii* or *B afzelii*) in morphea and lichen sclerosus et atrophicus tissues of German and Japanese but not of US patients. *Arch Dermatol* 133:41–44; 1997.

Goodlad JR, Davidson MM, Gordon P, Billington R, Ho-Yen DO: Morphoea and *Borrelia burgdorferi*: results from the Scottish Highlands in the context of the world literature. *Mol Pathol* 55:374–378; 2002.

Gordillo-Perez G, Torres J, Solorzano-Santos F, De Martino S, Lipsker D, Velazquez E, Ramon G, Onofre M, Jaulhac B: *Borrelia burgdorferi* infection and cutaneous Lyme disease, Mexico. *Emerg Infect Dis* 13:1556–1558; 2007.

Granter SR, Barnhill RL, Hewins ME, Duray PH: Identification of *Borrelia burgdorferi* in diffuse fasciitis with peripheral eosinophilia: borrelial fasciitis. *JAMA* 272:1283–1285; 1994.

Hauser W: [Zur Kenntnis der akrodermatitis chronica atrophicans]. *Arch Dermatol Syph* 199:350–393; 1955.

Herxheimer K, Hartmann K: [Uber acrodermatitis chronica atrophicans]. *Arch Dermatol Syph* 61:57–76; 1902.

Hoesly JM, Mertz LE, Winkelmann RK: Localized scleroderma (morphea) and antibody to *Borrelia burgdorferi*. *J Am Acad Dermatol* 17:455–458; 1987.

Hovmark A, Asbrink E, Olsson I: The spirochetal etiology of lymphadenosis benigna cutis solitaria. *Acta Derm Venereol* 66:479–484; 1986.

Jessner M: Zur Kenntnis der acrodermatitis chronica atrophicans. *Arch Dermatol Syph* 134:478–487; 1921.

Kaufman LD, Gruber BL, Phillips ME, Benach JL: Late cutaneous Lyme disease: Acrodermatitis chronica atrophicans. *Am J Med* 86:828–830; 1989.

Kaufmann-Wolf M: [Uber guartige lymphocytare Neubildungen der Scrotalhaut des Kindes]. *Arch f Dermatol u Syph (Berlin)* 130:425–435; 1921.

Kindstrand E, Nilsson BY, Hovmark A, Nennesmo I, Pirskanen R, Solders G, Asbrink E: Polyneuropathy in late Lyme borreliosis. A clinical, neurophysiological and morphological description. *Acta Neurol Scand* 101:47–52; 2000.

Kindstrand E, Nilsson BY, Hovmark A, Pirskanen R, Asbrink E: Peripheral neuropathy in acrodermatitis chronica atrophicans. A late *Borrelia* manifestation. *Acta Neurol Scand* 95:338–345; 1997.

Lavoie PE, Wilson AJ, Tuffanelli DL: Acrodermatitis chronica atrophicans with antecedent Lyme disease in a California. Case report. *Zentralbl Bakteriol Mikrobiol Hyg [A]*, 263:262–265; 1986.

Lenormand C, Jaulhac B, De Martino S, Barthel C, Lipsker D: Species of *Borrelia burgdorferi* complex that cause borrelial lymphocytoma in France. *Br J Dermatol* 161:174–176; 2009.

Lunemann JD, Zarmas S, Priem S, Franz J, Zschenderlein R, Aberer E, Klein R, Schouls L, Burmester GR, Krause A: Rapid typing of *Borrelia burgdorferi* sensu lato species in specimens from patients with different manifestations of Lyme borreliosis. *J Clin Microbiol* 39:1130–1133; 2001.

Maraspin V, Cimperman J, Lotric-Furlan S, Ruzic-Sabljic E, Jurca T, Picken RN, Strle F: Solitary borrelial lymphocytoma in adult patients. *Wien Klin Wochenschr* 114:515–523; 2002.

Müllegger RR: Clinical aspects and diagnosis of erythema migrans and borrelial lymphocytoma. *Acta Dermatovenerol Alp Panonica Adriat* 10:152–158; 2001.

Müllegger RR: Dermatological manifestations of Lyme borreliosis. *Eur J Dermatol* 14:296–309; 2004.

Müllegger RR, Glatz M: Is serological follow-up useful for patients with cutaneous Lyme borreliosis? *Curr Probl Dermatol* 37:178–182; 2009.

Müllegger RR, Means TK, Shin JJ, Lee M, Jones KL, Glickstein LJ, Luster AD, Steere AC: Chemokine signatures in the skin disorders of Lyme borreliosis in Europe. Predominance of CXCL9 and CXCL10 in erythema migrans and acrodermatitis and CXCL13 in lymphocytoma. *Infect Immun* 75:4621–4628; 2007.

Nadal D, Gundelfinger R, Flueler U, Boltshauser E: Acrodermatitis chronica atrophicans. *Arch Dis Child* 63:72–74; 1988.

Nygard K, Brantsaeter AB, Mehl R: Disseminated and chronic Lyme borreliosis in Norway, 1995–2004. *Euro Surveill* 10:235–238; 2005.

Ohlenbusch A, Matuschka FR, Richter D, Christen HJ, Thomssen R, Spielman A, Eiffert H: Etiology of the acrodermatitis chronica atrophicans lesion in Lyme disease. *J Infect Dis* 174:421–423; 1996.

Pick PJ: Uber eine neue Krankheit "Erythromelie." *Verh Ges Dtsch Naturf* 66:336; 1895.

Picken MM, Picken RN, Han D, Cheng Y, Ruzic-Sabljic E, Cimperman J, Maraspin V, Lotric-Furlan S, Strle F: A two year prospective study to compare culture and polymerase chain reaction amplification for the detection and diagnosis of Lyme borreliosis. *Mol Pathol* 50:186–193; 1997a.

Picken RN, Strle F, Ruzic-Sabljic E, Maraspin V, Lotric-Furlan S, Cimperman J, Cheng Y, Picken MM: Molecular subtyping of *Borrelia burgdorferi* sensu lato isolates from five patients with solitary lymphocytoma. *J Invest Dermatol* 108:92–97; 1997b.

Picken RN, Strle F, Picken MM, Ruzic-Sabljic E, Maraspin V, Lotric-Furlan S, Cimperman J: Identification of three species of *Borrelia burgdorferi* sensu lato (*B. burgdorferi* sensu stricto, *B. garinii*, and *B. afzelii*) among isolates from acrodermatitis chronica atrophicans lesions. *J Invest Dermatol* 110:211–214; 1998.

Pohl-Koppe A, Wilske B, Weiss M, Schmidt H: *Borrelia* lymphocytoma in childhood. *Pediatr Infect Dis J* 17:423–426; 1998.

Raguin G, Boisnic S, Souteyrand P, Baranton G, Piette JC, Godeau P, Frances C: No evidence for a spirochaetal origin of localized scleroderma. *Br J Dermatol* 127:218–220; 1992.

Rijpkema SG, Tazelaar DJ, Molkenboer MJ, Noorhoek GT, Plantinga G, Schouls LM, Schellekens JF: Detection of *Borrelia afzelii*, *Borrelia burgdorferi* sensu stricto, *Borrelia garinii* and group VS116 by PCR in skin biopsies of patients with erythema migrans and acrodermatitis chronica atrophicans. *Clin Microbiol Infect* 3:109–116; 1997.

Smetanick MT, Zellis SL, Ermolovich T: Acrodermatitis chronica atrophicans: A case report and review of the literature. *Cutis* 85:247–252; 2010.

Sommer A, Gambichler T, Bacharach-Buhles M, von Rothenburg T, Altmeyer P, Kreuter A: Clinical and serological characteristics of progressive facial hemiatrophy: a case series of 12 patients. *J Am Acad Dermatol* 54:227–233; 2006.

Spiegler E: Über die sogenannte Sarkomatosis cutis. *Archiv für Dermatologie und Syphilis* 27:163–174; 1894.

Stern HS, Elliott LF, Beegle PH Jr: Progressive hemifacial atrophy associated with Lyme disease. *Plast Reconstr Surg* 90:479–483; 1992.

Strle F, Pleterski-Rigler D, Stanek G, Pejovnik-Pustinek A, Ruzic E, Cimperman J: Solitary borrelial lymphocytoma: report of 36 cases. *Infection* 20:201–206; 1992.

Strle F, Picken RN, Cheng Y, Cimperman J, Maraspin V, Lotric-Furlan S, Ruzic-Sabljic E, Picken MM: Clinical findings for patients with Lyme borreliosis caused by *Borrelia burgdorferi* sensu lato with genotypic and phenotypic similarities to strain 25015. *Clin Infect Dis* 25:273–280; 1997.

Svarts N: Penicillinbehandling vid dermatitis atrophicans Herxheimer. *Nord Med* 32:2783; 1946.

Weber K, Preac-Mursic V, Reimers CD: Spirochetes isolated from two patients with morphea. *Infection* 16:25–26; 1988.

Weide B, Walz T, Garbe C: Is morphoea caused by *Borrelia burgdorferi*? A review. *Br J Dermatol* 142:636–644: 2000.

Wienecke R, Zochling N, Neubert U, Schlupen EM, Meurer M, Volkenandt M: Molecular subtyping of *Borrelia burgdorferi* in erythema migrans and acrodermatitis chronica atrophicans. *J Invest Dermatol* 103:19–22; 1994.

Wormser GP, Dattwyler RJ, Shapiro ED, Halperin JJ, Steere AC, Klempner MS, Krause PJ, Bakken JS, Strle F, Stanek G, Bockenstedt L, Fish D, Dumler JS, Nadelman RB: The clinical assessment, treatment, and prevention of Lyme disease, human granulocytic anaplasmosis, and babesiosis. Clinical practice guidelines by the Infectious Diseases Society of America. *Clin Infect Dis* 43:1089–1134; 2006.

Zalaudek I, Leinweber B, Kerl H, Müllegger RR: Acrodermatitis chronica atrophicans in a 15-year-old girl misdiagnosed as venous insufficiency for 6 years. *J Am Acad Dermatol* 52:1091–1094; 2005.

8

LYME BORRELIOSIS COINFECTIONS WITH ANAPLASMA AND BABESIA

Paul M. Lantos and Peter J. Krause

Lyme disease, human babesiosis, and human granulocytic anaplasmosis (HGA) are transmitted by the same *Ixodes* vector ticks and share the same mammalian reservoir hosts (Piesman et al., 1986; Telford et al., 1996; Schwartz et al., 1997; Fish and Childs, 2009). Simultaneous infection may occur in ticks, reservoir hosts, and people. Although human coinfection with one or more of these agents only recently has been recognized, studies have shown that concurrent infection has important implications for the natural course of disease, diagnostic evaluation, and appropriate antimicrobial therapy (Krause et al., 1996; Belongia et al., 1999; Thompson et al., 2001; Steere et al., 2003).

ECOLOGY

The microbial agents of Lyme disease, babesiosis, and HGA are biologically diverse. Three pathogenic *Borrelia* genospecies have been shown to cause Lyme disease in people, *Borrelia burgdorferi* sensu stricto, *Borrelia garinii*, and *Borrelia afzelii* (Steere, 2001; Wormser, 2006). *Babesia microti* causes the majority of cases of babesiosis, but other *Babesia* species have been found to cause disease in humans including *Babesia divergens, Babesia divergens*-like, *Babesia duncani* [WA-1], *Babesia venatorum* [EU-1], TW-1

Lyme Borreliosis in Europe and North America: Epidemiology and Clinical Practice, First Edition. Edited by Sunil K. Sood

[Taiwan 1], and KO-1 [Korea 1](Herwaldt et al., 2004; Swanson et al., 2006; Hunfeld et al., 2008). HGA is caused by the rickettsial organism *Anaplasma phagocytophilum* (Telford et al., 1996; Belongia et al., 1999).

The vectors for Lyme disease, babesiosis, and HGA are small, hard bodied ticks in the *Ixodes ricinus* complex. *Ixodes scapularis* (also known as *Ixodes dammini*) is the vector in eastern and midwestern North America. *Ixodes pacificus* is the vector in California and the Pacific Northwest, while *Ixodes ricinus* is the primary vector in Europe (Piesman et al., 1986; Telford et al., 1996; Schwartz et al., 1997; Fish and Childs, 2009). There is wide variation in the percentage of infected *Ixodes* ticks collected from different endemic areas: *B. burgdorferi* between 4% and 66%, *A. phagocytophilum* between 2% and 53%, and *B. microti* between 1% and 23% (Piesman et al., 1986; Telford et al., 1996; Schwartz et al., 1997; Swanson et al., 2006). The percentage of ticks infected with *B. burgdorferi* is usually at least two- to threefold greater than that of the other two pathogens. These infection rates are similar in Europe and in the United States (Baumgarten et al., 1999; Leutenegger et al., 1999; Swanson et al., 2006). The proportion of coinfected ticks generally is less than that of any single infection, while ticks infected by all three pathogens seldom are reported. For example, respective rates of infection of *I. scapularis* and *I. ricinus* ticks in Massachusetts and Poland are *B. burdorferi* 36% and 25%, *A. phagocytophila* 11% and 10%, *B. microti* 9% and 19%, two pathogens 4% and 5%, and three pathogens 0% and 1% (Telford et al., 1996; Skotarczak et al., 2003). Similarly the percentage of *I. ricinus* ticks in central Germany coinfected with *B. burgdorferi* and *A. phagocytophilum* (<1%) is less than the percentage infected by *B. burgdorferi* alone (11%) or *A. phagocytophilum* alone (2%) (Hildebrandt et al., 2003). The primary reservoir host of *B. burgdorferi*, *A. phagocytophilum*, and *B. microti* in North America is the white-footed mouse (*Peromyscus leucopus*). Limited studies suggest that infection prevalence in mice is much higher than in ticks or humans, at times exceeding 75% for *B. burgdorferi* or *B. microti*. At least 30% of mice have been found to be coinfected with *B. burgdorferi* and either *A. phagocytophilum* or *B. microti*, or *A. phagocytophilum* and *B. microti*, or all three pathogens, in areas endemic for all three pathogens (Anderson et al., 1986; Stafford et al., 1999; Fish and Childs, 2009). In Europe the meadow vole (*Microtus agrestis*) and the bank vole (*Clethrionomys glareolus*) are the principal reservoir hosts of *B. microti* (Gray and Weiss, 2007). Information on European *A. phagocytophilum* reservoirs is limited. Most strains are found in ruminants, especially sheep, but some strains may be harbored by rodents (Stuen, 2007).

EPIDEMIOLOGY OF HUMAN INFECTION

Lyme disease is far more commonly reported than babesiosis or HGA, with about 20,000 cases recorded each year in the United States by the Centers for Disease Control and Prevention (CDC, 2010). Several factors account for this higher incidence. *Borrelia burgdorferi* has a broader geographic distribution than either *A. phagocytophilum* or *B. microti*. Lyme disease is highly endemic in the northeastern and upper midwestern states of the United States with all but a tenth of Lyme disease cases reported from the coastal northeast between Maryland and Maine (Krause et al., 2002). In contrast, cases of babesiosis and HGA generally occur in more concentrated foci within Lyme disease endemic areas. *Borrelia burgdorferi* infection is more commonly found in ticks and rodents than *A. phagocytophilum* or *B. microti* in regions where all three infections are endemic (Swanson et al., 2006). Unlike Lyme disease, babesiosis is not a nationally reportable disease and HGA was not designated as such until 1998. Finally, Lyme disease is better recognized and more easily diagnosed than babesiosis or HGA, primarily because of the characteristic erythema migrans rash, whereas symptoms and signs of babesiosis and HGA are nonspecific and easily mistaken for a viral illness (Krause et al., 2002).

Results of a detailed epidemiologic study of Lyme disease and babesiosis suggest that the disparity in the frequency of these infections on the southern New England coast is less than would be expected from current epidemiologic data (Krause et al., 2003b). Furthermore both babesiosis and HGA may be increasing in incidence relative to Lyme disease. In the early 1990s on Block Island, Rhode Island, the *B. microti* incidence increased approximately fourfold while that of *B. burgdorferi* remained essentially unchanged. Nationally more than twice as many cases of HGA were reported to the CDC in 2002 than just three years previously (Demma et al., 2005).

The frequency of Lyme disease, babesiosis, and HGA coinfection has been determined by use of seroprevalence and prospective epidemiologic studies. Seroprevalence rates provide an estimate of exposure risk to one or more tick-borne pathogens but do not easily distinguish between sequential infection and simultaneous infection. Furthermore antibody titers may wane and disappear with time. Nonetheless, seroprevalence rates do suggest that coinfection is less common than single infection and that Lyme disease coinfection with babesiosis or HGA is more common than babesiosis—HGA coinfection (Magnarelli et al., 1998; Swanson et al., 2006). *Borrelia burgdorferi* and *B. microti* seroreactivity rates are 7% and 5%, respectively, on Block Island while only about 1% of the inhabitants have serologic evidence of exposure to both pathogens (Krause et al., 1996). Of 671 serosurvey subjects from New York, seroprevalence rates were 4% for the agent of Lyme disease, 3% for the agent of HGA, 1% for the agent of babesiosis, and 0.1% for both the agents of Lyme disease and HGA (Hilton et al., 1999).

Prospective case-finding studies using clinical, serological, and DNA amplification by polymerase chain reaction (PCR) offer a better means of determining the true incidence of coinfection than seroprevalence studies. The first epidemiologic and clinical study of coinfection was carried out in southern New England between 1990 and 1994 where 26 of 240 (11%) patients who experienced acute Lyme disease had evidence of concurrent babesiosis (Krause et al., 1996). In a related study, Lyme disease–babesiosis coinfections represented about 15% of all Lyme disease cases and 19% of all babesiosis cases (Krause et al., 2002). Overall, between 2% and 38% of Lyme disease patients have been found to be coinfected with babesiosis in epidemiologic studies (Meldrum et al., 1992; Krause et al., 1996; Belongia et al., 1999; Thompson et al., 2001; Steere et al., 2003; Swanson et al., 2006). A similar percentage of Lyme disease patients experience concurrent HGA infection with a range of 3% to 22% (Belongia et al., 1999; Belongia et al., 2001; Bjoersdorff et al., 2002; Steere et al., 2003; Arnez et al., 2003; Hermanowska-Szpakowicz et al., 2004). The heterogeneity in the reported frequency of coinfection can be attributed to temporal and geographical differences in the incidence of individual and coincident infections, as well as methodological differences such as case definition, inclusion criteria, and laboratory diagnostic assays. These differences are apparent when data are analyzed from different studies for the frequency of babesiosis and HGA coinfection among patients experiencing Lyme disease (Table 8.1).

TABLE 8.1 Babesiosis and HGA coinfection among patients experiencing Lyme disease

Geographic Region	Date	Reference	Study Population Criteria	Lyme Disease Patients Studied	Patients (%) with LD/HGA	LD/B	LD/B/HGA
Wisconsin	1997–1998	Belognia et al. (1999)	Unexplained febrile illness	9	2 (22%)		
Sweden	1998	Bjoersdorff et al. (2002)	Tick-associated febrile illness	15	3 (20%)		
Wisconsin	1996–1997	Belognia et al. (2001)	Lyme disease or HGA	94	11 (12%)		
Poland	2002–2004	Hermanowska-Szpakowicz et al. (2004)	Lyme disease or HGA	74	8 (11%)		
Slovenia	2001	Arnez et al. (2003)	Unexplained febrile illness	13	1 (8%)		
Rhode Island (Block Island)	1997–2000	Krause et al. (2002)	Erythema migrans rash or unexplained febrile illness	76	2 (3%)	16 (21%)	1 (1%)
Rhode Island (Block Island)	1990–1994	Krause et al. (1996)	Lyme disease or babesiosis	240		26 (11%)	
Connecticut and Rhode Island (mainland)	1998–2001	Steere et al. (2003)	Erythema migrans rash	93	2 (2%)	2 (2%)	0 (0%)

Note: LD Lyme disease, B Babesiosis, HGA Human granulocytic anaplasmosis.

CLINICAL PRESENTATION

Lyme disease is associated with an array of clinical features that generally allows for prompt diagnosis. Chief among these is the characteristic erythema migrans rash that appears within a month of tick bite (Wormser, 2006). Signs and symptoms of disseminated Lyme disease may occur during the acute infection or may appear many months later. The best recognized syndromes include multiple erythema migrans lesions, aseptic meningitis, cranial and peripheral neuropathies, pseudotumor cerebri, monoarticular or pauciarticular arthritis of large joints, and atrioventricular conduction block (Steere, 2001). In contrast, human babesiosis results in a viral-like illness characterized by fevers, chills, and constitutional symptoms (Krause et al., 1996, 2008). The onset of symptoms occurs 1 to 9 weeks after exposure. HGA produces symptoms within 2 weeks of transmission, and nearly all patients experience fever, chills, headaches, and myalgias (Bakken et al., 1994, Aguero-Rosenfeld et al., 1996, Bakken et al., 1996; Blanco and Oteo, 2002, Hermanowska-Szpakowicz et al., 2004). A similar viral-like illness also can occur in early Lyme disease, but this is uncommon and usually is accompanied by an erythema migrans rash (Feder et al., 1993; Steere, 2001; Wormser, 2006). Most cases of babesiosis and HGA result in mild to moderate illness that respond well to antimicrobial therapy, although each infection can result in multi-organ complications that end in death in about 3% to 20% of cases depending on immune status (Bakken et al., 1994; Aguero-Rosenfeld et al., 1996; Bakken et al., 1996; Blanco and Oteo, 2002; Stuen, 2007; Krause et al., 2008).

Patients who are coinfected with *B. burgdorferi* and *B. microti* and/or *A. phagocytophilum* generally have a more severe and protracted course of illness than those infected solely with *B. burgdorferi*. Fatigue, headache, chills, sweats, emotional lability, nausea, conjunctivitis, and splenomegaly were all found to be significantly more frequent in patients experiencing Lyme disease and babesiosis than Lyme disease alone (Krause et al., 1996). Symptoms persisted for longer than 3 months in about half of these coinfected patients compared to 4% of patients who experienced Lyme disease without concurrent infection. Similarly a greater number of symptoms with longer duration are noted in patients who have Lyme disease and HGA coinfection compared to those who have Lyme disease alone (Belongia et al., 1999; Krause et al., 2002). In contrast, a similar frequency of acute dissemination of Lyme spirochetes to the skin, heart, or the central nervous system appears to occur in Lyme disease patients with or without concurrent babesiosis (Krause et al., 2002). Coinfection with *B. burgdorferi* and *B. microti* does not appear to cause more long-term complications than with either infection alone (Wang et al., 2000; Stuen, 2007).

DIAGNOSIS

Physicians who are considering a diagnosis of Lyme disease, babesiosis, or HGA coinfection should have knowledge of the frequency of these diseases in the areas where their patients live and travel. Coinfection with babesiosis or HGA should be considered in any Lyme disease patient who experiences more severe or prolonged disease than expected, especially if they have fever, chills, and headache (Krause et al., 1996; Belongia et al., 1999; Krause et al., 2002). Routine blood studies tend to be normal in patients with Lyme disease, whereas there are characteristic hematologic and biochemical abnormalities associated with both babesiosis and HGA (Bakken et al., 1996; Krause et al., 2002). Anemia is suggestive of babesiosis, and leucopenia or neutropenia are common features of HGA. Thrombocytopenia may be present in both babesiosis and HGA. A complete blood count (CBC) is therefore a quick and useful way to screen for coinfection. Elevated bilirubin or lactate dehydrogenase (LDH), which are associated with hemolysis, may be seen in babesiosis. Transaminase elevation can be seen in HGA.

Specific diagnostic tests for coinfecting tick-transmitted diseases include blood smear, PCR, and serology. If the clinical picture and CBC are suggestive of babesiosis or HGA, a Giemsa-stained thin blood smear examination should be obtained. Intraerythrocytic parasitic forms are present in the blood of patients experiencing babesiosis while characteristic morulae can be visualized in the neutrophils of HGA patients (Bakken et al., 1996; Krause et al., 2002). Multiple blood smears should be performed if either disease is suspected, as blood smear examinations have poor sensitivity when the organism burden is low early in the course of disease. If blood smear examination fails to reveal babesiosis or HGA, amplification of anaplasma or babesial DNA by PCR and disease specific acute and convalescent serology should be obtained.

TREATMENT

Uncomplicated Lyme disease and HGA coinfection can be treated with doxycycline in patients 9 years and older (Wormser et al., 2006). For children younger than 9 years and pregnant women, it is preferable to treat Lyme disease with amoxicillin and consider the use of rifampin in young children for mild HGA in order to avoid exposure to doxycycline (Krause et al., 2003a). Lyme disease generally requires a treatment course of 2 to 3 weeks compared with 10 days for HGA. Treatment of Lyme disease and babesiosis coinfection consists of doxycycline or amoxicillin for Lyme disease and the combination of atovaquone and azithromycin for babesiosis (Krause et al., 2000; Wormser et al., 2006). Clindamycin and quinine can be used instead of atovaquone and azithromycin, but this combination is associated with significantly greater number of side effects and is no more effective in clearing infection. Clindamycin and quinine should be administered for severe babesial infection because there is a greater experience with its use in this setting. Highly immunocompromised patients, particularly those with asplenia, malignancy, HIV infection, and on immunosuppressive medication, generally experience severe babesiosis and may relapse after conventional courses of therapy. Such patients have required repeated or prolonged courses of antibabesial therapy with post-treatment monitoring for relapse (Krause et al., 2008). A complete summary of appropriate therapy for Lyme disease, babesiosis, and HGA and for coinfection can be found in the 2006 practice guideline from the Infectious Disease Society of America (Wormser et al., 2006).

REFERENCES

Aguero-Rosenfeld ME, Horowitz HW, Wormser GP, McKenna DF, Nowakowski J, Munoz J, Dumler JS: Human granulocytic ehrlichiosis. A case series from a medical center in New York State. *Ann Intern Med* 125:904–908; 1996.

Anderson JF, Johnson RC, Magnarelli LA, Hyde FW, Myers JE: *Peromyscus leucopus* and *Microtus pennsylvanicus* simultaneously infected with *Borrelia burgdorferi* and *Babesia microti*. *J Clin Microbiol* 23:135–137; 1986.

Arnez M, Luznik-Bufon T, Avsic-Zupanc T, Ruzic-Sabljic E, Petrovec M, Lotric-Furlan S, Strle F: Causes of febrile illnesses after a tick bite in Slovenian children. *Pediatr Infect Dis J* 22:1078–1083; 2003.

Bakken JS, Dumler JS, Chen SM, Eckman MR, van Etta LL, Walker DH: Human granulocytic ehrlichiosis in the upper Midwest United States. A new species emerging? *JAMA* 272:212–218; 1994.

Bakken JS, Krueth J, Wilson-Nordskog C, Tilden RL, Asanovich K, Dumler JS: Clinical and laboratory characteristics of human granulocytic ehrlichiosis. *JAMA* 275:199–205; 1996.

Baumgarten BU, Rollinghoff M, Bogdan C: Prevalence of *Borrelia burgdorferi* and granulocytic and monocytic ehrlichiae in *Ixodes ricinus* ticks from southern Germany. *J Clin Microbiol* 37:3448–3451; 1999.

Belongia EA, Reed KD, Mitchell PD, Chyou PH, Mueller-Rizner N, Finkel MF, Schriefer ME: Clinical and epidemiological features of early Lyme disease and human granulocytic ehrlichiosis in Wisconsin. *Clin Infect Dis* 29:1472–1477; 1999.

Belongia EA, Reed KD, Mitchell PD, Mueller-Rizner N, Vandermause M, Finkel MF, Kazmierczak JJ: Tickborne infections as a cause of nonspecific febrile illness in Wisconsin. *Clin Infect Dis* 32:1434–1439; 2001.

Bjoersdorff A, Wittesjo B, Berglun J, Massung RF, Eliasson I: Human granulocytic ehrlichiosis as a common cause of tick-associated fever in Southeast Sweden. Report from a prospective clinical study. *Scand J Infect Dis* 34:187–91; 2002.

Blanco JR, Oteo JA: Human granulocytic ehrlichiosis in Europe. *Clin Microbiol Infect* 8:763–772; 2002.

CDC: *Lyme disease* [online]. Available: http://www.cdc.gov/ncidod/dvbid/lyme/index.htm [Accessed April 26, 2010].

Demma LJ, Holman RC, McQuiston JH, Krebs JW, Swerdlow DL: Epidemiology of human ehrlichiosis and anaplasmosis in the United States, 2001–2002. *Am J Trop Med Hyg* 73:400–409; 2005.

Feder HM Jr, Gerber MA, Krause PJ, Ryan R, Shapiro ED: Early Lyme disease: A flu-like illness without erythema migrans. *Pediatrics* 91:456–459; 1993.

Fish D, Childs JE: Community-based prevention of Lyme disease and other tick-borne diseases through topical application of acaricide to white-tailed deer: Background and rationale. *Vector Borne Zoonotic Dis* 9:357–364; 2009.

Gray JS, Weiss LM: *Babesia microti*. *In* Khan NA (ed): *Emerging Protozoan Pathogens*. Abingdon, UK, Taylor and Francis; 2007.

Hermanowska-Szpakowicz T, Skotarczak B, Kondrusik M, Rymaszewska A, Sawczuk M, Maciejewska A, Adamska M, Pancewicz S, Zajkowska J: Detecting DNAs of *Anaplasma phagocytophilum* and *Babesia* in the blood of patients suspected of Lyme disease. *Ann Agric Environ Med* 11:351–354; 2004.

Herwaldt BL, De Bruyn G, Pieniazek NJ, Homer M, Lofy KH, Slemenda SB, Fritsche TR, Persing DH, Limaye AP: *Babesia divergens*-like infection, Washington State. *Emerg Infect Dis* 10:622–629; 2004.

Hildebrandt A, Schmidt KH, Wilske B, Dorn W, Straube E, Fingerle V: Prevalence of four species of *Borrelia burgdorferi* sensu lato and coinfection with *Anaplasma phagocytophila* in *Ixodes ricinus* ticks in central Germany. *Eur J Clin Microbiol Infect Dis* 22:364–367; 2003.

Hilton E, Devoti J, Benach JL, Halluska ML, White DJ, Paxton H, Dumler JS: Seroprevalence and seroconversion for tick-borne diseases in a high-risk population in the northeast United States. *Am J Med* 106:404–409; 1999.

Hunfeld KP, Hildebrandt A, Gray JS: Babesiosis. Recent insights into an ancient disease. *Int J Parasitol* 38:1219–1237; 2008.

Krause PJ, Telford S.R. III, Spielman A, Sikand V, Ryan R, Christianson D, Burke G, Brassard P, Pollack R, Peck J, Persing DH: Concurrent Lyme disease and babesiosis. Evidence for increased severity and duration of illness. *JAMA* 275:1657–1660; 1996.

Krause PJ, Lepore T, Sikand VK, Gadbaw J Jr, Burke G, Telford SR III, Brassard P, Pearl D, Azlanzadeh J, Christianson D, McGrath D, Spielman A: Atovaquone and azithromycin for the treatment of babesiosis. *N Engl J Med* 343:1454–1458; 2000.

Krause PJ, McKay K, Thompson CA, Sikand VK, Lentz R, Lepore T, Closter L, Christianson D, Telford SR, Persing D, Radolf JD, Spielman A: Disease-specific diagnosis of coinfecting tickborne zoonoses. Babesiosis, human granulocytic ehrlichiosis, and Lyme disease. *Clin Infect Dis* 34:1184–1191; 2002.

Krause PJ, Corrow CL, Bakken JS: Successful treatment of human granulocytic ehrlichiosis in children using rifampin. *Pediatrics* 112:e252–e253; 2003a.

Krause PJ, McKay K, Gadbaw J, Christianson D, Closter L, Lepore T, Telford SR III, Sikand V, Ryan R, Persing D, Radolf JD, Spielman A: Increasing health burden of human babesiosis in endemic sites. *Am J Trop Med Hyg* 68:431–436; 2003b.

Krause PJ, Gewurz BE, Hill D, Marty FM, Vannier E, Foppa IM, Furman RR, Neuhaus E, Skowron G, Gupta S, McCalla C, Pesanti EL, Young M, Heiman D, Hsue G, Gelfand JA, Wormser GP, Dickason J, Bia FJ, Hartman B, Telford SR III, Christianson D, Dardick K, Coleman M, Girotto JE, Spielman A: Persistent and relapsing babesiosis in immunocompromised patients. *Clin Infect Dis* 46:370–376; 2008.

Leutenegger CM, Pusterla N, Mislin CN, Weber R, Lutz H: Molecular evidence of coinfection of ticks with *Borrelia burgdorferi* sensu lato and the human granulocytic ehrlichiosis agent in Switzerland. *J Clin Microbiol* 37:3390–3391; 1999.

Magnarelli LA, Ijdo JW, Anderson JF, Padula SJ, Flavell RA, Fikrig E: Human exposure to a granulocytic *Ehrlichia* and other tick-borne agents in Connecticut. *J Clin Microbiol* 36:2823–2827; 1998.

Meldrum SC, Birkhead GS, White DJ, Benach JL, Morse DL: Human babesiosis in New York State. An epidemiological description of 136 cases. *Clin Infect Dis* 15:1019–1023; 1992.

Piesman J, Mather TN, Telford S.R. III, Spielman A: Concurrent *Borrelia burgdorferi* and *Babesia microti* infection in nymphal *Ixodes dammini*. *J Clin Microbiol* 24:446–447; 1986.

Schwartz I, Fish D, Daniels TJ: Prevalence of the rickettsial agent of human granulocytic ehrlichiosis in ticks from a hyperendemic focus of Lyme disease. *N Engl J Med* 337:49–50; 1997.

Skotarczak B, Rymaszewska A, Wodecka B, Sawczuk M: Molecular evidence of coinfection of *Borrelia burgdorferi* sensu lato, human granulocytic ehrlichiosis agent, and *Babesia microti* in ticks from northwestern Poland. *J Parasitol* 89:194–196; 2003.

Stafford KC III, Massung RF, Magnarelli LA, Ijdo JW, Anderson JF: Infection with agents of human granulocytic ehrlichiosis, Lyme disease, and babesiosis in wild white-footed mice (*Peromyscus leucopus*) in Connecticut. *J Clin Microbiol* 37:2887–2892; 1999.

Steere AC: Lyme disease. *N Engl J Med* 345:115–125; 2001.

Steere AC, McHugh G, Suarez C, Hoitt J, Damle N, Sikand VK: Prospective study of coinfection in patients with erythema migrans. *Clin Infect Dis* 36:1078–1081; 2003.

Stuen S: *Anaplasma phagocytophilum*. The most widespread tick-borne infection in animals in Europe. *Vet Res Commun* 31(suppl 1): 79–84; 2007.

Swanson SJ, Neitzel D, Reed KD, Belongia EA: Coinfections acquired from *Ixodes* ticks. *Clin Microbiol Rev* 19:708–727; 2006.

Telford SR III, Dawson JE, Katavolos P, Warner CK, Kolbert CP, Persing DH: Perpetuation of the agent of human granulocytic ehrlichiosis in a deer tick-rodent cycle. *Proc Natl Acad Sci USA* 93:6209–6214; 1996.

Thompson C, Spielman A, Krause PJ: Coinfecting deer-associated zoonoses. Lyme disease, babesiosis, and ehrlichiosis. *Clin Infect Dis* 33:676–685; 2001.

Wang TJ, Liang MH, Sangha O, Phillips CB, Lew RA, Wright EA, Berardi V, Fossel AH, Shadick NA: Coexposure to *Borrelia burgdorferi* and *Babesia microti* does not worsen the long-term outcome of Lyme disease. *Clin Infect Dis* 31:1149–1154; 2000.

Wormser GP: Clinical practice. Early Lyme disease. *N Engl J Med* 354:2794–2801; 2006.

Wormser GP, Dattwyler RJ, Shapiro ED, Halperin JJ, Steere AC, Klempner MS, Krause PJ, Bakken JS, Strle F, Stanek G, Bockenstedt L, Fish D, Dumler JS, Nadelman RB: The clinical assessment, treatment, and prevention of Lyme disease, human granulocytic anaplasmosis, and babesiosis. Clinical practice guidelines by the Infectious Diseases Society of America. *Clin Infect Dis* 43:1089–1134; 2006.

9

THE ROLE OF CULTURE AND NUCLEIC ACID AMPLIFICATION IN DIAGNOSIS OF LYME BORRELIOSIS

Gary P. Wormser and Guiqing Wang

Success in cultivation of Lyme borrelia (herein the term Lyme borrelia refers to *Borrelia burgdorferi* sensu lato; *Borrelia burgdorferi* sensu stricto is referred to herein as *B. burgdorferi*) was first reported in 1982 when the spirochete was recovered from pooled mid-gut contents of four *Ixodes scapularis* vector ticks (Burgdorfer et al., 1982; Barbour, 1984), using a complex, highly fortified liquid medium, originally developed for growing relapsing fever borrelia (Kelly, 1971). Lyme borrelia were subsequently recovered using similar culture methods from reservoir animals (Bosler et al., 1983; Anderson et al., 1983, 1987) and humans with Lyme disease (Benach et al., 1983; Steere et al., 1983b; Berger et al., 1983). This chapter, which is adapted from our general review of diagnostic methods for Lyme borreliosis (Aguero-Rosenfeld et al., 2005), will specifically discuss the role of culture and polymerase chain reaction (PCR) methods.

CULTURE OF LYME BORRELIA

Culture Techniques

The liquid media currently used to grow Lyme borrelia were derived from the original Kelly medium (Kelly, 1971) through various modifications made over time (Stoenner, 1974;

Lyme Borreliosis in Europe and North America: Epidemiology and Clinical Practice, First Edition. Edited by Sunil K. Sood

TABLE 9.1 Selected features of various modifications of Kelly medium

Stoenner modification
Addition of Yeastolate and CMRL 1066, without glutamine and without sodium bicarbonate (Stoenner et al., 1982).
Barbour modification (BSK II)
Use of CMRL 1066 without glutamine; Yeastolate; neopeptone as the peptone preparation; and HEPES as a buffer (Barbour, 1984).
Preac-Mursic modification (MKP[a])
Removal of Yeastolate; different proportions of certain ingredients (Preac-Mursic et al., 1986).
BSK–H
Deletion of gelatin; different proportions of certain ingredients (Pollack et al., 1993).

[a]Also referred to as the Pettenkofer modification (Picken et al., 1997).

Stoenner et al., 1982; Barbour, 1984; Berger et al., 1985; Preac-Mursic et al., 1986). Current versions of this medium—Barbour–Stoenner–Kelly II medium (BSK II, Barbour, 1984), BSK-H (Pollack et al., 1993), and Kelly medium Preac-Mursic (MKP; Preac-Mursic et al., 1986)—are better able to support growth of Lyme borrelia in terms of recovery from low inocula, shorter generation times of the spirochete, and maximal concentration of spirochetes in culture ($\sim 10^8$–10^9/mL) (Table 9.1). Key ingredients of these liquid formulations include CMRL-1066 (which is a standard medium used for growing various types of mammalian cells), bovine serum albumin-fraction V (which serves as a rich source of protein and to stabilize the pH), *N*-acetylglucosamine (a precursor for bacterial cell wall biosynthesis), rabbit serum, citrate, pyruvate, among many others (Table 9.1). Why such an enriched medium is required is now better understood in light of information learned through sequencing the entire genome of a representative strain of *Borrelia burgdorferi* (B31 strain) (Fraser et al., 1997), an isolate derived from the first successful cultivation of *B. burgdorferi* (Barbour, 1984). *Borrelia burgdorferi* lacks recognized genes that encode enzymes required for synthesis of most amino acids, fatty acids, enzyme co-factors and nucleotides; it also does not have the genes for tricarboxylic acid cycle enzymes or for compounds of the electron transport system (Fraser et al., 1997; Wang et al., 2001). Therefore the availability of a wide variety of nutrients is necessary for growth.

The growth-promoting capability of a particular batch of liquid medium depends on the careful selection of certain key components that may be highly variable in composition according to their source (Pollack et al., 1993), particularly the preparations of BSA (Callister et al., 1990) and rabbit serum (Pollack et al., 1993). For example, a minority of preparations of rabbit serum contain antispirochetal antibodies and inclusion of such preparations in the medium will reduce or entirely abrogate growth of Lyme borrelia (Pollack et al., 1993). Aside from its effects on overall growth promotion, the quality of the BSA also influences *B. burgdorferi* gene expression (Yang et al., 2001). Consequently, as a necessary quality control measure, each new batch of liquid medium must be tested for its ability to support adequately the growth of laboratory-adapted strains of Lyme borrelia.

BSK-H preparations when frozen at −20°C remain stable for at least 8 months (Pollack et al., 1993).

Cultures in liquid medium are optimally incubated at 30° to 34°C under microaerophilic conditions (Barbour, 1984; Preac-Mursic et al., 1986; Yang et al., 2001). Incubation at temperatures of 39°C or higher may reduce or prevent growth (Yang et al., 2001). Depending on the starting inoculum, cultures are incubated for up to 8 to 12 weeks, which is much longer than is necessary to grow most other human bacterial pathogens, due in part to the spirochete's prolonged generation time of 7 to >24 hours during log phase growth (Barbour, 1984; Preac-Mursic et al., 1991; Wang et al., 2001). Clinical isolates of Lyme borrelia tend to have much longer generation times than laboratory-adapted strains that have been in long-term culture. Detection of growth is done by periodic examination of an aliquot of culture supernatant to look for the presence of spirochetes by dark-field microscopy or by fluorescence microscopy after staining with the fluorochrome dye acridine orange or a specific fluorescein-tagged antibody (Pavia and Niederbuhl, 1985; Wormser et al., 2000a; Reed, 2002). Visualized spirochete-like structures should be confirmed as Lyme borrelia by demonstration of reactivity with specific monoclonal antibodies or by detection of specific DNA sequences using PCR methodology (Stanek et al., 1990; Nadelman et al., 1996; Wormser et al., 2000; Wang et al., 2001). Lack of experience in the microscopic detection of Lyme borrelia can lead to false-positive readings, as other structures such as cellular debris may appear thread-like and thus be mistaken for Lyme borrelia.

Lyme borrelia can also be grown on solid media using agarose to solidify the liquid media discussed above (or with slight modifications) and incubation under microaerophilic or anaerobic conditions (Barbour, 1984; Kurtti et al., 1987; Preac-Mursic et al., 1991). An advantage of using solid media is that individual colonies can be identified as a means to select out particular clonal strains of Lyme borrelia. Such colonies, however, are much smaller and less recognizable than those occurring with the more readily cultivable Gram-positive and Gram-negative bacterial pathogens, rendering the method impractical.

Laboratory propagated strains of Lyme borrelia can be successfully co-cultivated with various tick cell lines (Kurtti et al., 1988; Munderloh et al., 1994; Obonyo et al., 1999) and with certain mammalian cell lines (Hechemy et al., 1992; Tylewska-Wierzbanowska and Chmielewski, 1997; Speck et al., 2002). Co-cultivation techniques have been used for primary isolation of Lyme borrelia from clinical specimens as well (Tylewska-Wierzbanowska and Chmielewski, 1997; Speck et al., 2002) but have not been put into clinical microbiologic practice because of the technical challenge.

Culture Contamination

In performing borrelial cultures, contamination with other bacteria and with fungi may arise for several reasons. One is that disinfection of some types of specimens, especially skin biopsy samples or ticks, may be insufficient in a minority of cases to render them free of contaminating microorganisms. Another contributing factor is that the richness of BSK II, as well as other similar liquid media (Table 9.1), makes them excellent growth media for many other microorganisms besides borrelia. Further the process of identifying positive cultures requires repeated sampling of the media, and the more often this occurs, the greater the opportunity for contamination.

Steps to limit potential contamination include meticulous disinfection of the specimens to be cultured, inoculating specimens and sampling the cultures in a laminar-flow biohazard hood, and adding antimicrobial drugs to the media. Examples of drugs with relatively selective activity against contaminating microorganisms that have been added to liquid media as either single agents or in combination, include rifampin, ciprofloxacin, nalidixic acid, 5-fluorouracil, trimethroprim-sulfamethoxazole, amikacin, spectinomycin, gentamicin, kanamycin, fosfomycin, nystatin, and amphotericin B (Barbour, 1984; Johnson et al., 1984; Neubert et al., 1986; Preac-Mursic et al., 1986; Nelson et al., 1991; Preac-Mursic et al., 1991; Berger et al., 1992; Morshed et al., 1993). Although the activity of these drugs is regarded as poor against Lyme borrelia, especially at concentrations below 100 mcg/ml, inclusion of any antimicrobial agent raises concerns that this intervention will prevent growth of at least some strains of Lyme borrelia or alternatively may contribute to slower growth rates and delay time to culture positivity.

If contamination should occur, recovery of Lyme borrelia may still be possible by sequential filtration of the media first through a 0.45-μm pore-size filter followed by a 0.2-μm pore-size filter (Jobe et al., 1993); borrelia may be able to traverse these filters because of their more narrow width compared with other bacteria or fungi (Wang et al., 2001). If filtration proves ineffective, then another strategy that can be tried is to introduce an antibiotic with selective antimicrobial activity appropriate for the contaminant, as discussed above (Barbour, 1984). If neither of these approaches is effective, then detection of culture positivity may still be possible by PCR based on amplification of specific Lyme borrelia DNA (Schwartz et al., 1993). A disadvantage of PCR detection of culture positivity under these circumstances is that subculture of Lyme borrelia would be impossible.

Culture of Clinical Specimens

Lyme borrelia can be recovered from various tissues and body fluids of patients with Lyme disease, including biopsy (Steere et al., 1983b; Asbrink and Hovmark, 1985; Berger et al., 1985; Neubert et al., 1986; Preac-Mursic et al., 1986; Berger et al., 1992a; Schwartz et al., 1992; Wormser et al., 1992; Melski et al., 1993; Mitchell et al., 1993; Nadelman et al., 1993; van Dam et al., 1993; Strle et al., 1996; Picken et al., 1997; Brettschneider et al., 1998; Jurca et al., 1998; Steere et al., 1998; Logar et al., 1999; Lebech et al., 2000; Nowakowski et al., 2001; Oksi et al., 2001; Ornstein et al., 2001; Zore et al., 2002; Carlsson et al., 2003) and lavage (Wormser et al., 1992) specimens of erythema migrans skin lesions (EM), biopsy specimens of acrodermatitis chronica atrophicans skin lesions (ACA) (Asbrink and Hovmark, 1985; Neubert et al., 1986; Preac-Mursic et al., 1986; van Dam et al., 1993; Picken et al., 1998), biopsy specimens of borrelial lymphocytoma skin lesions (Maraspin et al., 2002), cerebrospinal fluid specimens (Steere et al., 1983b; Preac-Mursic et al., 1986; Karlsson et al., 1990; van Dam et al., 1993; Cimperman et al., 1999; Ornstein et al., 2001) and blood specimens (Benach et al., 1983; Steere et al., 1983a, 1984; Neubert et al., 1986; Nadelman et al., 1990; Wormser et al., 1998, 2000, 2001a; Arnez et al., 2001; Maraspin et al., 2001; Oksi et al., 2001) (Table 9.2). Anecdotally, recovery of Lyme borrelia has also been reported from other tissue or fluid specimens (Maraspin et al., 2001), such as synovial fluid (Schmidli et al., 1988; Marlovits et al., 2004), cardiac tissue (Stanek et al., 1990), and iris (Preac-Mursic et al., 1993).

Aside from the late cutaneous manifestation ACA, from which Lyme borrelia have been recovered more than 10 years after onset of the skin lesion (Asbrink and Hovmark, 1985),

TABLE 9.2 Cultivation of Lyme Borrelia from clinical samples

Site	Representative Culture Yield	
	USA (ref)	Europe (ref)
	Skin	
Erythema migrans	> 50%[a] Berger et al., 1992; Schwartz et al., 1992; Wormser et al., ; Mitchell et al., 1993; Melski et al., 1993; Nadelman et al., 1993; Steere et al., 1998; Nowakowski et al., 2001	≥ 40%[b] Asbrink and Hovmark, 1985; van Dam et al., 1993; Moter et al., 1994; Strle et al., 1996; Picken et al., 1997; Brettschneider et al., 1998; Jurca et al., 1998; Lebech et al., 2000; Ornstein et al., 2001; Zore et al., 2002; Carlsson et al., 2003
Acrodermatitis chronica atrophicans	ND	≥ 22%[c] Asbrink and Hovmark, 1985; van Dam et al., 1993; Picken et al., 1998
Borrelial lymphocytoma	ND	24% Maraspin et al., 2002
	Cerebrospinal fluid	
	anecdotal*	10%[d] Karlsson et al., 1990; van Dam et al., 1993; Cimperman et al., 1999; Ornstein et al., 2001
	Synovial fluid	
	anecdotal	anecdotal
	Blood	
	> 40%** Wormser et al., 2000a, 2001	1.2%*** to 9%**** Arnez et al., 2001; Maraspin et al., 2001; Oksi et al., 2001

[a]Highest reported yield 86% (Berger et al., 1992a).
[b]Highest reported yield 88% (van Dam et al., 1993).
[c]Highest reported yield 60% (van Dam et al., 1993)
[d]Highest reported yield 17% (van Dam et al., 1993).
*CSF (1 ml in 9 ml medium with no air pocket) in 2 children with meningitis (Sood SK, unpublished);
** plasma (high-volume, ≥9 ml) of untreated adult United States patients with erythema migrans; ***plasma (low-volume, ≤3 ml) of European adults with erythema migrans; ****plasma (low-volume, <1 ml) of untreated European children with erythema migrans. ND = no data available.

the vast majority of successful isolations of borrelia have been from untreated patients with early disease (EM or early neuroborreliosis) (Karlsson et al., 1990; Schwartz et al., 1992; Nadelman and Wormser, 1998; Wang et al., 1999; Wilske, 2003). Lyme borrelia have only rarely been recovered from specimens of synovial fluid or synovial tissues in patients with Lyme arthritis, the most frequent late extracutaneous manifestation of this spirochetal infection in the United States (Steere et al., 1983a, 1984; Marques et al., 2000; Stanek and Strle, 2003).

Erythema Migrans

Recovery of Lyme borrelia from 2- to 4-mm skin biopsy samples of an EM skin lesion can typically be achieved in at least 40% of untreated patients (Table 9.2). The highest reported success rates were 86% in a small United States study of 21 patients for whom 4-mm skin biopsy specimens were cultured (Berger et al., 1992a) and 88% in a study from the Netherlands of 57 patients who underwent a 4-mm skin biopsy (van Dam et al., 1993). Lyme borrelia can be recovered from both primary (site of tick bite) and secondary EM lesions (that arise by hematogenous dissemination) (Mitchell et al., 1993; Melski et al., 1993). Despite the clinical tradition of biopsying the advancing border of an EM lesion, a recent systematic study of this practice conducted in Europe found comparable yields from biopsy specimens taken from the EM center (Jurca et al., 1998). According to one report, positive cultures can also be obtained from clinically normal appearing skin 4 mm beyond the EM border (Berger et al., 1992a).

Lyme borrelia can also be grown from culture of saline injected into and then withdrawn from an EM lesion. In one study of a group of United States patients with EM, cultures were established for both a 2-mm skin biopsy sample and for a lavage sample in which nonbacteriostatic sterile saline was injected into the same EM lesion and then recovered using a novel 2-needle technique (Wormser et al., 1992). A version of this technique had previously been found to be successful in recovering Lyme borrelia from the skin of infected animals (Piesman et al., 1991). In the clinical study, excluding contaminated samples, *B. burgdorferi* was recovered from 20 (74%) of the 27 skin biopsy specimens, compared with 12 (40%) of the 30 lavage samples ($p < 0.05$) (Wormser et al., 1992). Although less sensitive, cutaneous lavage has the advantage of being less invasive.

Recovery of *B. burgdorferi* from solitary EM lesions is significantly more likely in United States patients with skin lesions of shorter duration (Nadelman et al., 1993), suggesting that the patient's immune response is usually effective in clearing the spirochete from that skin site over a relatively short time interval. Consistent with this premise are the results of a recent study, in which the number of spirochetes in 2-mm skin biopsy samples of the advancing border of an EM skin lesion was enumerated using a quantitative PCR technique (qPCR) (Liveris et al., 2002). This study demonstrated that significantly fewer spirochetes were present in older or larger EM lesions (in the United States the size of an EM lesion correlates directly with its duration) (Berger, 1989; Nadelman et al., 1993, 1996). The same phenomenon probably explains a much earlier clinical observation that in the absence of antibiotic therapy, EM lesions will nevertheless resolve in a median time period of approximately four weeks (Steere et al., 1983a). Clearance of spirochetes from the skin in the absence of antibiotic treatment has also been documented in a rhesus macaque model of *B. burgdorferi* infection (Philipp et al., 1993). Persistence of spirochetes in skin after spontaneous resolution of EM, however, has been reported in a European study (Kuiper et al., 1994).

Borrelia burgdorferi usually cannot be recovered on culture of EM lesions of patients already receiving appropriate antibiotic treatment (Wormser et al., 2000b) and rarely, if ever, from the prior site of a resolved EM lesion in US patients who have completed a course of appropriate antimicrobial therapy (Berger et al., 1992b; Nadelman et al., 1993). *Borrelia burgdorferi* has been recovered, however, from cultures of EM lesions of patients treated with the first-generation cephalosporin, cephalexin, an antibiotic that is inactive in vitro against Lyme borrelia and ineffective clinically (Agger et al., 1992; Nowakowski et al., 2000). In Europe, Lyme borrelia have been recovered from skin and sometimes other sites during or following a course of antibiotic therapy in a small percentage of cases (Preac-Mursic et al., 1989; Logar et al., 1999). The explanation for the apparent disparity with the experience in the United States is unknown.

Whole Blood, Serum, Plasma

The rate of recovery of Lyme borrelia from blood or blood components of untreated patients with EM had generally been 5% or less (Benach et al., 1983; Steere et al., 1983b; Wallach et al., 1993; Goodman et al., 1995), and until recently this source of culture material was largely abandoned. In past studies on the sensitivity of blood cultures for recovery of Lyme borrelia, only a very small volume of under 1 ml of blood or blood components was cultured (Benach et al., 1983; Steere et al., 1983b, 1984; Nadelman et al., 1990; Wallach et al., 1993; Nadelman et al., 1994; Goodman et al., 1995). In other bacterial infections, however, the volume of blood cultured is an important determinant of yield (Washington and Ilstrup, 1986; Mermel and Maki, 1993; Weinstein, 1996). The reason for this is that with more conventional pathogens the number of cultivable bacteria per milliliter of whole blood is less than 1 in 50% of bacteremic patients and less than 0.1 in nearly 20% (Dorn et al., 1976; Kellogg et al., 1984). Therefore, in view of the recommendation to culture quantities of blood as large as 20 to 30 ml in other bacterial infections (Weinstein, 1996), the rationale of culturing much smaller volumes for Lyme disease patients was open to challenge.

In a series of recent experiments in adult patients with EM from the United States, it was demonstrated that recovery of *B. burgdorferi* was better from serum than from an identical volume of whole blood (Wormser et al., 1998), and that the yield from plasma was significantly greater than that from serum ($p = 0.005$) (Wormser et al., 2000a). Yield directly correlated with the volume of material cultured. Recovery of *B. burgdorferi* from high-volume cultures of 9 ml of plasma inoculated into a modified BSK II preparation devoid of antimicrobials and gelatin, with a 20:1 ratio of medium to plasma, was consistently above 40% (Wormser et al., 2000a, 2001). Unfortunately, high-volume plasma cultures are not appropriate for young children, since obtaining such a large quantity of blood would be unacceptable. Reported recovery rates from blood of patients with EM in Europe have been <10% (Arnez et al., 2001; Maraspin et al., 2001; Oksi et al., 2001). This may be due to a low frequency of hematogenous dissemination of *B. afzelii*, the principal cause of EM in Europe (Wang et al., 1999), or to culturing an inadequate volume of blood.

Plausible explanations for why plasma or serum would be a better source for recovery of *B. burgdorferi* than whole blood, if relatively small volumes are cultured, are that Lyme borrelia are not intracellular pathogens (Barthold, 2000) and in particular are not known to be associated with erythrocytes. An explanation of why plasma is a better source of culture material than serum (Wormser et al., 2000a, Goodman et al., 1995) is that a larger number of spirochetes appear to become trapped in a blood clot than in centrifuged erythrocytes. This hypothesis follows from an in vitro study in which known concentrations of *B. burgdorferi* were introduced into blood tubes with and without EDTA anticoagulant (Wormser et al., 2000a). In that study a greater than 40-fold reduction in spirochete number was observed in serum compared with plasma. Whether spirochete trapping during clot formation is merely a mechanical event or is related to binding of *B. burgdorferi* to activated platelets (Coburn et al., 1993) or to another clot component is unknown.

A study that addressed further increasing the volume of plasma from 9 ml to 18 ml in adult patients with EM found only a small increment in culture yield of approximately 10% (Wormser et al., 2001), suggesting that if substantially greater yields from blood cultures are still possible, it will be by further enriching the culture medium rather than by increasing the volume of plasma cultured. In that study it was estimated that the number of cultivable *B. burgdorferi* cells per milliliter of whole blood was approximately 0.1, which, if correct, would explain why blood cultures had such a consistently low yield in former studies in which the volume of blood or blood components cultured was extremely small (Wormser et al., 2001).

Although less extensively studied, the culture of blood samples is rarely positive in patients with any objective clinical manifestation of Lyme disease other than EM (Nadelman et al., 1990; Marques et al., 2000; J. Nowakowski, 2009). Blood cultures are also negative in patients with persistent subjective symptoms following completion of an appropriate course of antibiotic treatment (Marques et al., 2000; Klempner et al., 2001). These findings suggest that spirochetemia is transient and only occurs early during the course of infection.

Cerebrospinal Fluid

Evaluation of the sensitivity of culture of cerebrospinal fluid specimens in patients regarded as having neuroborreliosis by clinical and/or other laboratory test methods (e.g., intrathecal production of antibody to borrelia) has been reported principally from Europe (Karlsson et al., 1990; van Dam et al., 1993; Cimperman et al., 1999; Ornstein et al., 2001). The sensitivity of culture was approximately 10% (Table 9.2). The quantity of cerebrospinal fluid that was cultured varied from 0.2 to 5 ml (Karlsson et al., 1990; van Dam et al., 1993; Ornstein et al., 2001). None of the studies systematically compared the yields of culture of different volumes of cerebrospinal fluid. The highest yields for *B. garinii* (the principal cause of neuroborreliosis in Europe) were associated with shorter duration of illness (usually <14 days).

Sensitivity

Although as few as one spirochete can be recovered on culture using laboratory adapted and continuously propagated strains of *B. burgdorferi* (Barbour, 1984; Philipp et al., 1993; Pollack et al., 1993; Straubinger et al., 2000), the sensitivity of culture for clinical specimens is undefined. Compared to PCR for detection of spirochetes in cutaneous specimens of EM lesions, culture has proved to be slightly more sensitive in some studies but not in others (Moter et al., 1994; Picken et al., 1997; Brettschneider et al., 1998; Jurca et al., 1998; Steere et al., 1998; Lebech et al., 2000; Nowakowski et al., 2001; Oksi et al., 2001; Zore et al., 2002; Carlsson et al., 2003). Such disparate results are likely to be attributable to differences in the PCR protocols employed, including type of PCR, primer selection, and/or method of tissue preservation, as well as differences in culture techniques including size of the skin biopsy sample cultured and/or choice of culture medium. In a recent US study of skin biopsy samples of 47 untreated adult patients with EM lesions, culture grew *B. burgdorferi* in 51% compared with a 81% detection rate using a qPCR method ($p = 0.004$ by Fisher's exact test, two-tailed), and a 64% detection rate using a nested PCR ($p = 0.3$) (Table 9.3) (Nowakowski et al., 2001). In that study, culture of skin biopsy samples was more sensitive than serology

TABLE 9.3 Comparison of the sensitivity of culture versus other diagnostic methods for 47 adult patients with erythema migrans

Diagnostic Method	Sensitivity
Culture	
Skin biopsy of EM	51%
Plasma	45%
PCR on skin biopsy of EM	
Nested	64%
Quantitative	81%
Two-stage conditional serologic testing	
Acute phase	40%
Convalescent phase	66%

Source: Modified from reference Nowakowski et al. (2001).
Note: Evaluated in the year 2000 at the Lyme Disease Diagnostic Center in Valhalla, New York.

done on acute phase serum samples (Table 9.3), which is similar to what has been observed by other investigators (Strle et al., 1996; Steere et al., 1998).

Although all of the different Lyme borrelia species and subspecies recognized to cause human infection can be cultivated, it is not clear whether the sensitivity of culture is identical for each. In one study, subtyping of *B. burgdorferi* was performed directly on 51 skin biopsy samples of patients with EM using PCR-restriction fragment length polymorphism (RFLP) of the 16S-23S ribosomal DNA intergenic spacer region and also on the strains of *B. burgdorferi* that grew from culture of the same biopsy samples (Liveris et al., 1999). No significant difference in the rate of recovery of any single subtype was observed. In another study, however, culture of *I. spinipalpis* ticks from Colorado, in comparison to PCR testing of DNA extracted directly from infected ticks, appeared to select for specific genotypes of *B. burgdorferi* (Norris et al., 1997). Clearly, further investigation of this question is needed.

Practical Considerations

Culture has been principally used as a diagnostic modality in research studies and has enabled a better understanding of the clinical, laboratory, and pathogenetic aspects of Lyme borreliosis through identification of a group of culture-authenticated patients (Aguero-Rosenfeld et al., 1996; Nadelman et al., 1996; Strle et al., 1996, 1999; Logar et al., 1999; Smith et al., 2002; Carlsson et al., 2003). For example, the recognition that substantive differences exist in the clinical manifestations of patients with EM caused by *B. burgdorferi* compared with those caused by *B. afzelii* was based on analysis of culture-confirmed cases (Strle et al., 1999). In addition, culturing of ticks, EM skin lesions, and blood samples was instrumental to demonstrating that different subtypes of *B. burgdorferi* vary in their invasiveness and their potential to spread to extracutaneous sites (Seinost et al., 1999; Wormser et al., 1999). Patients with culture-confirmed Lyme disease have also been a valuable source of specimens to assess the accuracy of other diagnostic tests (Mitchell et al., 1994; Aguero-Rosenfeld et al., 1996; Vaz et al., 2001). Such well-defined patient populations have also played an important role in studying therapeutic regimens (Wormser et al., 2003) and vaccines (Steere et al., 1998).

Culture, however, has not been used in routine clinical practice as a diagnostic test for several reasons. One reason has been the lack of consistent availability of high-quality (i.e., borrelial growth promoting) lots of liquid medium for growing Lyme borrelia. Until fairly recently this medium was not distributed commercially, and although BSK-H is now available, it has periodically been in short supply.

A second reason is that by most conventional bacteriologic standards, borrelial cultures are more labor intensive, more expensive, and much slower requiring up to 8 to 12 weeks of incubation before being considered negative. The rapidity of identifying a positive culture, however, is directly dependent on the frequency with which the culture supernatant is examined microscopically, since macroscopic changes in the appearance of the culture medium tend to occur later, if at all. In our research studies, in which borrelial cultures are usually only first examined at 2 weeks, approximately 70% of positive cultures of skin biopsy samples of EM lesions and approximately 85% of positive cultures of plasma from EM patients were identified as positive at 2 weeks and approximately 95% of each type of sample by 4 weeks (Aguero-Rosenfeld et al., 2005). Time to detection of a positive specimen can be reduced to a clinically relevant time frame if cultures are examined on a daily basis (Mitchell et al., 1994). For example, the Marshfield Laboratories identified 74 (82%) of 90 positive cultures within the first 7 days of incubation and 32 (35%) within the first 3 days (Reed, 2002). In the experience of that laboratory the longest time to detection of a positive culture was 16 days. Culture positivity might be detected even more quickly if aliquots of culture supernatant were examined by PCR, rather than microscopy, to detect Lyme borrelia DNA (Schwartz et al., 1993; Chmielewski et al., 2003), and in the future it is conceivable that such an approach might be adaptable to automation.

A third limiting factor is that culture is only useful for untreated patients, at least in the United States. Culture positivity may be rapidly aborted by even a few doses of an appropriate antibiotic treatment (Berger et al., 1985; Schwartz et al., 1992; Nadelman et al., 1993).

Perhaps the most fundamental limitation is that culture is far too insensitive in patients with extracutaneous manifestations of Lyme disease, which is unfortunately the group of patients who pose the greatest diagnostic confusion (Nadelman and Wormser, 1998; Stanek and Strle, 2003). Culture has been most successful for patients with early Lyme disease who have EM, but visual recognition of the characteristic appearance of the skin lesion is usually sufficient for an accurate diagnosis, and no laboratory testing is indicated (Nadelman and Wormser, 1995, 1998). Culture would only be helpful in a minority of cases in which the rash may be atypical or the patient was not known to have had tick exposure in a Lyme borreliosis endemic area. In summary, culture is not recommended for diagnostic use in routine clinical practice.

NUCLEIC ACID AMPLIFICATION OF LYME BORRELIA DNA

Nucleic acid-based molecular methods offer a potential diagnostic tool for rapid, sensitive and specific identification of Lyme borrelia infection in patients with Lyme borreliosis. The first application of PCR, in which a portion of the chromosome of *B. burgdorferi* was targeted, was reported in 1989 (Rosa and Schwan, 1989). Since then, a variety of PCR assays aimed to detect Lyme borrelia DNA in clinical specimens have been developed and evaluated for their diagnostic value in patients with different clinical manifestations of Lyme borreliosis. Many technical details and applications of PCR assays were addressed in several recently published reviews (Schmidt, 1997; Bunikis and Barbour, 2002; Wang, 2002; Dumler, 2003; Wilske, 2003; Aguero-Rosenfeld et al., 2005).

Nucleic Acid Amplification Techniques

Nucleic acid-based techniques include hybridization probe-based and nucleic acid amplification-based approaches. For laboratory diagnosis of Lyme borreliosis, mainly nucleic acid amplification-based techniques are currently employed and will be discussed in this chapter.

A variety of clinical specimens from patients with suspected Lyme borreliosis have been analyzed by PCR assays (Schmidt, 1997; Aguero-Rosenfeld et al., 2005). Of these, skin biopsy samples taken from patients with EM were the most frequently tested specimens (Schwartz et al., 1992; Wienecke et al., 1993; Muellegger et al., 1995, 1996; von Stedingk et al., 1995; Picken et al., 1997; Rijpkema et al., 1997; Brettschneider et al., 1998; Oksi et al., 2001; Liveris et al., 2002; Wang, 2002). Other commonly used clinical specimens for PCR analysis include whole blood (Liebling et al., 1993), serum (Wallach et al., 1993; Demaerschalck et al., 1995) or plasma specimens (Goodman et al., 1995; Oksi et al., ; Oksi et al., 2001), cerebrospinal fluid from patients with neuroborreliosis (Debue et al., 1991; Keller et al., 1992; Luft et al., 1992; Liebling et al., 1993; Pachner and Delaney, 1993; Zbinden et al., 1994; Christen et al., 1995; Eiffert et al., 1995; Nocton et al., 1996; Priem et al., 1997; Oksi et al., ; Schwaiger et al., 2001; Ornstein et al., 2002), and synovial fluid/tissue from patients with Lyme arthritis (Debue et al., 1991; Liebling et al., 1993; Bradley et al., 1994; Persing et al., 1994; Jaulhac et al., 1996; Nocton et al., 1996; Priem et al., 1997; Eiffert et al., 1998; van der Heijden et al., 1999; Schwaiger et al., 2001; Schnarr et al., 2001). One study suggested that plasma may be the blood component most efficient for PCR analysis (Goodman et al., 1995).

Due to the extremely small amount of spirochetal DNA present in the typical volume of patient samples analyzed (Goodman et al., 1995; Wormser et al., 2001; Liveris et al., 2002) and the potential for the presence of host PCR inhibitors (Cogswell et al., 1996; Schwartz et al., 1997; Bergmann et al., 2002), appropriate specimens and procedures for sample collection, transport, and DNA preparation are critical for yielding reliable and consistent PCR results. While many published papers have reported the optimization and comparison of PCR protocols for various target genes of Lyme borrelia, less information is available addressing specimen processing for optimal DNA recovery prior to amplification. Clinical specimens collected from patients should be subjected to DNA extraction and PCR analysis shortly after collection, or they should be kept frozen. Studies on infected animal tissues suggest that PCR with DNA prepared from fresh frozen tissues has higher yields than that from paraffin-embedded, formalin-fixed tissues (Lebech et al., 1995).

PCR results can be qualitative (conventional PCR and nested PCR) or quantitative (qPCR) (competitive PCR and real-time PCR). Although many Lyme borrelia genes have been amplified and analyzed by PCR in research laboratories, only a few of these target genes have been utilized for detection of Lyme borrelia DNA in clinical specimens. Among these are the chromosomally encoded ribosomal DNA, *flaB*, *recA*, and *p66* and the plasmid-encoded *ospA* (Schmidt, 1997).

Several real-time PCR instruments are now commercially available (Wolk et al., 2001); each of these integrates the thermocycling, fluorescence detection and quantification in a single platform. Real-time PCR has been used for quantification of spirochetes in various biological specimens of patients with Lyme borreliosis (Schwaiger et al., 2001; Liveris et al., 2002), and in Europe, for typing of the three pathogenic Lyme borrelia species in ticks and EM patients (Pietila et al., 2000; Mommert et al., 2001; Rauter et al., 2002).

PCR Analysis of Clinical Specimens

Skin Biopsy

Skin biopsy specimens from patients with EM and ACA have been evaluated by PCR for diagnosis of Lyme borrelia infection. The PCR targets that have been employed for detection of Lyme borrelia DNA in skin biopsy specimens include *p66* (Wienecke et al., 1993; von Stedingk et al., 1995; Muellegger et al., 1995, 1996; Brettschneider et al., 1998), *rrs* (Schwartz et al., 1992; Schwaiger et al., 2001), *fla* (Picken et al., 1997; Oksi et al., 2001; Liveris et al., 2002), *rrl* (Brettschneider et al., 1998), *rrf-rrl* spacer (Rijpkema et al., 1997), *recA* (Liveris et al., 2002), and *ospA* (Moter et al., 1994; Rijpkema et al., 1997; Steere et al., 1998).

The sensitivity of PCR for detection of Lyme borrelia DNA in EM lesions is usually high, ranging from 50% to 70% in most studies (Dumler, ; Aguero-Rosenfeld et al., 2005). A prospective study in the United States showed that 85 of 132 (64%) skin biopsies taken from EM patients during a phase III vaccine trial were positive by PCR (Steere et al., 1998). Lyme borrelia-specific DNA has been detected in 54% to 100% of skin biopsy samples from patients with ACA in Europe (Table 9.4). Sensitivity of PCR for detection of Lyme borrelia in skin biopsy samples from patients appears to be dependent on the target sequences selected (Rijpkema et al., 1997; Brettschneider et al., 1998; Zore et al., 2002).

Blood Specimens

Lyme borrelia DNA has been detected by PCR in blood samples from patients with EM (Goodman et al., 1995; Oksi et al., 2001) or early disseminated disease such as neuroborreliosis and carditis (Liebling et al., 1993; Demaerschalck et al., 1995). In a prospective study, *B. burgdorferi* DNA was detected by PCR in 14 of 76 (18.4%) plasma samples from patients with EM in the United States; moreover PCR-documented spirochetemia in patients with EM was correlated with symptomatic illness and/or with the presence of multiple EM lesions (Goodman et al., 1995).

While the yield of blood culture approaches 50% in patients with EM with the use of high-volume plasma specimens (Wormser et al., 2000a, 2001), the sensitivity of PCR for detection of Lyme borrelia infection in blood, plasma, or serum samples remains low (Table 9.4). This discrepancy may be due to too small a test volume (usually 0.1 to 1 ml) of blood and/or the presence of PCR inhibitors in host blood (Cogswell et al., 1996; Al-Soud and Radstrom, 2001).

None of 78 patients with post-Lyme disease syndrome (arthralgias or myalgia, neurocognitive symptoms, dysesthesia, fatigue or malaise, headache, or sleep disturbance) had

TABLE 9.4 PCR sensitivity and specificity for detection of Lyme borrelia DNA in clinical specimens from patients with Lyme borreliosis

Clinical Specimen	Number of Studies Included	Median Sensitivity (% range)	Reported Specificity (% range)
	Skin biopsy, EM		
United States	4	64 (59–67)	98–100
Europe	12	73 (36–88)	100
	Skin biopsy, ACA		
Europe	8	76 (54–100)	100
	Blood/plasma/serum		
United States	3	18 (0–59)	100
Europe	3	10 (4–100)	
	CSF		
United States	6	73 (25–93)	93–100
Europe	10	23 (12–100)	98–100
	Synovial fluid		
United States	4	88 (44–100)	100
Europe	4	65 (42–85)	100

Source: Adapted from reference Aguero-Rosenfeld et al. (2005).
Note: EM: erythema migrans; ACA: acrodermatitis chronica atrophicans; CSF: cerebrospinal fluid.

detectable DNA in blood specimens, despite seropositivity by Western blot for IgG antibodies against *B. burgdorferi* in 39 of these patients (Klempner et al., 2001).

Cerebrospinal Fluid Specimens

Lyme borrelia DNA has been detected by PCR in cerebrospinal fluid specimens from patients with a variety of neurological symptoms in the United States and in Europe. However, the lack of a gold standard method to support the diagnosis of neuroborreliosis makes it difficult to assess the performance of PCR on cerebrospinal fluid. Sensitivity of PCR on cerebrospinal fluid specimens seems to be dependent on type of clinical presentation, disease duration, and whether antibiotic treatment was given. In a study of 60 patients with neuroborreliosis (16 with acute and 44 with chronic neuroborreliosis), the sensitivity of PCR in cerebrospinal fluid was 38% in acute and 25% in late neuroborreliosis, and an inverse correlation was found between duration of antimicrobial treatment and PCR results (Nocton et al., 1996). In another study 7 of 14 (50%) neuroborreliosis patients with disease duration of less than 2 weeks yielded a positive PCR result, compared with only 2 of 16 (13%) patients in whom the illness duration was greater than 2 weeks ($P = 0.045$) (Lebech et al., 2000). Lyme borrelia DNA was detectable in cerebrospinal fluid specimens of patients in a study from Sweden only if cerebrospinal fluid pleocytosis was present (7/36, 19.4%); none of 29 patients with clinical signs of Lyme borreliosis (EM, cranial neuritis and/or radiculoneuritis) without cerebrospinal fluid pleocytosis were PCR positive (Ornstein et al., 2002).

Synovial Fluid

PCR analysis of synovial fluid is a much more sensitive approach than culture for detection of Lyme borrelia in affected joints of patients with Lyme arthritis (Liebling et al., 1993; Bradley et al., 1994; Nocton et al., 1994; Persing et al., 1994; Jaulhac et al., 1996; Priem et al., 1997; Eiffert et al., 1998). In a US study of 88 patients, *B. burgdorferi* DNA was detected in synovial fluid samples of 75 (85%) patients with Lyme arthritis (Nocton et al., 1994). The PCR positivity rate was lower in patients who had received antibiotic therapy compared with untreated patients. Of 73 patients who were untreated or treated with only short courses of oral antibiotics, 70 (96%) had a positive PCR in synovial fluid samples. In contrast, *B. burgdorferi* DNA was demonstrated in only 7 of 19 (37%) patients who had received either a course of parenteral antibiotics or ≥ 1 month of oral antibiotic therapy (Nocton et al., 1994). The yield of PCR to detect Lyme borrelia DNA in synovial fluid samples appears to be dependent on the primer-probe set (s) selected. For example, of the patients with PCR positive results in the above-mentioned study, the most sensitive primer-probe set detected *B. burgdorferi* DNA in 89% versus 56% for the least sensitive set.

Target imbalance of *B. burgdorferi* chromosomal versus plasmid DNA has been observed in PCR analysis of synovial fluid specimens; higher sensitivity was reported in PCR with primers targeting *B. burgdorferi* plasmid-encoded *ospA* compared with chromosome-encoded 16S ribosomal RNA genes (Nocton et al., 1994; Persing et al., 1994). It has been speculated that *B. burgdorferi* present in the synovium may shed ospA DNA segments into the synovial fluid.

There have been a number of anecdotal reports of detection of Lyme borrelia DNA by PCR in urine specimens from patients with EM (Lebech and Hansen, 1992; Schmidt et al., 1995; Schmidt et al., 1996; Bergmann et al., 2002), neuroborreliosis (Lebech and Hansen, 1992; Huppertz et al., 1993; Liebling et al., 1993; Karch et al., 1994; Maiwald et al., 1995; Priem et al., 1997) and Lyme arthritis (Karch et al., 1994; Priem et al., 1997), but the reported sensitivity of urine PCR has been highly variable. In addition nonspecific amplification in urine PCR using several different targets has been documented (Liebling et al., 1993; Karch et al., 1994; Schmidt et al., 1996; Brettschneider et al., 1998). Thus it does not appear to be appropriate to use urine PCR alone for the laboratory diagnosis of Lyme borreliosis.

PCR Sensitivity and Specificity

Table 9.4 summarizes the reported sensitivity and specificity of PCR assays for detection of Lyme borrelia infection in various clinical samples, based on studies published in MEDLINE-indexed periodicals during the years 1991 to 2003. Of the studies in which Lyme borrelia DNA in skin biopsies was examined, sensitivity of the PCR assays varied from 36% to 88% for patients with EM and from 54% to 100% for patients with ACA in individual studies. The median sensitivities of the reported PCR assays for detection of Lyme borrelia DNA in skin biopsies from patients with EM was 64% in the United States and 73% in Europe.

The overall sensitivity of PCR for detection of Lyme borrelia in whole blood (plasma or serum) and cerebrospinal fluid specimens is low (Table 9.4). Higher PCR positivity rates were reported on blood specimens from patients with Lyme borreliosis in the United States than in Europe (18% vs. 10%, $P < 0.01$), which is in accordance with the more likely occurrence of multiple EMs (a clinical indication of hematogenous dissemination) in US patients (Strle et al., 1999). The positivity rate of PCR for detection of Lyme borrelia in cerebrospinal fluid specimens from patients in the United States was also higher than that in Europe. Possibly, *B. burgdorferi* infection results in a greater number of spirochetes in cerebrospinal fluid compared with *B. garinii* infection (*B. garinii* is the principal etiologic agent of neuroborreliosis in Europe), or different clinical criteria may have been employed for evaluation of suspected cases. The reported median sensitivity of PCR assays for identification of Lyme borrelia in patients with Lyme arthritis was 88% and 65% in North America and Europe, respectively (Table 9.4) (Aguero-Rosenfeld et al., 2005). A meta-analysis of PCR for detection of Lyme borrelia DNA in clinical specimens reported similar results to that found in Table 9.4 (Dumler, 2001).

Applications and Limitations

PCR is a promising technique for providing laboratory evidence to confirm Lyme borrelia infection in selected patients with Lyme borreliosis. An advantage over culture is that both viable and nonviable organisms can be detected; PCR also provides a result much more quickly than culture. A disadvantage compared to culture is that positive PCR results do not establish whether the infection is active. Furthermore, if testing conditions are not strictly controlled, PCR may be falsely positive due to laboratory contamination (Molloy et al., 2001). Therefore positive PCR results for Lyme borrelia nucleic acids obtained in samples from patients with extracutaneous manifestations of Lyme borreliosis in the absence of serological evidence of Lyme borrelia infection should be interpreted with caution. Conversely, PCR may be falsely negative due to inhibitors present in various biological samples (blood, urine, synovial fluid, or cerebrospinal fluid) obtained from patients with Lyme borreliosis (Molloy et al., 2001). Co-amplification of an internal control target and inclusion of both positive and negative controls in each PCR run are recommended to assist in recognition of false positive or false negative results in clinical specimens.

Several genotypes of the single species *B. burgdorferi* in the United States (Liveris et al., 1999; Seinost et al., 1999; Wormser et al., 1999) and multiple genotypes of three pathogenic Lyme borrelial species, *B. burgdorferi*, *B. garinii*, or *B. afzelii,* in Europe (Wang et al., 1999) are responsible for causing human disease. Infections with distinct species or genotypes of Lyme borrelia are correlated with different clinical manifestations of Lyme borreliosis (van Dam et al., 1993; Seinost et al., 1999; Wang et al., 1999). Genotyping of the infecting Lyme borrelia will, therefore, provide useful information for elucidation of pathogen–disease associations (Wang et al., 1999). PCR-based techniques have been utilized for direct typing of the infecting Lyme borrelia strains in clinical specimens from patients with EM (Rijpkema et al., 1997; Liveris et al., 1999), neuroborreliosis (Demaerschalck et al., 1995; Lebech et al., 1995) and Lyme arthritis (Eiffert et al., 1998). Real-time PCR assays have been developed to differentiate the species of Lyme borrelia that are clinically relevant in Europe (Pietila et al., 2000; Mommert et al., 2001; Rauter et al., 2002). A multiplex PCR with potential to detect coinfection of Lyme borrelia with other vector-borne pathogens in clinical specimens has been described (Courtney et al., 2004).

Recently the number of spirochetes in clinical specimens of patients with Lyme borreliosis was determined by real-time qPCR assays. In one study, in which *B. burgdorferi*-specific *recA* DNA was detected by a Lightcycler qPCR assay, the number of spirochetes in a 2-mm biopsy of an EM skin lesion ranged from 10 to 11,000, with a mean number of 2462 spirochetes (Liveris et al., 2002). A significantly larger number of spirochetes was detected in culture-positive than in culture-negative specimens (3940 vs. 1642 spirochetes, $P < 0.01$). In another study, Lyme borrelia *fla* was detected using a TaqMan™ probe in 5 of 28 (17.9%) synovial fluid specimens and one of five (20%) synovial membrane biopsies obtained from 31 patients with arthropathies in Switzerland (Schwaiger et al., 2001). The numbers of spirochetes varied from 20 to 41,000/ml of synovial fluid. Given its high sensitivity, specificity and potential automation in DNA preparation (Wolk et al., 2001; Exner and Lewinski, 2003), increased use of real-time PCR may be expected in the laboratory diagnosis of Lyme borreliosis.

SUMMARY

Culture is most successful for detection of Lyme borrelia when applied to skin biopsy specimens of EM or ACA lesions and to plasma blood samples of United States patients with EM. At present this diagnostic modality is principally regarded as a research tool. Nucleic amplification techniques such as PCR have comparable or slightly better sensitivity than culture for detection of Lyme borrelia in skin biopsy samples, but this usage is restricted to research studies. For clinical purposes the principal role of PCR is in testing synovial fluid samples to support the diagnosis of Lyme arthritis in *Borrelia* IgG antibody seropositive patients with joint swelling. Amplification of Lyme borrelia DNA by PCR on cerebrospinal fluid specimens may also provide support for the diagnosis of neuroborreliosis, but most hospitals refer the specimen to a referral laboratory at great expense. Considering the very low yield, this is not a cost-effective diagnostic modality. With PCR testing, special emphasis needs to be placed on meticulous quality control to avoid DNA contamination leading to false-positive test results.

ACKNOWLEDGMENTS

The authors thank Drs. Maria Aguero-Rosenfeld and Ira Schwartz for critically reviewing the manuscript and Ms. Lisa Giarratano for assistance.

REFERENCES

Agger WA, Callister SM, Jobe DA: In vitro susceptibilities of *Borrelia burgdorferi* to five oral cephalosporins and ceftriaxone. *Antimicrob Agents Chemother* 36:1788–1790; 1992.

Aguero-Rosenfeld ME, Nowakowski J, Bittker S, Cooper D, Nadelman RB, Wormser GP: Evolution of the serologic response to *Borrelia burgdorferi* in treated patients with culture-confirmed erythema migrans. *J Clin Microbiol* 34:1–9; 1996.

Aguero-Rosenfeld ME, Wang G, Schwartz I, Wormser GP: Diagnosis of Lyme borreliosis. *Clin Microbiol Rev* 18:484–509; 2005.

Al-Soud WA, Radstrom P: Purification and characterization of PCR-inhibitory components in blood cells. *J Clin Microbiol* 39:485–493; 2001.

Anderson JF, Magnarelli LA, Burgdorfer W, Barbour AG: Spirochetes in *Ixodes dammini* and mammals from Connecticut. *Am J Trop Med Hyg* 32:818–824; 1983.

Anderson JF, Duray PH, Magnarelli LA: Prevalence of *Borrelia burgdorferi* in white-footed mice and *Ixodes dammini* at Fort McCoy. *Wis. J Clin Microbiol* 25:1495–1497; 1987.

Arnez M, Ruzic-Sabljic E, Ahcan J, Radsel-Medvescek A, Pleterski-Rigler D, Strle F: Isolation of *Borrelia burgdorferi* sensu lato from blood of children with solitary erythema migrans. *Pediatr Infect Dis J* 20:251–255; 2001.

Asbrink E, Hovmark A: Successful cultivation of spirochetes from skin lesions of patients with erythema chronicum migrans Afzelius and acrodermatitis chronica atrophicans. *Acta Pathol Microbiol Immunol Scand [B]* 93:161–163; 1985.

Barbour AG: Isolation and cultivation of Lyme disease spirochetes. *Yale J Biol Med* 57:521–525; 1984.

Barthold SW: Lyme Borreliosis. *In* Nataro JP, Blaser MJ, Cunningham-Rundles S. (eds): *Persistent Bacterial Infections*. Washington, DC, ASM Press; 2000.

Benach JL, Bosler EM, Hanrahan JP, Coleman JL, Habicht GS, Bast TF, Cameron DJ, Ziegler JL, Barbour AG, Burgdorfer W, Edelman R, Kaslow RA: Spirochetes isolated from the blood of two patients with Lyme disease. *N Engl J Med* 308:740–742; 1983.

Berger BW: Dermatologic manifestations of Lyme disease. *Rev Infect Dis* 11(suppl 6)**:** S1475–S1481; 1989.

Berger BW, Clemmensen OJ, Ackerman AB: Lyme disease is a spirochetosis. A review of the disease and evidence for its cause. *Am J Dermatopathol* 5:111–124; 1983.

Berger BW, Kaplan MH, Rothenberg IR, Barbour AG: Isolation and characterization of the Lyme disease spirochete from the skin of patients with erythema chronicum migrans. *J Am Acad Dermatol* 13:444–449; 1985.

Berger BW, Johnson RC, Kodner C, Coleman L: Cultivation of *Borrelia burgdorferi* from erythema migrans lesions and perilesional skin. *J Clin Microbiol* 30:359–361; 1992a.

Berger BW, Johnson RC, Kodner C, Coleman L: Failure of *Borrelia burgdorferi* to survive in the skin of patients with antibiotic-treated Lyme disease. *J Am Acad Dermatol* 27:34–37; 1992b.

Bergmann AR, Schmidt BL, Derler AM, Aberer E: Importance of sample preparation for molecular diagnosis of Lyme borreliosis from urine. *J Clin Microbiol* 40:4581–4584; 2002.

Bosler EM, Coleman JL, Benach JL, Massey DA, Hanrahan JP, Burgdorfer W, Barbour AG: Natural distribution of the *Ixodes dammini* spirochete. *Science* 220:321–322; 1983.

Bradley JF, Johnson RC, Goodman JL: The persistence of spirochetal nucleic acids in active Lyme arthritis. *Ann Intern Med* 120:487–489; 1994.

Brettschneider S, Bruckbauer H, Klugbauer N, Hofmann H: Diagnostic value of PCR for detection of *Borrelia burgdorferi* in skin biopsy and urine samples from patients with skin borreliosis. *J Clin Microbiol* 36:2658–2665; 1998.

Bunikis J, Barbour AG: Laboratory testing for suspected Lyme disease. *Med Clin North Am* 86:311–340; 2002.

Burgdorfer W, Barbour AG, Hayes SF, Benach JL, Grunwaldt E, Davis JP: Lyme disease-a tick-borne spirochetosis? *Science* 216:1317–1319; 1982.

Callister SM, Case KL, Agger WA, Schell RF, Johnson RC, Ellingson JL: Effects of bovine serum albumin on the ability of Barbour–Stoenner–Kelly medium to detect *Borrelia burgdorferi*. *J Clin Microbiol* 28:363–365; 1990.

Carlsson SA, Granlund H, Jansson C, Nyman D, Wahlberg P: Characteristics of erythema migrans in *Borrelia afzelii* and *Borrelia garinii* infections. *Scand J Infect Dis* 35:31–33; 2003.

Chmielewski T, Fiett J, Gniadkowski M, Tylewska-Wierzbanowska S: Improvement in the laboratory recognition of Lyme borreliosis with the combination of culture and PCR methods. *Mol Diagn* 7:155–62; 2003.

Christen HJ, Eiffert H, Ohlenbusch A, Hanefeld F: Evaluation of the polymerase chain reaction for the detection of *Borrelia burgdorferi* in cerebrospinal fluid of children with acute peripheral facial palsy. *Eur J Pediatr* 154:374–377; 1995.

Cimperman J, Maraspin V, Lotric-Furlan S, Ruzic-Sabljic E, Strle F: Lyme meningitis. A one-year follow up controlled study. *Wien Klin Wochenschr* 111:961–963; 1999.

Coburn J, Leong JM, Erban JK: Integrin alpha IIb beta 3 mediates binding of the Lyme disease agent *Borrelia burgdorferi* to human platelets. *Proc Natl Acad Sci USA* 90:7059–7063; 1993.

Cogswell FB, Bantar CE, Hughes TG, Gu Y, Philipp MT: Host DNA can interfere with detection of *Borrelia burgdorferi* in skin biopsy specimens by PCR. *J Clin Microbiol* 34:980–982; 1996.

Courtney JW, Kostelnik LM, Zeidner NS, Massung RF: Multiplex real-time PCR for detection of *Anaplasma phagocytophilum* and *Borrelia burgdorferi*. *J Clin Microbiol* 42:3164–3168; 2004.

Debue M, Gautier P, Hackel C, van Elsen A, Herzog A, Bigaignon G, Bollen A: Detection of *Borrelia burgdorferi* in biological samples using the polymerase chain reaction assay. *Res Microbiol* 142:565–572; 1991.

Demaerschalck I, Ben Messaoud A, De Kesel M, Hoyois B, Lobet Y, Hoet P, Bigaignon G, Bollen A, Godfroid E: Simultaneous presence of different *Borrelia burgdorferi* genospecies in biological fluids of Lyme disease patients. *J Clin Microbiol* 33:602–608; 1995.

Dorn GL, Burson GG, Haynes JR: Blood culture technique based on centrifugation: clinical evaluation. *J Clin Microbiol* 3:258–263; 1976.

Dumler JS: Molecular diagnosis of Lyme disease. Review and meta-analysis. *Mol Diagn* 6:1–11; 2001.

Dumler JS: Molecular methods for ehrlichiosis and Lyme disease. *Clin Lab Med* 23:867–884, vi; 2003.

Eiffert H, Ohlenbusch A, Christen HJ, Thomssen R, Spielmen A, Matuschka FR: Nondifferentiation between Lyme disease spirochetes from vector ticks and human cerebrospinal fluid. *J Infect Dis* 171:476–479; 1995.

Eiffert H, Karsten A, Thomssen R, Christen HJ: Characterization of *Borrelia burgdorferi* strains in Lyme arthritis. *Scand J Infect Dis* 30:265–268; 1998.

Exner MM, Lewinski MA: Isolation and detection of *Borrelia burgdorferi* DNA from cerebral spinal fluid, synovial fluid, blood, urine, and ticks using the Roche MagNA Pure system and real-time PCR. *Diagn Microbiol Infect Dis* 46:235–240; 2003.

Fraser CM, Casjens S, Huang WM, Sutton GG, Clayton R, Lathigra R, White O, Ketchum KA, Dodson R, Hickey EK, Gwinn M, Dougherty B, Tomb JF, Fleischmann RD, Richardson D, Peterson J, Kerlavage AR, Quackenbush J., Salzberg S, Hanson M, van Vugt R, Palmer N, Adams MD, Gocayne J, Weidman J, Utterback T, Watthey L, McDonald L, Artiach P, Bowman C, Garland S, Fuji C, Cotton MD, Horst K, Roberts K, Hatch B, Smith HO, Venter JC: Genomic sequence of a Lyme disease spirochaete, *Borrelia burgdorferi*. *Nature* 390:580–586; 1997.

Goodman JL, Bradley JF, Ross AE, Goellner P, Lagus A, Vitale B, Berger BW, Luger S, Johnson RC: Bloodstream invasion in early Lyme disease. Results from a prospective, controlled, blinded study using the polymerase chain reaction. *Am J Med* 99:6–12; 1995.

Hechemy KE, Samsonoff WA, Harris HL, McKee M: Adherence and entry of *Borrelia burgdorferi* in Vero cells. *J Med Microbiol* 36:229–238; 1992.

Huppertz HI, Schmidt H, Karch H: Detection of *Borrelia burgdorferi* by nested polymerase chain reaction in cerebrospinal fluid and urine of children with neuroborreliosis. *Eur J Pediatr* 152:414–417; 1993.

Jaulhac B, Chary-Valckenaere I, Sibilia J, Javier RM, Piemont Y, Kuntz JL, Monteil H, Pourel J: Detection of *Borrelia burgdorferi* by DNA amplification in synovial tissue samples from patients with Lyme arthritis. *Arthritis Rheum* 39:736–745; 1996.

Jobe DA, Callister SM, Schell RF: Recovery of *Borrelia burgdorferi* by filtration. *J Clin Microbiol* 31:1896–1898; 1993.

Johnson SE, Klein GC, Schmid GP, Bowen GS, Feeley JC, Schulze T: Lyme disease. A selective medium for isolation of the suspected etiological agent, a spirochete. *J Clin Microbiol* 19:81–82; 1984.

Jurca T, Ruzic-Sabljic E, Lotric-Furlan S, Maraspin V, Cimperman J, Picken RN, Strle F: Comparison of peripheral and central biopsy sites for the isolation of *Borrelia burgdorferi* sensu lato from erythema migrans skin lesions. *Clin Infect Dis* 27:636–638; 1998.

Karch H, Huppertz HI, Bohme M, Schmidt H, Wiebecke D, Schwarzkopf A: Demonstration of *Borrelia burgdorferi* DNA in urine samples from healthy humans whose sera contain *B. burgdorferi*-specific antibodies. *J Clin Microbiol* 32:2312–2314; 1994.

Karlsson M, Hovind-Hougen K, Svenungsson B, Stiernstedt G: Cultivation and characterization of spirochetes from cerebrospinal fluid of patients with Lyme borreliosis. *J Clin Microbiol* 28:473–479; 1990.

Keller TL, Halperin JJ, Whitman M: PCR detection of *Borrelia burgdorferi* DNA in cerebrospinal fluid of Lyme neuroborreliosis patients. *Neurology* 42:32–42; 1992.

Kellogg JA, Manzella JP, McConville JH: Clinical laboratory comparison of the 10-ml isolator blood culture system with BACTEC radiometric blood culture media. *J Clin Microbiol* 20:618–623; 1984.

Kelly R: Cultivation of *Borrelia hermsi. Science* 173:443–444; 1971.

Klempner MS, Hu LT, Evans J, Schmid CH, Johnson GM, Trevino RP, Norton D, Levy L, Wall D, McCall J, Kosinski M, Weinstein A: Two controlled trials of antibiotic treatment in patients with persistent symptoms and a history of Lyme disease. *N Engl J Med* 345:85–92; 2001.

Kuiper H, van Dam AP, Spanjaard L, De Jongh BM, Widjojokusumo A, Ramselaar TC, Cairo I, Vos K, Dankert J: Isolation of *Borrelia burgdorferi* from biopsy specimens taken from healthy-looking skin of patients with Lyme borreliosis. *J Clin Microbiol* 32:715–720; 1994.

Kurtti TJ, Munderloh UG, Johnson RC, Ahlstrand GG: Colony formation and morphology in *Borrelia burgdorferi. J Clin Microbiol* 25:2054–2058; 1987.

Kurtti TJ, Munderloh UG, Ahlstrand GG, Johnson RC: *Borrelia burgdorferi* in tick cell culture. Growth and cellular adherence. *J Med Entomol* 25:256–261; 1988.

Lebech AM, Hansen K: Detection of *Borrelia burgdorferi* DNA in urine samples and cerebrospinal fluid samples from patients with early and late Lyme neuroborreliosis by polymerase chain reaction. *J Clin Microbiol* 30:1646–1653; 1992.

Lebech AM, Clemmensen O, Hansen K: Comparison of in vitro culture, immunohistochemical staining, and PCR for detection of *Borrelia burgdorferi* in tissue from experimentally infected animals. *J Clin Microbiol* 33:2328–2333; 1995.

Lebech AM, Hansen K, Brandrup F, Clemmensen O, Halkier-Sorensen L: Diagnostic value of PCR for detection of *Borrelia burgdorferi* DNA in clinical specimens from patients with erythema migrans and Lyme neuroborreliosis. *Mol Diagn* 5:139–150; 2000.

Liebling MR, Nishio MJ, Rodriguez A, Sigal LH, Jin T, Louie JS: The polymerase chain reaction for the detection of *Borrelia burgdorferi* in human body fluids. *Arthritis Rheum* 36:665–675; 1993.

Liveris D, Varde S, Iyer R, Koenig S, Bittker S, Cooper D, McKenna D, Nowakowski J, Nadelman R., Wormser GP, Schwartz I: Genetic diversity of *Borrelia burgdorferi* in Lyme disease patients as determined by culture versus direct PCR with clinical specimens. *J Clin Microbiol* 37:565–569; 1999.

Liveris D, Wang G, Girao G, Byrne DW, Nowakowski J, McKenna D, Nadelman R, Wormser GP, Schwartz I: Quantitative detection of *Borrelia burgdorferi* in 2-millimeter skin samples of erythema migrans lesions. Correlation of results with clinical and laboratory findings. *J Clin Microbiol* 40:1249–1253; 2002.

Logar M, Lotric-Furlan S, Maraspin V, Cimperman J, Jurca T, Ruzic-Sabljic E, Strle F: Has the presence or absence of *Borrelia burgdorferi* sensu lato as detected by skin culture any influence on the course of erythema migrans? *Wien Klin Wochenschr* 111:945–950; 1999.

Luft BJ, Steinman CR, Neimark HC, Muralidhar B, Rush T, Finkel MF, Kunkel M, Dattwyler RJ: Invasion of the central nervous system by *Borrelia burgdorferi* in acute disseminated infection. *JAMA* 267:1364–1367; 1992.

Maiwald M, Stockinger C, Hassler D, von Knebel Doeberitz M, Sonntag HG: Evaluation of the detection of *Borrelia burgdorferi* DNA in urine samples by polymerase chain reaction. *Infection* 23:173–179; 1995.

Maraspin V, Ruzic-Sabljic E, Cimperman J, Lotric-Furlan S, Jurca T, Picken RN, Strle F: Isolation of *Borrelia burgdorferi* sensu lato from blood of patients with erythema migrans. *Infection* 29:65–70; 2001.

Maraspin V, Cimperman J, Lotric-Furlan S, Ruzic-Sabljic E, Jurca T, Picken RN, Strle F: Solitary borrelial lymphocytoma in adult patients. *Wien Klin Wochenschr* 114:515–523; 2002.

Marlovits S, Khanakah G, Striessnig G, Vecsei V, Stanek G: Emergence of Lyme arthritis after autologous chondrocyte transplantation. *Arthritis Rheum* 50:259–264; 2004.

Marques AR, Stock F, Gill V: Evaluation of a new culture medium for *Borrelia burgdorferi*. *J Clin Microbiol* 38:4239–4241; 2000.

Melski JW, Reed KD, Mitchell PD, Barth GD: Primary and secondary erythema migrans in central Wisconsin. *Arch Dermatol* 129:709–716; 1993.

Mermel LA, Maki DG: Detection of bacteremia in adults: consequences of culturing an inadequate volume of blood. *Ann Intern Med* 119:270–272; 1993.

Mitchell PD, Reed KD, Vandermause MF, Melski JW: Isolation of *Borrelia burgdorferi* from skin biopsy specimens of patients with erythema migrans. *Am J Clin Pathol* 99:104–107; 1993.

Mitchell PD, Reed KD, Aspeslet TL, Vandermause MF, Melski JW: Comparison of four immunoserologic assays for detection of antibodies to *Borrelia burgdorferi* in patients with culture-positive erythema migrans. *J Clin Microbiol* 32:1958–1962; 1994.

Molloy PJ, Persing DH, Berardi VP: False-positive results of PCR testing for Lyme disease. *Clin Infect Dis* 33:412–413; 2001.

Mommert S, Gutzmer R, Kapp A, Werfel T: Sensitive detection of *Borrelia burgdorferi* sensu lato DNA and differentiation of *Borrelia* species by LightCycler PCR. *J Clin Microbiol* 39:2663–2667; 2001.

Morshed MG, Konishi H, Nishimura T, Nakazawa T: Evaluation of agents for use in medium for selective isolation of Lyme disease and relapsing fever *Borrelia* species. *Eur J Clin Microbiol Infect Dis* 12:512–518; 1993.

Moter SE, Hofmann H, Wallich R, Simon MM, Kramer MD: Detection of *Borrelia burgdorferi* sensu lato in lesional skin of patients with erythema migrans and acrodermatitis chronica atrophicans by ospA-specific PCR. *J Clin Microbiol* 32:2980–2988; 1994.

Muellegger R, Zoechling N, Schluepen EM, Soyer HP, Hoedl S, Kerl H, Volkenandt M: Polymerase chain reaction control of antibiotic treatment in dermatoborreliosis. *Infection* 24:76–79; 1996.

Muellegger RR, Zoechling N, Soyer HP, Hoedl S, Wienecke R, Volkenandt M, Kerl H: No detection of *Borrelia burgdorferi*-specific DNA in erythema migrans lesions after minocycline treatment. *Arch Dermatol* 131:678–682; 1995.

Munderloh UG, Liu Y, Wang M, Chen C, Kurtti TJ: Establishment, maintenance and description of cell lines from the tick *Ixodes scapularis*. *J Parasitol* 80:533–543; 1994.

Nadelman RB, Wormser GP: Erythema migrans and early Lyme disease. *Am J Med* 98:15S–23S; discussion 23S–24S; 1995.

Nadelman RB, Wormser GP: Lyme borreliosis. *Lancet* 352:557–565; 1998.

Nadelman RB, Pavia CS, Magnarelli LA, Wormser GP: Isolation of *Borrelia burgdorferi* from the blood of seven patients with Lyme disease. *Am J Med* 88:21–26; 1990.

Nadelman RB, Nowakowski J, Forseter G, Bittker S, Cooper D, Goldberg N, McKenna D, Wormser GP: Failure to isolate *Borrelia burgdorferi* after antimicrobial therapy in culture-documented Lyme borreliosis associated with erythema migrans: report of a prospective study. *Am J Med* 94:583–588; 1993.

Nadelman RB, Schwartz I, Wormser GP: Detecting *Borrelia burgdorferi* in blood from patients with Lyme disease. *J Infect Dis* 169:1410–1411; 1994.

Nadelman RB, Nowakowski J, Forseter G, Goldberg NS, Bittker S, Cooper D, Aguero-Rosenfeld M, Wormser GP: The clinical spectrum of early Lyme borreliosis in patients with culture-confirmed erythema migrans. *Am J Med* 100:502–8; 1996.

Nelson JA, Bouseman JK, Kitron U, Callister SM, Harrison B, Bankowski MJ, Peeples ME, Newton BJ, Anderson JF: Isolation and characterization of *Borrelia burgdorferi* from Illinois *Ixodes dammini*. *J Clin Microbiol* 29:1732–1734; 1991.

Neubert U, Krampitz HE, Engl H: Microbiological findings in erythema (chronicum) migrans and related disorders. *Zentralbl Bakteriol Mikrobiol Hyg [A]* 263:237–252; 1986.

Nocton JJ, Dressler F, Rutledge BJ, Rys PN, Persing DH, Steere AC: Detection of *Borrelia burgdorferi* DNA by polymerase chain reaction in synovial fluid from patients with Lyme arthritis. *N Engl J Med* 330:229–234; 1994.

Nocton JJ, Bloom BJ, Rutledge BJ, Persing DH, Logigian EL, Schmid CH, Steere AC: Detection of *Borrelia burgdorferi* DNA by polymerase chain reaction in cerebrospinal fluid in Lyme neuroborreliosis. *J Infect Dis* 174:623–627; 1996.

Norris DE, Johnson BJ, Piesman J, Maupin GO, Clark JL, Black WCT: Culturing selects for specific genotypes of *Borrelia burgdorferi* in an enzootic cycle in Colorado. *J Clin Microbiol* 35:2359–2364; 1997.

Nowakowski J, McKenna D, Nadelman RB, Cooper D, Bittker S, Holmgren D, Pavia C, Johnson RC, Wormser GP: Failure of treatment with cephalexin for Lyme disease. *Arch Fam Med* 9:563–567; 2000.

Nowakowski J, Schwartz I, Liveris D, Wang G, Aguero-Rosenfeld ME, Girao G, McKenna D, Nadelman RB, Cavaliere LF, Wormser GP: Laboratory diagnostic techniques for patients with early Lyme disease associated with erythema migrans: a comparison of different techniques. *Clin Infect Dis* 33:2023–2027; 2001.

Nowakowski J, McKenna D, Nadelman RB, Bittker S, Cooper D, Pavia C, Holmgren D, Visintainer P, Wormser GP: Blood cultures for patients with extracutaneous manifestations of Lyme disease in the United States. *Clin Infect Dis*. 1;49(11):1733–1735; 2009.

Obonyo M, Munderloh UG, Fingerle V, Wilske B, Kurtti TJ: *Borrelia burgdorferi* in tick cell culture modulates expression of outer surface proteins A and C in response to temperature. *J Clin Microbiol* 37:2137–2141; 1999.

Oksi J, Marjamaki M, Nikoskelainen J, Viljanen MK: *Borrelia burgdorferi* detected by culture and PCR in clinical relapse of disseminated Lyme borreliosis. *Ann Med* 31:225–232; 1999.

Oksi J, Marttila H, Soini H, Aho H, Uksila J, Viljanen MK: Early dissemination of *Borrelia burgdorferi* without generalized symptoms in patients with erythema migrans. *APMIS* 109:581–588; 2001.

Ornstein K, Berglund J, Nilsson I, Norrby R, Bergstrom S: Characterization of Lyme borreliosis isolates from patients with erythema migrans and neuroborreliosis in southern Sweden. *J Clin Microbiol* 39:1294–1298; 2001.

Ornstein K, Berglund J, Bergstrom S, Norrby R, Barbour AG: Three major Lyme *Borrelia* genospecies (*Borrelia burgdorferi* sensu stricto, *B. afzelii* and *B. garinii*) identified by PCR in cerebrospinal fluid from patients with neuroborreliosis in Sweden. *Scand J Infect Dis* 34:341–346; 2002.

Pachner AR, Delaney E: The polymerase chain reaction in the diagnosis of Lyme neuroborreliosis. *Ann Neurol* 34:544–550; 1993.

Pavia CS, Niederbuhl CJ: Experimental infection of inbred guinea pigs with *Treponema pallidum*: development of lesions and formation of antibodies. *Genitourin Med* 61:75–81; 1985.

Persing DH, Rutledge BJ, Rys PN, Podzorski DS, Mitchell PD, Reed KD, Liu B, Fikrig E, Malawista SE: Target imbalance. Disparity of *Borrelia burgdorferi* genetic material in synovial fluid from Lyme arthritis patients. *J Infect Dis* 169:668–672; 1994.

Philipp MT, Aydintug MK, Bohm RP Jr, Cogswell FB, Dennis VA, Lanners HN, Lowrie RC Jr, Roberts ED, Conway MD, Karacorlu M, Peyman GA, Gubler DJ, Johnson BJ, Piesman J, Gu Y: Early and early disseminated phases of Lyme disease in the rhesus monkey. A model for infection in humans. *Infect Immun* 61:3047–3059; 1993.

Picken MM, Picken RN, Han D, Cheng Y, Ruzic-Sabljic E, Cimperman J, Maraspin V, Lotric-Furlan S, Strle F: A two year prospective study to compare culture and polymerase chain reaction amplification for the detection and diagnosis of Lyme borreliosis. *Mol Pathol* 50:186–193; 1997.

Picken RN, Strle F, Picken MM, Ruzic-Sabljic E, Maraspin V, Lotric-Furlan S, Cimperman J: Identification of three species of *Borrelia burgdorferi* sensu lato (*B. burgdorferi* sensu stricto, *B. garinii,* and *B. afzelii*) among isolates from acrodermatitis chronica atrophicans lesions. *J Invest Dermatol* 110:211–214; 1998.

Piesman J, Maupin GO, Campos EG, Happ CM: Duration of adult female *Ixodes dammini* attachment and transmission of *Borrelia burgdorferi,* with description of a needle aspiration isolation method. *J Infect Dis* 163:895–897; 1991.

Pietila J, He Q, Oksi J, Viljanen MK: Rapid differentiation of *Borrelia garinii* from *Borrelia afzelii* and *Borrelia burgdorferi* sensu stricto by LightCycler fluorescence melting curve analysis of a PCR product of the recA gene. *J Clin Microbiol* 38:2756–2759; 2000.

Pollack RJ, Telford S.R. III, Spielman A: Standardization of medium for culturing Lyme disease spirochetes. *J Clin Microbiol* 31:1251–1255; 1993.

Preac-Mursic V, Wilske B, Schierz G: European *Borrelia burgdorferi* isolated from humans and ticks culture conditions and antibiotic susceptibility. *Zentralbl Bakteriol Mikrobiol Hyg [A]* 263:112–118; 1986.

Preac-Mursic V, Weber K, Pfister HW, Wilske B, Gross B, Baumann A, Prokop J: Survival of *Borrelia burgdorferi* in antibiotically treated patients with Lyme borreliosis. *Infection* 17:355–359; 1989.

Preac-Mursic V, Wilske B, Reinhardt S: Culture of *Borrelia burgdorferi* on six solid media. *Eur J Clin Microbiol Infect Dis* 10:1076–1079; 1991.

Preac-Mursic V, Pfister HW, Spiegel H, Burk R, Wilske B, Reinhardt S, Bohmer R: First isolation of *Borrelia burgdorferi* from an iris biopsy. *J Clin Neuroophthalmol* 13:155–61; discussion 162; 1993.

Priem S, Rittig MG, Kamradt T, Burmester GR, Krause A: An optimized PCR leads to rapid and highly sensitive detection of *Borrelia burgdorferi* in patients with Lyme borreliosis. *J Clin Microbiol* 35:685–690; 1997.

Rauter C, Oehme R, Diterich I, Engele M, Hartung T: Distribution of clinically relevant *Borrelia* genospecies in ticks assessed by a novel, single-run, real-time PCR. *J Clin Microbiol* 40:36–43; 2002.

Reed KD: Laboratory testing for Lyme disease: Possibilities and practicalities. *J Clin Microbiol* 40:319–324; 2002.

Rijpkema SG, Tazelaar DJ, Molkenboer MJ, Noordhoek GT, Plantinga G, Schouls LM, Schellekens JF: Detection of *Borrelia afzelii, Borrelia burgdorferi* sensu stricto, *Borrelia garinii* and group

VS116 by PCR in skin biopsies of patients with erythema migrans and acrodermatitis chronica atrophicans. *Clin Microbiol Infect* 3:109–116; 1997.

Rosa PA, Schwan TG: A specific and sensitive assay for the Lyme disease spirochete *Borrelia burgdorferi* using the polymerase chain reaction. *J Infect Dis* 160:1018–1029; 1989.

Schmidli J, Hunziker T, Moesli P, Schaad UB: Cultivation of *Borrelia burgdorferi* from joint fluid three months after treatment of facial palsy due to Lyme borreliosis. *J Infect Dis* 158:905–906; 1988.

Schmidt B, Muellegger RR, Stockenhuber C, Soyer HP, Hoedl S, Luger A, Kerl H: Detection of *Borrelia burgdorferi*-specific DNA in urine specimens from patients with erythema migrans before and after antibiotic therapy. *J Clin Microbiol* 34:1359–1363; 1996.

Schmidt BL: PCR in laboratory diagnosis of human *Borrelia burgdorferi* infections. *Clin Microbiol Rev* 10:185–201; 1997.

Schmidt BL, Aberer E, Stockenhuber C, Klade H, Breier F, Luger A: Detection of *Borrelia burgdorferi* DNA by polymerase chain reaction in the urine and breast milk of patients with Lyme borreliosis. *Diagn Microbiol Infect Dis* 21:121–128; 1995.

Schnarr S, Putschky N, Jendro MC, Zeidler H, Hammer M, Kuipers JG, Wollenhaupt J: *Chlamydia* and *Borrelia* DNA in synovial fluid of patients with early undifferentiated oligoarthritis. Results of a prospective study. *Arthritis Rheum* 44:2679–2685; 2001.

Schwaiger M, Peter O, Cassinotti P: Routine diagnosis of *Borrelia burgdorferi* (sensu lato) infections using a real-time PCR assay. *Clin Microbiol Infect* 7:461–469; 2001.

Schwartz I, Wormser GP, Schwartz JJ, Cooper D, Weissensee P, Gazumyan A, Zimmermann E, Goldberg NS, Bittker S, Campbell GL, Pavia CS: Diagnosis of early Lyme disease by polymerase chain reaction amplification and culture of skin biopsies from erythema migrans lesions. *J Clin Microbiol* 30:3082–3088; 1992.

Schwartz I, Bittker S, Bowen SL, Cooper D, Pavia C, Wormser GP: Polymerase chain reaction amplification of culture supernatants for rapid detection of *Borrelia burgdorferi*. *Eur J Clin Microbiol Infect Dis* 12:879–882; 1993.

Schwartz I, Varde S, Nadelman RB, Wormser GP, Fish D: Inhibition of efficient polymerase chain reaction amplification of *Borrelia burgdorferi* DNA in blood-fed ticks. *Am J Trop Med Hyg* 56:339–342; 1997.

Seinost G, Dykhuizen DE, Dattwyler RJ, Golde WT, Dunn JJ, Wang IN, Wormser GP, Schriefer ME, Luft BJ: Four clones of *Borrelia burgdorferi* sensu stricto cause invasive infection in humans. *Infect Immun* 67:3518–3524; 1999.

Smith RP, Schoen RT, Rahn DW, Sikand VK, Nowakowski J, Parenti DL, Holman MS, Persing DH, Steere AC: Clinical characteristics and treatment outcome of early Lyme disease in patients with microbiologically confirmed erythema migrans. *Ann Intern Med* 136:421–428; 2002.

Speck S, Failing K, Reiner B, Wittenbrink MM: Evaluation of different media and a BGM cell culture assay for isolation of *Borrelia burgdorferi* sensu lato from ticks and dogs. *Vet Microbiol* 89:291–302; 2002.

Stanek G, Klein J, Bittner R, Glogar D: Isolation of *Borrelia burgdorferi* from the myocardium of a patient with longstanding cardiomyopathy. *N Engl J Med* 322:249–252; 1990.

Stanek G, Strle F: Lyme borreliosis. *Lancet* 362:1639–1647; 2003.

Steere AC, Bartenhagen NH, Craft JE, Hutchinson GJ, Newman JH, Rahn DW, Sigal LH, Spieler PN, Stenn KS, Malawista SE: The early clinical manifestations of Lyme disease. *Ann Intern Med* 99:76–82; 1983a.

Steere AC, Grodzicki RL, Kornblatt AN, Craft JE, Barbour AG, Burgdorfer W, Schmid GP, Johnson E, Malawista SE: The spirochetal etiology of Lyme disease. *N Engl J Med* 308:733–740; 1983b.

Steere AC, Grodzicki RL, Craft JE, Shrestha M, Kornblatt AN, Malawista SE: Recovery of Lyme disease spirochetes from patients. *Yale J Biol Med* 57:557–560; 1984.

Steere AC, Sikand VK, Meurice F, Parenti DL, Fikrig E, Schoen RT, Nowakowski J, Schmid CH, Laukamp S, Buscarino C, Krause DS: Vaccination against Lyme disease with recombinant *Borrelia burgdorferi* outer-surface lipoprotein A with adjuvant. Lyme Disease Vaccine Study Group. *N Engl J Med* 339:209–215; 1998.

Stoenner HG: Biology of *Borrelia hermsii* in Kelly medium. *Appl Microbiol* 28:540–543; 1974.

Stoenner HG, Dodd T, Larsen C: Antigenic variation of *Borrelia hermsii*. *J Exp Med* 156:1297–1311; 1982.

Straubinger RK, Straubinger AF, Summers BA, Jacobson RH: Status of *Borrelia burgdorferi* infection after antibiotic treatment and the effects of corticosteroids. An experimental study. *J Infect Dis* 181:1069–1081; 2000.

Strle F, Nelson JA, Ruzic-Sabljic E, Cimperman J, Maraspin V, Lotric-Furlan S, Cheng Y, Picken MM, Trenholme GM, Picken RN: European Lyme borreliosis. 231 culture-confirmed cases involving patients with erythema migrans. *Clin Infect Dis* 23:61–65; 1996.

Strle F, Nadelman RB, Cimperman J, Nowakowski J, Picken RN, Schwartz I, Maraspin V, Aguero-Rosenfeld ME, Varde S, Lotric-Furlan S, Wormser GP: Comparison of culture-confirmed erythema migrans caused by *Borrelia burgdorferi* sensu stricto in New York State and by *Borrelia afzelii* in Slovenia. *Ann Intern Med* 130:32–36; 1999.

Tylewska-Wierzbanowska S, Chmielewski T: The isolation of *Borrelia burgdorferi* spirochetes from clinical material in cell line cultures. *Zentralbl Bakteriol* 286:363–370; 1997.

Van Dam AP, Kuiper H, Vos K, Widjojokusumo A, De Jongh BM, Spanjaard L, Ramselaar AC, Kramer MD, Dankert J: Different genospecies of *Borrelia burgdorferi* are associated with distinct clinical manifestations of Lyme borreliosis. *Clin Infect Dis* 17:708–717; 1993.

Van der Heijden IM, Wilbrink B, Rijpkema SG, Schouls LM, Heymans PH, van Embden JD, Breedveld FC, Tak PP: Detection of *Borrelia burgdorferi* sensu stricto by reverse line blot in the joints of Dutch patients with Lyme arthritis. *Arthritis Rheum* 42:1473–1480; 1999.

Vaz A, Glickstein L, Field JA, McHugh G, Sikand VK, Damle N, Steere AC: Cellular and humoral immune responses to *Borrelia burgdorferi* antigens in patients with culture-positive early Lyme disease. *Infect Immun* 69:7437–7444; 2001.

Von Stedingk LV, Olsson I, Hanson HS, Asbrink E, Hovmark A: Polymerase chain reaction for detection of *Borrelia burgdorferi* DNA in skin lesions of early and late Lyme borreliosis. *Eur J Clin Microbiol Infect Dis* 14:1–5; 1995.

Wallach FR, Forni AL, Hariprashad J, Stoeckle MY, Steinberg CR, Fisher L, Malawista SE, Murray HW: Circulating *Borrelia burgdorferi* in patients with acute Lyme disease: results of blood cultures and serum DNA analysis. *J Infect Dis* 168:1541–1543; 1993.

Wang G: Direct detection methods for Lyme *Borrelia,* including the use of quantitative assays. *Vector Borne Zoonotic Dis* 2:223–231; 2002.

Wang G, van Dam AP, Schwartz I, Dankert J: Molecular typing of *Borrelia burgdorferi* sensu lato. Taxonomic, epidemiological, and clinical implications. *Clin Microbiol Rev* 12:633–653; 1999.

Wang G, Wormser GP, Schwartz I: *Borrelia burgdorferi. In* Sussman M (ed.): *Molecular Medical Microbiology. London*, Academic Press; 2001.

Washington JA II, Ilstrup DM: 1986. Blood cultures. Issues and controversies. *Rev Infect Dis* 8:792–802; 1986.

Weinstein MP: Current blood culture methods and systems. Clinical concepts, technology, and interpretation of results. *Clin Infect Dis* 23:40–46; 1996.

Wienecke R, Neubert U, Volkenandt M: Molecular detection of *Borrelia burgdorferi* in formalin-fixed, paraffin-embedded lesions of Lyme disease. *J Cutan Pathol* 20:385–388; 1993.

Wilske B: Diagnosis of Lyme borreliosis in Europe. *Vector Borne Zoonotic Dis* 3:215–227; 2003.

Wolk D, Mitchell S, Patel R: Principles of molecular microbiology testing methods. *Infect Dis Clin North Am* 15:1157–1204; 2001.

Wormser GP, Forseter G, Cooper D, Nowakowski J, Nadelman RB, Horowitz H, Schwartz I, Bowen SL, Campbell GL, Goldberg NS: Use of a novel technique of cutaneous lavage for diagnosis of Lyme disease associated with erythema migrans. *JAMA* 268:1311–1313; 1992.

Wormser GP, Nowakowski J, Nadelman RB, Bittker S, Cooper D, Pavia C: Improving the yield of blood cultures for patients with early Lyme disease. *J Clin Microbiol* 36:296–298; 1998.

Wormser GP, Liveris D, Nowakowski J, Nadelman RB, Cavaliere LF, McKenna D, Holmgren D, Schwartz I: Association of specific subtypes of *Borrelia burgdorferi* with hematogenous dissemination in early Lyme disease. *J Infect Dis* 180:720–725; 1999.

Wormser GP, Bittker S, Cooper D, Nowakowski J, Nadelman RB, Pavia C: Comparison of the yields of blood cultures using serum or plasma from patients with early Lyme disease. *J Clin Microbiol* 38:1648–1650; 2000a.

Wormser GP, Nadelman RB, Dattwyler RJ, Dennis DT, Shapiro ED, Steere AC, Rush TJ, Rahn DW, Coyle PK, Persing DH, Fish D, Luft BJ: Practice guidelines for the treatment of Lyme disease. The Infectious Diseases Society of America. *Clin Infect Dis* 31(suppl 1): 1–14; 2000b.

Wormser GP, Bittker S, Cooper D, Nowakowski J, Nadelman RB, Pavia C: Yield of large-volume blood cultures in patients with early Lyme disease. *J Infect Dis* 184:1070–1072; 2001.

Wormser GP, Ramanathan R, Nowakowski J, McKenna D, Holmgren D, Visintainer P, Dornbush R, Singh B, Nadelman RB: Duration of antibiotic therapy for early Lyme disease. A randomized, double-blind, placebo-controlled trial. *Ann Intern Med* 138:697–704; 2003.

Yang X, Popova TG, Goldberg MS, Norgard MV: Influence of cultivation media on genetic regulatory patterns in *Borrelia burgdorferi*. *Infect Immun* 69:4159–4163; 2001.

Zbinden R, Goldenberger D, Lucchini GM, Altwegg M: Comparison of two methods for detecting intrathecal synthesis of *Borrelia burgdorferi*-specific antibodies and PCR for diagnosis of Lyme neuroborreliosis. *J Clin Microbiol* 32:1795–1798; 1994.

Zore A, Ruzic-Sabljic E, Maraspin V, Cimperman J, Lotric-Furlan S, Pikelj A, Jurca T, Logar M, Strle F: Sensitivity of culture and polymerase chain reaction for the etiologic diagnosis of erythema migrans. *Wien Klin Wochenschr* 114:606–609; 2002.

10

SERODIAGNOSIS OF LYME BORRELIOSIS

Barbara J. B. Johnson, Maria E. Aguero-Rosenfeld, and Bettina Wilske

Serology is currently the mainstay of laboratory testing to support the clinical diagnosis of Lyme borreliosis. Serologic assays provide indirect evidence of *Borrelia burgdorferi* infection by detecting the humoral immune response, usually immunoglobulins M and G, to antigens of the organism. Assays of the immune responses to an infectious agent do not detect the agent itself, of course, and may be negative when an infected individual has not yet had time to develop antibodies. Serologic assays alone cannot answer the question, Does this patient have Lyme disease? Tests may be positive due to exposure to cross-reacting antigens or to the persistence of *B. burgdorferi* antibodies after a previous infection unrelated to a current illness. The clinical relevance of a test result reporting antibodies to *B. burgdorferi* depends on the pretest probability that the patient has Lyme disease, as well as on the sensitivity and specificity of the assay used. When these characteristics are understood and taken into account, serology is the most useful tool for assessing exposure to *B. burgdorferi* in all stages of Lyme disease after the first 2 to 3 weeks of infection (Aguero-Rosenfeld et al., 2005; Johnson, 2006; Wilske et al., 2007a).

The findings and conclusions in this report are those of the authors and do not necessarily represent the official position of the Centers for Disease Control and Prevention (CDC). The use of trade names is for information purposes only and does not constitute endorsement by the CDC.

Lyme Borreliosis in Europe and North America: Epidemiology and Clinical Practice, First Edition. Edited by Sunil K. Sood

TWO-TIERED SEROLOGY: A FIRST STANDARD FOR SERODIAGNOSIS IN THE UNITED STATES

After *B. burgdorferi* sensu stricto was detected in ticks of the genus *Ixodes* and cultivated in vitro in 1981, the first serologic assays for Lyme disease were developed (Burgdorfer et al., 1982; Barbour, 1984; Russell et al., 1984). The number of assays in use proliferated, but the performance characteristics of many tests were inadequate to serve the needs of either clinicians or epidemiologists. These tests lacked specificity, and the sensitivity and reproducibility of various tests were poorly understood (Magnarelli, 1989; Bakken et al., 1997). Few laboratories had evaluated these tests using serum samples from patients with clinically well-characterized Lyme disease, or from patients with culture-confirmed *B. burgdorferi* infection or seroconversion demonstrated in serially drawn specimens (ASTPHLD, 1991).

In the early 1990s efforts were made to ameliorate this unacceptable testing situation by investigators in clinical reference centers, public health agencies, and private industry. A two-test approach for Lyme disease serology had been adopted by several academic laboratories serving major clinical referral practices. When these laboratories participated in a multicenter evaluation of serodiagnostic assays by testing blind-coded samples from clinically well-characterized Lyme disease patients and healthy blood donors, the three reference centers that used Western immunoblotting to supplement their enzyme immunoassay (EIA) results performed much better than the three that used EIAs alone (Craven et al., 1996). These results provided part of the foundation for the initial standardization of serology. Criteria for the scoring and interpretation of both IgM and IgG immunoblots were derived and evaluated (Dressler et al., 1993; Engstrom et al., 1995). In late 1994 the Association of State and Territorial Public Health Laboratory Directors (ASTPHLD), the Centers for Disease Control and Prevention (CDC), and other agencies recommended that a two-step approach (commonly called "two-tiered serology") be adopted for testing serum specimens (ASTPHLD, 1995; CDC, 1995). The first commercial immunoblot devices (kits) for Lyme disease serology were cleared by the US Food and Drug Administration (FDA) in 1996 (www.fda.gov, product code LSR).

The public health community advocated two-tiered testing not only as a means to improve care of individual patients and epidemiologic surveillance for Lyme disease but also to establish a standard against which new, potentially improved, serologic methods could be evaluated. The FDA adopted the position that before new tests could be cleared as alternatives to two-tiered testing, test performance should be equal to or better than the recommended two-test procedures (Brown et al., 1999)

The essential features of two-tiered serology are illustrated in Figure 10.1. The first tier consists of a sensitive initial serologic test or tests that detect class-specific antibodies (IgM and IgG, either together or separately) by an EIA or, less commonly, an immunofluorescent assay (IFA). If the first-tier assay result is negative, the serum is reported to be negative for antibodies to *B. burgdorferi* and is not tested further. Serum samples that are found to be reactive ("positive") or indeterminate (called "equivocal" or "borderline" in some tests) are tested by supplemental standardized Western immunoblotting. If an IgG immunoblot is scored as positive, two-tiered testing is reported as positive. If an IgM immunoblot is scored as positive, Lyme disease serology is reported as positive with the caveat that this finding is clinically relevant only in early disease, that is, in the first month of illness (CDC, 1995).

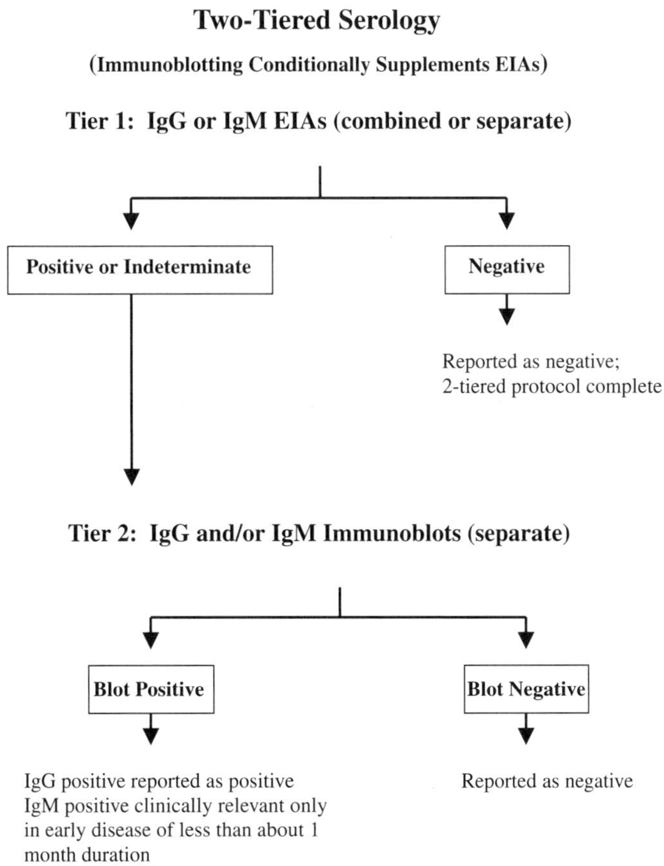

Figure 10.1 Two-tiered serology for Lyme disease. The first tier is shown as an EIA. Immunofluorescent assays (IFAs) may be substituted, but they are uncommonly used since they require a skilled microscopist and generally cannot be scored objectively. When a serologic result is negative and early Lyme disease is still suspected on clinical grounds, a second sample may be tested 2 to 3 weeks later, preferably paired with the original specimen.

It is important to appreciate that the first and second tier tests are not independent indicators of exposure to *B. burgdorferi* (Wormser et al., 2000). A Western blot cannot appropriately be said to "confirm" the results of a first tier test. The initial and supplementary tests usually are constructed with essentially the same antigens—whole-cell antigens of bacteria grown in culture—but they are processed differently. EIAs provide an estimate of the magnitude of the IgG/IgM humoral antibody response to all of the antigens that are expressed under the culture conditions used to produce the antigen. EIA results are objective and quantitative. They can be correlated with antibody titers. Immunoblotting techniques, in contrast, separate the many bacterial antigens spatially on a solid support so that the specificity and complexity of the antibody responses are revealed. The rationale for determining IgM and IgG antibody profiles is to learn whether the antibodies recognize proteins of *B. burgdorferi* that have been established to be more predictive of Lyme disease than other components of the bacteria. Many antigens have similarities to those of other organisms, such as proteins involved in motility (e.g., flagellin) and responses to stress (e.g., "heat shock" proteins). Recognition of one or more antigens from this set by serum antibodies is not necessarily indicative of exposure to *B. burgdorferi*, although these reactions contribute to the signal strength measured in an EIA. Immunoblots usually contain variable amounts of each protein (reflecting the relative expression of each of them in culture) and are qualitative, not quantitative tests.

The protein "bands" selected for scoring were chosen from all of the immunogenic proteins detected in immunoblots. The frequency of recognition of each protein was compared between serum samples from clinically characterized Lyme disease patients and samples from healthy donors (Engstrom et al., 1995) or patients with other neurologic, rheumatologic, or infectious illnesses (Dressler et al., 1993). Proteins that were more frequently recognized by serum samples from Lyme disease patients compared with controls, as judged by tests of statistical significance, were ranked and evaluated in combinations. Early in infection, IgM responses predominate and relatively fewer antibodies of any class are detectable compared with infections of longer duration. IgM blots are scored as positive if at least 2 out of 3 diagnostically significant bands (that were determined by chi-square analysis) are present (Engstrom et al., 1995). For IgG, the number of the most common bands selected for scoring was chosen by receiver operating characteristic (ROC) analysis, a technique that maximizes the area under a graph of test sensitivity versus (1-specificity). IgG blots are scored as positive if at least 5 out of 10 designated bands are present (Dressler et al., 1993). Examples of immunoblots are shown in Figure 10.2.

An immunoblot is scored with reference to a calibration control (positive control) that identifies the positions of diagnostically significant bands. In commercial blots, this calibrator is usually a polyclonal serum sample that has a well-characterized pattern of reactivity, often determined by use of monoclonal antibodies developed to identify specific proteins. Monoclonal antibodies themselves may be used as calibrators.

In addition a control for reaction strength (sometimes called a "weak-positive" control) is necessary to aid in deciding whether a band has sufficient color density to be scored. This decision is a major source of difficulty in the interpretation of immunoblots. The problem is that there is an inherent low level of "stickiness" between proteins, a background against which significant antibody–antigen interactions must be judged. In general, IgM antibodies are more nonspecifically "sticky" than IgG antibodies, owing to their pentameric (rather than monomeric) structure. Faint bands, particularly in IgM blots, may not be diagnostically significant even for so-called specific antigens. Unfortunately, data describing the validation of the "weak-positive" controls in commercial tests are not published. There is unease among specialists in some academic and government reference laboratories that it is not uncommon for samples to show "significant" IgM bands of an intensity greater than the weak-positive control that probably reflect nonspecific reactivity. Manufacturers should make an effort to demonstrate in the scientific literature that their reaction strength controls produce valid results. If health care providers adhere to the recommendation to demonstrate that antibodies are present at a positive or indeterminate level by a first-tier test before ordering an immunoblot, the risk of an erroneously positive serology based on scoring faint bands is reduced, but not eliminated.

Assays conditions influence whether nonspecific stickiness will result in a detectable band. These conditions include such variables as the concentrations of salts, detergent, and detecting reagents; assay temperature; and lengths of time allowed for antibodies to interact with antigens and for development of blot signal (usually color). Since assay designs differ among commercial products and "in-house" tests, a well-validated reaction strength control

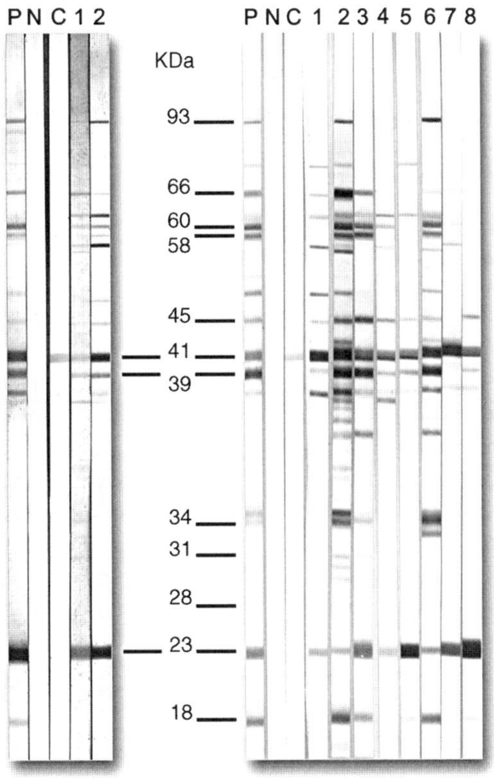

Figure 10.2 Examples of conventional IgM and IgG immunoblots. (*Left panel*) IgM blots; (*right panel*) IgG blots. *P*, positive control serum; *N*, negative control serum; *C*, calibration control (weak positive control); kDa, molecular mass in kilodaltons. Calibration control bands are typically light and reproduce poorly, so they have been digitally enhanced to be more visible. The arrows identify the bands that are recommended for scoring when a patient has been exposed to *B. burgdorferi* in the United States. Two additional bands are labeled in the IgG blot (outer surface proteins A and B at 31 and 34 kDa, respectively). IgM blots profiles are for a patient with acute EM (lane 1) and for the same patient at convalescence (lane 2). IgG lanes 1 to 8 show the profiles of 8 patients with later manifestations of Lyme borreliosis. The antigen was *B. burgdorferi* sensu stricto strain B31.

is test-specific.[1] Even when a reaction strength control is valid, the scoring of blots involves some subjectivity. The knowledge and experience of the reader may influence the result. Densitometers are used with some blot kits in attempt to minimize this problem, but operator judgment is still involved.

A negative control is required for each group of immunoblot strips run at the same time. This control serum may have some faint bands, for the reasons above, but should give a negative result when scored by the blot interpretation criteria.

[1] The rate of color development by the reaction strength control must be linear over the same time frame as the bands in the test serum sample. Difficulties can arise when the control develops full color before the patient's sample. The ratio of signal strength in a patient's sample compared with the reaction strength control will go up with length of time allowed for color development. If development time is excessive, the outcome will be a false-positive test result.

Most serologic assays currently in use (first- and second-step assays) employ antigen preparations obtained from *B. burgdorferi* cultured in vitro that do not contain all antigens presented to the immune system during active infection. During mammalian infection, borreliae express many antigens that are absent (or present at only low levels) in cells grown in laboratory cultures. Some newer serologic assays use antigens that are expressed preferentially in vivo. They are produced by recombinant DNA techniques or other synthetic means.

Performance Characteristics of First-Tier Tests

Types of First-Tier Tests Available Commercially

Although 52 different first-tier tests developed by 21 companies were approved by the FDA between 1987 and 2009, many of the cleared assays are no longer marketed (http://www.accessdata.fda.gov/scripts/cdrh/cfdocs/cfPMN/pmn.cfm, product code LSR, accessed 3/26/2010). Two-thirds (35/52) of these tests were approved before the era of two-tiered serology (1994), when whole-cell antigen EIAs and IFAs were designed to stand alone. Many were inadequately sensitive in order to achieve a modicum of specificity (Bakken et al., 1997). Currently a relatively small number of whole-cell antigen EIAs that have been tuned to optimize sensitivity are in widespread commercial use, and unlike some early tests, they are suitable for use in a two-tiered testing scheme. FDA-authorized first-tier tests made by five companies were used by about three-quarters of the nearly 400 laboratories that participated in the 2007 College of American Pathologists proficiency surveys; the EIA of one company was used for more than 40% of the results reported (CAP, 2007).

First-tiered tests based on synthetic or recombinant antigens, rather than lysates of whole cells, recently have been approved by the FDA. They are based on an immunodominant antigen, VlsE. VlsE is expressed well by borreliae in mammalian hosts but is produced at a very low level in the culture medium usually used for growth of organisms in the laboratory. In consequence this diagnostically useful antigen is effectively lacking in traditional two-tiered assays. The gene encoding the VlsE protein undergoes rapid recombination in vivo, resulting in a large repertoire of antigenic variants, but maintains certain invariant regions (Zhang et al., 1997). One small peptide of VlsE, a 25-amino acid portion of the sixth invariant region (IR6) plus a cysteine to aid in assay design, has proven to be remarkably useful as a diagnostic antigen (Liang et al., 1999). The prototype test is called the C6 assay. A version of the C6 assay designed and produced by Immunetics, Inc. was authorized by the FDA for commercial use in 2001. In this assay the peptide reproduces the IR6 found in *B. burgdorferi* sensu stricto strain B31. A diagnostic assay containing entire VlsE molecules expressed as recombinant proteins from both *B. burgdorferi* and *Borrelia garinii*, a species of Lyme disease *Borrelia* found only in Eurasia, became available as a first-tiered test in 2007 (Diasorin Liaison, www.fda.gov).

Sensitivity of First-Tier Tests by Stage of Lyme Disease

The antibody response to *B. burgdorferi* develops slowly over the first few weeks after the spirochete is introduced into the body. Since ticks bites often are not noticed, the course of development of serum immune responses generally is studied as a function of time after the first appearance of erythema migrans (EM) (Aguero-Rosenfeld et al., 1993, 1996). Patients with EM are often seronegative at the time of presentation (Table 10.1). The probability of seroreactivity is low during the first week after EM becomes visible. It increases with duration of EM and with the development of signs of disseminated disease. By convalescence, however, up to 80% of treated EM patients are seropositive. The optimal time for detecting antibodies in treated EM patients is 8 to 14 days after the start of antibiotic therapy (Engstrom et al., 1995; Aguero-Rosenfeld et al., 1996). Most of the treated patients who failed to seroconvert at convalescence in the studies in Table 10.1 were those who had a single localized EM lesion without evidence of disseminated infection.

From about 2 to 6 weeks after initial infection, antibodies rise in titer, recognize an increasing number of borrelial antigens, and switch classes from predominantly IgM responses to IgG. Because the antibody responses are evolving during the first weeks of infection, some patients with clinical presentations compatible with early Lyme disease may not yet be seropositive. In this situation serologic evidence of infection is best obtained by testing paired samples that are obtained several weeks apart. If paired samples are tested in parallel, increasing titers can support the clinical diagnosis of Lyme disease, but unfortunately this serologic tool is seldom used in routine clinical practice.

The evolution of the immune responses during early infection is illustrated by the serologic findings in patients with early neurologic disease. In a study of patients with facial paralysis, 87% had diagnostic levels of IgM antibodies, 66% were IgG positive, and all were seropositive for at least one antibody class (Peltomaa et al., 2004) (Table 10.1). This profile of antibody reactivity by class (i.e., greater frequency of positive IgM responses than IgG, with many people seropositive for both classes) also is seen in patients with other manifestations of early neurologic disease, typically meningitis and/or radiculoneuritis (Roux et al., 2007). Fewer data are available for less common manifestations of infection of the nervous system such as parenchymal inflammation of the brain or spinal cord or radiculopathy. Physicians should be aware that patients with early neurologic Lyme disease commonly have a history of recent EM. Lyme facial paralysis, for example, was associated with EM in 72% to 87% of patients, depending on the study (Peltomaa et al., 2004).

Another possible presentation of Lyme disease during the early weeks of infection is carditis, which manifests primarily as atrioventricular block. The median time from onset of EM to carditis is about 3 weeks (range 4–83 days) (Steere et al., 1980). Lyme carditis is uncommon, occurring in 0.5% to 2% of Lyme disease patients in the United States. It appears to have even lower incidence in Europe (Haddad and Nadelman, 2003). In consequence few serum samples from these patients have been available in retrospective or prospective evaluations of serologic tests. The vast majority of carditis cases are reported to be seropositive at presentation (Wormser et al., 2006). Some patients develop cardiac manifestations after a short duration of infection and may not yet be seropositive, underscoring the diagnostic importance of finding other signs and symptoms of Lyme disease. Lyme carditis typically occurs in patients with previous or concurrent EM (>80%) or sometimes early neurologic Lyme disease.

By the time patients develop later manifestations of Lyme disease, they are almost universally seropositive (Table 10.1). Numerous studies with robust samples sizes have been published about the immune responses in Lyme arthritis. Patients with Lyme arthritis typically have high IgG titers, higher than those seen in any of the various manifestations of Lyme disease, and waning IgM responses (Dressler et al., 1993; Akin et al., 1999; Kannian et al., 2007). Although an IgM response to a protein of 34 kDa (known as outer surface protein B or OspB) has been observed to develop late in infection in patients with prolonged disease, this new response occurs in the context of a robust IgG response to a large number of antigens. IgM responses in the absence of diagnostic levels

TABLE 10.1 Sensitivity of first-tier tests for antibodies to *B. burgdorferi* in U.S. patients by clinical manifestation of infection

		Seropositivity (%)			
		Acute Erythema Migrans (Days from Onset)		Acute Stage of Other Manifestations	Convalescent
	Reference	≤7 Days	>7 Days	At Presentation	Post-treatment
Erythema migrans					
WC ELISA 1, IgG + IgM[a]	Aguero-Rosenfeld et al., 1996	10	71		84[c]
WC ELISA 2, IgG + IgM[b]	Johnson et al., 2006; Bacon et al., 2003	31	89		95[d]
C6 kinetic ELISA, IgG[b]	Johnson et al., 2006; Bacon et al., 2003	30	52		75[d]
Early neurologic disease					
WC ELISA 2, IgG + IgM[e]	Johnson et al., 2006			100	
WC ELISA 2, IgG + IgM[e]	Johnson et al., 2006				100
WC ELISA 3, IgM[f]	Peltomaa et al., 2004			87	
WC ELISA 3, IgG[f]	Peltomaa et al., 2004			66	
WC ELISA 3, IgM or IgG[f]	Peltomaa et al., 2004			100	
C6 ELISA, IgG[f]	Peltomaa et al., 2004			100	

Lyme arthritis			
WC ELISA 3, IgM[g]	Dressler et al., 1993	16	
WC ELISA 3, IgG[g]	Dressler et al., 1993	100	
WC ELISA 2, IgG + IgM[h]	Johnson et al., 2006	97	
WC ELISA 2, IgG + IgM[h]	Johnson et al., 2006		100
WC ELISA 3, IgG[i]	Kannian et al., 2007	100	
WC ELISA 3, IgG[i]	Kannian et al., 2007		100
C6 ELISA, IgG[i]	Kannian et al., 2007	100	
C6 ELISA, IgG[i]	Kannian et al., 2007		93
Late neurologic disease			
WC ELISA 3, IgM[j]	Dressler et al., 1993	4	
WC ELISA 3, IgG[j]	Dressler et al., 1993	84	
WC ELISA 2, IgG + IgM[k]	Johnson et al., 2006	100	

[a]WC = whole cell antigens. All 46 EM cases confirmed by culture of *B. burgdorferi*. Calculated from Aguero-Rosenfeld et al., 1996.
[b]EM ($n = 80$) confirmed by culture ($n = 38$) or by evidence of disseminated infection ($n = 35$). Calculated from Bacon et al., 2003; Johnson, 2006, and Johnson unpublished.
[c]Obtained 8–14 days after the start of antibiotic therapy.
[d]Obtained 2–4 weeks after the start of antibiotic therapy.
[e]Acute and convalescent samples not paired. Acute samples from patients with meningitis (10/15), facial paralysis (8/15), and radiculoneuropathy (3/15); convalescent samples from patients with meningitis (5/11), facial paralysis (5/11), and radiculoneuropathy (2/11).
[f]Facial paralysis, commonly with recent EM (34/47); samples obtained within 6 weeks of onset of paralysis.
[g]Lyme arthritis ($n = 25$).
[h]Acute ($n = 33$) and convalescent ($n = 24$) samples not paired.
[i]Acute samples ($n = 23$) from patients with antibiotic-responsive arthritis; post-treatment samples ($n = 41$) from patients with antibiotic-refractory arthritis.
[j]Late neurologic disease ($n = 25$) manifested as encephalopathy or polyneuropathy; about half had received antibiotic therapy prior to a diagnosis of neurologic Lyme disease.
[k]Late neurologic disease manifested as encephalopathy (9/11) and polyneuropathy (3/11).

of IgG antibodies should not be used to support the diagnosis of any manifestation of late Lyme disease.

Late neurologic Lyme disease, presenting as encephalomyelitis, peripheral neuropathy, or encephalopathy, is rare (Wormser et al., 2006; Halperin et al., 2007). It has been speculated that late neuroborreliosis has become rarer in recent years due to earlier diagnosis and treatment, preventing progression to late-stage manifestations. Serum IgG antibodies have been consistently found in the patients who have been available for study. In the 2003 study summarized in Table 10.1, 100% of 11 late neurologic Lyme disease patients were seropositive (Bacon et al., 2003). These patients were classified as having late neurologic Lyme disease not only because of their neurologic findings but also because of antecedent other clinical manifestations of Lyme disease that were well documented. This demanding standard for admission to the study was necessary, since the signs of late neurologic Lyme disease, particularly encephalopathy, are not unique to infection by *B. burgdorferi*.

The serologic characteristics of patients who experience ongoing pain, fatigue, and/or memory difficulties after appropriate courses of antibiotic therapy for Lyme disease are beyond the scope of this review. This condition has been variously called post–Lyme disease syndrome, post-treatment Lyme disease syndrome, or "chronic Lyme disease." The preponderance of evidence indicates that these patients are no longer infected with *B. burgdorferi* (Feder et al., 2007). Serologic testing of patients with post–Lyme disease symptoms may be either positive or negative, depending on the clinical stage of Lyme disease when antibiotic therapy was started and the length of time that has passed since the infection was treated (Klempner et al., 2001).

Inadequate Specificity of First-Tier Tests Based on Whole-Cell Antigens

Although EIAs performed as first-tier serologic assays have excellent sensitivity after the first weeks of infection, alone they usually have inadequate specificity. Inadequate specificity is a characteristic of EIAs based on whole-cell antigens of *B. burgdorferi*, which are derived from cells grown in vitro. Whole-cell EIAs currently in common use have specificities of around 95% when used to evaluate healthy blood donors from North American areas that are not endemic for Lyme disease (Johnson, 2006). When healthy donors from endemic areas are tested, higher rates of reaction in EIAs are seen, owing to the persistence of antibodies years after active Lyme disease (Kalish et al., 2001) and seroconversion of exposed individuals who do not develop clinical illness (asymptomatic seroconversion rate of around 10%) (Steere et al., 1998). Since these latter positive reactions are true anti–*B. burgdorferi* antibodies, the specificities of EIAs are typically determined with samples from non-endemic areas.

High rates of false-positive EIA results (up to about 55%) are well documented in patients with other spirochetal illnesses, particularly syphilis, leptospirosis, and tick-borne relapsing fever, where cross-reactivity would be expected on biologic grounds (Johnson, 2006). Positive EIAs may occur with serum from patients with periodontal disease when treponemes are present in gingival pockets, although data are sparse. Samples from patients with other spirochetal infections are commonly tested by developers of serologic assays. Such samples provide a rigorous challenge of an assay's specificity since common antigenic motifs among spirochetes are well known. Furthermore some Lyme disease antibody assays have included other spirochetal antigens in their format as a means of adsorbing cross-reacting antibodies. Although the results of testing serum samples from patients with other spirochetal diseases are instructive to microbiologists, they are less pertinent to physicians who can distinguish these infections clinically from Lyme disease, with the possible exception of tertiary syphilis.

In patients with rheumatologic, neurologic, or other conditions within the differential diagnosis of Lyme disease, false-positive rates of around 10% have been observed, depending on the population (Johnson, 2006). This generalization applies to patients with antinuclear antibodies, rheumatoid factor, clinical rheumatoid arthritis, or multiple sclerosis. Studies are still needed of a larger number and wider array of patients with illness that may be difficult to distinguish clinically from Lyme disease.

The issue of false-positive Lyme disease serology reported in patients with human granulocytic anaplasmosis (HGA) is very difficult to study. Investigators usually cannot rule out coinfection or prior infections with *B. burgdorferi* (Wormser et al., 1997). Other reasons reported to give nonspecific reactivity in Lyme disease EIAs are polyclonal B cell activation, Epstein Barr virus (EBV) infections, or malaria (Kaell et al., 1993; Magnarelli, 1995; Burkot et al., 1997). There also have been reports of nonspecific reactions in tropical serum samples (Burkot et al., 1997).

Serum from people who received the recombinant OspA Lyme disease vaccine (approved by the FDA in 1999, but removed from the market in 2002) will react in whole-cell EIAs (Aguero-Rosenfeld et al., 1999). Although this potential source of false positivity does not affect a large percentage of the population, it is appropriate to inquire whether a patient received the OspA vaccine. Two-tiered testing will generally be negative, however, since the immunoblot reactivity of serum from vaccinees is distinctive and does not fulfill either the IgG or the IgM blot criteria.

The specificities of EIAs developed with a synthetic, immunodominant peptide of the VlsE molecule (C6 peptide) or with whole recombinant VlsE are superior to EIAs based on whole-cell antigens. These assays usually achieve specificities of 98% or higher, depending on the test and how the cutoff value for a diagnostically significant reaction was set (Liang et al., 1999; Bacon et al., 2003; Kannian et al., 2007).

Conditional Immunoblotting to Improve the Specificity of Serology

The specificity of serology is significantly improved when immunoblotting is added to the testing protocol. Blotting should be performed "conditionally," that is, depending on whether there is some evidence of the presence of antibodies to *B. burgdorferi* as determined by a first-tier test. When a first-tier test is positive or indeterminate, assessment of the reactivity profile of the antibody response on immunoblot permits discrimination between true and false positives. The utility of conditional blotting is illustrated by the retrospective study summarized in Table 10.2 (Bacon et al., 2003; Johnson, 2006). Whereas the specificity of the EIA was 96% for healthy blood donors, two-tiered testing improved specificity to 100%. For a panel of samples from patients with diverse other illnesses, both infectious and noninfectious, conditional blotting increased specificity from 85% to 98% (Table 10.2a).

Crude estimates of the number of serologic tests for Lyme disease performed annually in the United States range between 1 and 2 million assays. If these estimates are correct, each 1% improvement in test specificity saves 10,000 to 20,000 false-positive results. To put this number in context, in recent years about 20,000 cases of Lyme disease have been reported

TABLE 10.2 Sensitivity and specificity of two-tiered testing

a. Specificity of serology is improved when first-tier testing is supplemented by conditional immunoblotting.[a]

Non-Lyme disease	n	Specificity (%) EIA	Specificity (%) Two-Tier
Healthy U.S. donors	257	96	100
Conditions other than Lyme disease, total	292	85	98
Rheumatoid arthritis and/or rheumatoid factor positive	109	94	99
Anti-nuclear antibody positive	116	93	98
Other spirochetal diseases	67	58	97

b. Sensitivity of two-tiered testing is good for later stages of disease, but not for erythema migrans (EM).[a]

Stage of Lyme disease	n	Sensitivity (%) EIA	Sensitivity (%) Two-Tier
EM, acute	80	60	38
EM, convalescent	106	91	67
Early neurologic disease, acute	15	100	87
Lyme arthritis	33	97	97
Late neurologic disease	11	100	100

[a]Concepts illustrated with data from Johnson, 2006 and Bacon et al., 2003.

annually to the CDC as part of the US national system for surveillance of notifiable diseases (CDC, 1997, 2007).

Adequate specificity comes at a cost. A fundamental characteristic of diagnostic testing is that there is a trade-off between specificity and sensitivity. Serologic testing for antibodies to *B. burgdorferi* is no exception. The trade-off has the greatest consequence in early borreliosis, when antibody concentrations are still low. As illustrated in Table 10.2b, two-tiered testing of serum from patients with EM is much less sensitive than use of a whole-cell lysate EIA. EIAs detect the sum of interactions of antibodies with dozens of antigens, whereas blots are scored with respect to 3 (for IgM) and 10 (for IgG) specific proteins. In late Lyme borreliosis, such as Lyme arthritis or late neurologic disease, the immune system has had time to develop antibodies to more antigens and in higher concentrations, so the difference in sensitivity between EIAs and two-tiered results greatly diminishes or disappears.

The sensitivity of serologic testing of patients with EM is inadequate to be clinically useful. In acute EM, sensitivity is commonly less than 40% (Table 10.2b). In patients with a single EM and no symptoms of disseminated infection (e.g., headache, stiff neck, arthralgias), the sensitivity of two-tiered testing is only about 25% (Bacon et al., 2003). In patients with symptoms of disseminated infection or multiple EMs, sensitivity doubles to about

50%. Lower antibody detection rates have been reported in culture-positive European patients compared with patients from the United States, possibly due to differences in the causative agents (mainly *Borrelia afzelii* versus *B. burgdorferi*) and the fact that multiple EMs occur more often in the United States (Strle et al., 1999). It is appropriate to treat EM patients with antibiotics based on their clinical presentation and history of probable exposure to infected ticks in an endemic area. "Treat but don't test" has long been the position of an expert panel of the American College of Physicians that estimated that the pretest probability of Lyme disease in this circumstance is greater than 0.8 (Tugwell et al., 1997).

After the first weeks of infection and coincident with the development of signs of disseminated disease, the sensitivity of two-tiered testing is good (Table 10.2b). In early neurologic Lyme disease the sensitivity of two-tiered testing approaches 90%. Some patients with early neurologic Lyme disease may have an illness of 5 to 6 weeks' duration and yet not have an IgG response that meets blot criteria; they may, however, fulfill IgM blot criteria instead. It has been suggested that IgM testing may be useful until about 6 weeks after onset of Lyme borreliosis (Kannian et al., 2007), about 2 weeks longer than the period recognized in the 1995 recommendations (ASTPHLD, 1995; CDC, 1995). As discussed above, if serology is negative at the time that a patient is initially examined, it may be useful to test a second sample a few weeks later if Lyme disease is still suspected. In patients with Lyme arthritis or with late neurologic disease, the sensitivity of two-tiered testing is close to 100%.

Strengths and Weaknesses of Two-Tiered Testing

This diagnostic algorithm has been evaluated both retrospectively (see above) and prospectively (Steere et al., 2008). It has high specificity for determination of IgG antibodies to *B. burgdorferi*. Experienced laboratories with good quality control and quality assurance programs obtain consistent results (Bacon et al., 2003; Kannian et al., 2007; CAP, 2007). The specificity of IgM testing is not as good (Engstrom et al., 1995; Johnson et al., 1996), which accounts for the recommendation that IgM testing should be performed only in the first month of illness (ASTPHLD, 1995). Some investigators in reference laboratories believe that two-tiered IgM testing using current methods should not be done, both for reasons of specificity and because the duration of illness is often unclear or at least undocumented by good clinical information in requests for testing (unpublished Banbury conference summary, *The Laboratory Diagnosis of Lyme Disease*, September 2007). Recently an IgG immunoblot with VlsE band was described that eliminates the need for IgM testing (Branda et al., 2010). It provides superior sensitivity in acute neuroborreliosis and carditis, while maintaining high specificity.

Two-tiered testing is insensitive in acute EM and not useful in clinical practice. Sensitivity of standard two-tiered testing in early neurologic disease is less than ideal (Table 10.2b), although the new IgG algorithm incorporating VlsE increased sensitivity from 63% to 96% (Branda et al., 2010). The recommendation to obtain a second blood sample a few weeks after the initial one to seek evidence of seroconversion is inconvenient and costly, and causes delay in diagnosis. Furthermore commercial testing laboratories are generally not set up to save initial specimens. To obtain the most reliable results, initial and subsequent samples should be tested at the same time, but this is practical only in research or academic settings.

The antibody responses to *B. burgdorferi* increase in magnitude and diversity with duration of infection, as discussed earlier. In consequence immunoblotting band profiles increase in intensity and complexity with duration of infection as well. These characteristics can be diagnostically useful in specialized circumstances, such as when the results of serially drawn blood samples are available for the atypical patient who remains unwell after a standard course of antibiotic therapy. Expansion of the number and intensity of immunoblot bands is compatible with ongoing infection. In general, though, reporting of specific banding patterns (including those not considered to be "significant bands") is counterproductive. This practice gives rise to the erroneous concept of a "partially positive" or "nearly positive" blot, which causes diagnostic confusion particularly when a patient is tested despite a low pretest probability of Lyme disease (e.g., lacks objectives signs of borreliosis). Clinical laboratories sometimes prominently report banding patterns and give inadequate attention to the interpretation of these results. When this is done, health care providers may be confused and develop the mistaken idea that the presence of any number of bands is a significant finding. Specific bands, if they are reported at all, should be de-emphasized in the report.

Immunoblots are complex, technically demanding, and difficult to standardize. Some laboratories are inexperienced in properly using blot color development cutoff controls. The Clinical Laboratory Standards Institute (formerly known as National Committee for Clinical Laboratory Standards, NCCLS) notes that "The erroneous scoring of a faint band is a common reason for false-positive readings..." (NCCLS, 2000). IgM results are more affected by this problem than IgG blots (Johnson et al., 1996). Only 2 of 3 specified bands are required for an IgM blot to be reported as positive, whereas 5 of 10 bands are necessary for an IgG blot to be positive by the recommended blot interpretation criteria (CDC, 1995). A single erroneously scored faint band will affect IgM results more readily than IgG results, especially since about half of the population have antibodies that react with one of the IgM bands (FlaB, a protein of 41 kDa), regardless of Lyme disease status (Aguero-Rosenfeld et al., 1996). Densitometers may be used to assist with judging whether a given band meets the threshold for being reportable, but they will not help when underlying test design and color development problems are present.

In sum, two-tiered testing brought order to a chaotic testing environment in the early 1990s and improved the performance of serology for Lyme disease. It has worked well for determination of IgG antibodies after the first weeks of infection, despite its complexity, but works less well for determination of the IgM response. It also defines a standard against which new testing approaches can be judged.

HETEROGENEITY OF *B. burgdorferi* SENSU LATO IN EUROPE: IMPLICATIONS FOR SERODIAGNOSIS

The diversity of Lyme disease spirochetes, as well as the diversity and variability of their protein-encoding genes, impact laboratory diagnosis of Lyme borreliosis in Europe.

Heterogeneity of Causative Strains

In contrast to the United States where only one species, *B. burgdorferi* sensu stricto, causes Lyme disease, the human pathogenic strains in Europe belong to several different species

TABLE 10.3 Borrelia species in skin, CSF, or synovial fluid of European Lyme borreliosis patients

a. *Borrelia* species isolated from skin

Reference	Number	*B. burgdorferi* s.s.	*B. afzelii*	*B. garinii*	*B. spielmanii*
Ruzic-Sabeljic et al., 2000	87	1%	85%	14%	not done
Fingerle et al., 2008	160	6%	67%	24%	2.5%
Wilske et al., 1996b	68	6%	84%	10%	not done

b. *Borrelia* species detected in CSF

Reference	Method	Number	*B. burgdorferi* s.s.	*B. afzelii*	*B. garinii*
Eiffert et al., 1995	PCR	12	0%	33%	67%
Ruzic-Sabeljic el al., 2001	culture	40	2.5%	35%	62.5%
Wilske et al., 1996a	culture	37	11%	24%	65%

c. *Borrelia* species detected in synovial fluid

Reference	Method	Number	*B. burgdorferi* s.s.	*B. afzelii*	*B. garinii*
Fingerle et al., 2008	culture	6	2	2	2
Eiffert et al., 1998	PCR	7	3	1	3
Jaulhac et al., 2000	PCR	10	9	0	1
Vasliu et al., 1998	PCR	15	4	5	6

that vary in their distribution by geographic area. These species are *B. burgdorferi* sensu stricto, *Borrelia afzelii*, *Borrelia garinii* (various serotypes have been described for *B. garinii* [Wilske et al., 1993], and serotype 4 has been named *B. bavariensis* [Margos et al., 2009]), and *Borrelia spielmanii* (former genospecies A14S) (Wang et al., 1999; Richter et al., 2006). *Borrelia valaisiana* and *Borrelia lusitaniae* have been associated anecdotally with Lyme disease in some parts of Europe, particularly *B. lusitaniae* in Portugal. The major species have been associated with different clinical manifestations of the disease. *B. afzelii* has a high prevalence among isolates from human skin, especially those from patients with acrodermatitis chronica atrophicans (ACA), a chronic skin condition that has not been described in the United States (Canica et al., 1993; Ohlenbusch et al., 1996; Wilske et al., 1996b; Ruzic-Sabljic et al., 2000; Fingerle et al., 2008) (Table 10.3a). Isolates from cerebrospinal fluid most often belong to *B. garinii* (Wilske et al., 1993, 1996a,b; Eiffert et al., 1995; Ruzic-Sabljic et al., 2001; Fingerle et al., 2008) (Table 10.3b). Reports differ among authors on whether *B. burgdorferi* sensu stricto is preferentially associated with Lyme arthritis (Eiffert et al., 1998; Vasiliu et al., 1998; Jaulhac et al., 2000). With the exception of a study from France (Jaulhac et al., 2000), borreliae detected by PCR in synovial fluids from European patients with Lyme arthritis are highly heterogeneous. This high heterogeneity was confirmed by culture of three species of *Borrelia* from synovial fluids of Lyme arthritis patients (Fingerle et al., 2008) (Table 10.3c). To date, *B. spielmanii* has been isolated only from skin biopsy specimens (Fingerle et al., 2008).

TABLE 10.4 Sequence identities among major immmunodominant proteins from *B. burgdorferi* sensu stricto, *B. afzelii*, and *B. garinii* in Europe[a]

Protein	DNA Sequences Range (in %)	Amino Acid Sequences Range (in %)
DbpA[b]	51–63	40–44
VlsE	65–72	51–56
OspC[b]	61–77	54–68
OspA[b]	85–86	78–81
BmpA (p39)[b]	91–93	89–90
p58[b]	90–97	90–97
FlaB (flagellin)	94–95	96–97
FlaB fragment (aa 129-251)	92–93	92–96
p83/100[b]	81–87	87–89

[a]Strains analyzed were *B. burgdorferi* B31, *B. afzelii* PKo, and *B. garinii* PBi.
[b]Sequence identities were calculated without the leader sequence of the lipoproteins.

Molecular Heterogeneity of Immunodominant Proteins and Implications for Serodiagnosis

Amino acid sequence identities among major immunodominant proteins (DbpA, VlsE, OspC, OspA, BmpA, p83/100, p58, and flagellin) from the three main human pathogenic species range from 40–44% to 96–97% (Table 10.4). The most heterogeneous protein is DbpA (decorin binding protein A). Six distinct DbpA groups have been described (Schulte-Spechtel et al., 2006; Fingerle et al., 2008). Group I is comprised of *B. burgdorferi* s.s., and group II of *B. afzelii*. *B. garinii*, the most heterogeneous species, is divided into groups III and IV, whereas *B. spielmanii* strains form groups V and VI despite being homogeneous in OspA. OspA is not only heterogeneous among species but also rather heterogeneous among *B. garinii* strains (Wilske et al., 1996b). OspC has conserved epitopes primarily recognized by IgM antibodies, but also type-specific ones especially recognized by IgG antibodies (Wilske et al., 1996b). These factors make OspC a poor antigen for detection of IgG antibodies. In addition it is apparently downregulated during the course of the disease. Antigen diversity therefore has made the development of immunoblots for use in Europe far more challenging than in the United States.

Serodiagnosis

Strategies to improve serodiagnosis by using recombinant proteins derived from different strains have been successful, especially those expressed in vivo like OspC, DbpA, and VlsE. OspCs and DbpAs have been used for EIAs (Panelius et al., 2003). For commercial EIAs, recombinant VlsE has been added to increase the sensitivity of conventional EIAs (Wilske et al., 2007b), and an indirect chemiluminescent immunoassay (CLIA) using recombinant VlsE based on the European *B. garinii* stain PBi is available commercially as well (see also below).

As in the United States, a two-tiered procedure (Figure 10.1) is recommended for serodiagnosis in Europe (Wilske et al., 2000). However, the immunoblot interpretation criteria recommended by the CDC for use in the United States (ASTPHLD, 1995; CDC, 1995) are not applicable to European patients (Hauser et al., 1997; Wilske et al., 2007b). Detailed advice on serologic testing for Lyme borreliosis in Europe and guidelines for the interpretation of standardized immunoblots for the three main pathogenic species of borreliae can be found in (Wilske et al., 2000 and 2007b). Reference Wilske et al., 2000 is available online in English at http://nrz-borrelien.lmu.de/miq-lyme/index.html. Two presentations of Lyme borreliosis that are unique to European patients are *Borrelia* lymphocytoma, an uncommon skin manifestation that occurs early in infection, and ACA, a chronic late skin condition. The antibody detection rates in patients with lymphocytoma are 70% to 100% (Pohl-Koppe et al., 1998) and with ACA are 100% (Hansen and Asbrink, 1989).

Recombinant antigen immunoblots that have been used for years in Europe recently were improved significantly in sensitivity compared with the whole-cell lysate immunoblot by using a line blot technique and a broad panel of antigens (Wilske et al., 1999; Schulte-Spechtel et al., 2003; Goettner et al., 2005). For serodiagnosis of acute neuroborreliosis, a line blot showed a significant increase in sensitivity compared to a whole-cell lysate blot (Goettner et al., 2005). For this line blot, 7 different borrelial proteins were used. For 5 of the 7 proteins, 1 to 3 additional homologous proteins from different species were evaluated. Representative examples are shown in Figure 10.3. Combination of homologues derived

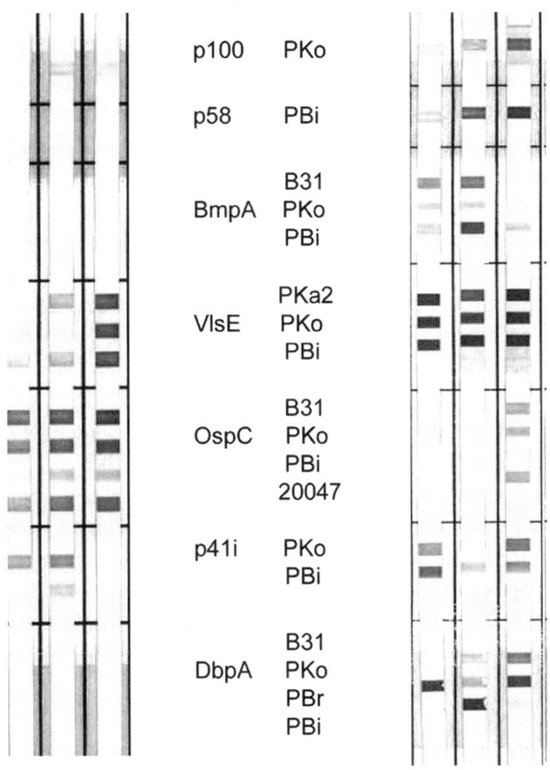

Figure 10.3 Examples of recombinant line IgM and IgG immunoblots. Serum samples are from three patients with early neuroborreliosis. *Borrelia* strains belong to the following species: B31 and PKa2 to *B. burgdorferi* s.s., PKo to *B. afzelii*, PBr to *B. garinii* OspA-type 3, PBi to *B. garinii* OspA-type 4, and 20047 to *B. garinii* of unknown OspA-type.

from different strains considerably increases the sensitivity of antibody detection, especially in the case of highly heterogeneous proteins like DbpA (Table 10.5). This is especially important in neuroborreliosis where causative strains are very heterogeneous (Panelius et al., 2003; Schulte-Spechtel et al., 2003; Goettner et al., 2005).

OspC has long been regarded to be the major protein recognized by IgM antibodies. The line blot study revealed that IgM antibodies reacted comparably well with VlsE derived from strain PBi. This was not seen with VlsE from other strains, suggesting that the source of the antigen is important in Europe. IgG antibodies reacted preferentially with VlsE of strain PBi in patients with EM or early neuroborreliosis (Table 10.5). In patients with late manifestations of Lyme borreliosis (ACA or Lyme arthritis), IgG antibodies reacted well with VlsE from either *B. garinii* or *B. burgdorferi* sensu stricto, but not with VlsE from *B. afzelii*, a phenomenon that is difficult to interpret.

NEWER ASSAYS AND FUTURE DIRECTIONS

Clinicians and their patients could all benefit from simpler, more objective, and less costly alternatives to two-tiered serology. There are many indications that this goal will be achieved in the not so distant future. The alternatives under consideration are diverse. They include "stand-alone" single-step EIAs, bead-based assays using peptides or purified recombinant antigens and luminometer technology to detect antibodies, and stand-alone immunoblots striped with defined antigens (either isolated from *Borrelia* or prepared as recombinants) and objectively scored by densitometry. New immunoblot interpretation criteria have been proposed for blots that include VlsE. New methods of data analysis are being developed to extract additional information that may be clinically useful from existing test results. Novel target antigens or combinations of antigens may be revealed by proteomic approaches that have the power to examine the diagnostic utility of each of the proteins encoded by *B. burgdorferi*.

At this time the most highly developed and evaluated alternatives to two-tiered serology are EIAs based on the C6 peptide of VlsE (Liang et al., 1999). The peer-reviewed scientific literature describes the performance of many C6 peptides assays developed by individual investigators in their own laboratories, although an increasing number of reports evaluate the commercial C6 test produced by Immunetics (Marangoni et al., 2005; Cinco and Murgia, 2006; Smismans et al., 2006; Tjernberg et al., 2007). Accordingly there are differences between C6 test designs and in the performance characteristics that have been reported. Depending in part on whether the developer envisioned a C6 EIA as a first-tier assay or as a stand-alone test that would not require supplementary immunoblotting, the specificity may be very high (99% or greater) or much lower (92%) (Liang et al., 1999; Bacon et al., 2003; Peltomaa et al., 2004; Smismans et al., 2006). Despite variability in tests, such as the cutoff value for a positive result, a consistent picture has emerged that C6 is a very important diagnostic antigen.

C6 EIAs have been reported to be significantly more sensitive in early acute Lyme disease in North American patients than conventional two-tiered serology and equivalent to it in sensitivity in later disease (Bacon et al., 2003, Tables 1 and 2; G. Wormser, personal communication, 2008). In the United Kingdom, unpublished work suggests that two-tiered IgM testing may be more sensitive than the commercial C6 assay in early disease (S. O'Connell, personal communication, 2008). Infections acquired in North America may

TABLE 10.5 Antibody reactivities with recombinant borrelial proteins in the line immunoblot

a. IgG reactivities with DbpA and VlsE (percent)

		DbpA					VlsE			
Diagnosis	Number	PBi *B. garinii*	PBr *B. garinii*	PKo *B. afzelii*	B31 *B. burgdorferi*	At least 1 DbpA	PBi *B. garinii*	PKo *B. afzelii*	PKa2 *B. burgdorferi*	At least 1 VlsE
EM[a]	15	0	13.3	26.7	6.7	33.3	80.0	60.0	40.0	80.0
Early neuroborreliosis	50	38.0	40.0	34.0	12.0	78.0	88.0	82.0	82.0	92.0
Acrodermatitis	10	10.0	0.0	80.0	10.0	80.0	100.0	0	100.0	100.0
Arthritis	10	70.0	10.0	90.0	20.0	100.0	100.0	20.0	90.0	100.0
Controls	110	1.8	1.8	0.0	0.0	3.6	0.9	2.7	0.0	3.6

b. IgM reactivities with OspC and VlsE (percent)

		OspC					VlsE			
Diagnosis	Number	20047 *B. garinii*	PBi *B. garinii*	PKo *B. afzelii*	B31 *B. burgdorferi*	At least 1 OspC	PBi *B. garinii*	PKo *B. afzelii*	PKa2 *B. burgdorferi*	At least 1 VlsE
EM[a]	15	60.0	13.3	73.3	80.0	80.0	53.3	26.7	20.0	53.3
Early neuroborreliosis	50	20.0	6.0	38.0	52.0	54.0	52.0	14.0	12.0	56.0
Controls	110	0.9	0	0.9	1.8	1.8	5.4	0	0	5.4

[a]Disease duration > 2 weeks.
[b]*B. g., B. garinii; B. a., B. afzelii; B. b., B. burgdorferi.*

stimulate a more brisk early antibody response than European infections. A C6 assay has been recommended as the most valuable testing option when early Lyme disease is suspected in a patient with a "flu-like" illness without EM, an uncommon but difficult to diagnose situation (Steere et al., 2004). Whether the commercial C6 EIA is approved by the FDA and adopted as an alternative to two-tiered testing in the United States likely will depend on whether its specificity is demonstrated to be high enough, especially in late disease (arthritis, carditis, or neuroborreliosis).

Some investigators are concerned about whether it is wise to rely on a single test antigen, especially in Europe where multiple species of *Borrelia* infect patients. Direct comparisons between the commercial C6 EIA and the leading multi-antigen assays, using suitably large and diverse serum panels, will be necessary to resolve this matter. In Europe the single-peptide C6 EIA should be compared with two-tiered serology that incorporates VlsE in the first-tier EIA and with immunoblots with VlsE and multiple antigens from different strains.

All three of the major pathogenic species of Lyme disease *Borrelia* induce antibodies that recognize the C6 peptide (Liang et al., 2000), despite some sequence differences between their respective VlsE IR6 regions. This sequence variation opens the question of whether C6-type assays can be improved by including IR6 variants, particularly for use in Europe. Some differences in sensitivity have been observed between EIAs constructed with IR6 variant antigens (Gomes-Solecki et al., 2007; Sillanpaa et al., 2007), but they have not been described as statistically significant. Indeed the specifics of test design were cited as a more decisive factor than antigen sequence variation in test results (Sillanpaa et al., 2007).

The titer of antibodies that recognize the C6 antigen declines more rapidly after antibiotic therapy than does the titer of antibodies detected by lysates of whole *Borrelia* (Philipp et al., 2001). In a study of antibody responses in patients with early localized or disseminated disease, a decrease in titer of four-fold or greater at six months after treatment or a negative C6 test result was highly associated with a successful outcome of therapy (Philipp et al., 2001, 2005). Similar observations were subsequently made using the full-length VlsE molecule as antigen (Marangoni et al., 2006). The distinctive time course of anti-C6 or anti-VlsE antibodies after antibiotic therapy for early Lyme disease could assist in the evaluation of patients who present much later with a new clinical sign compatible with Lyme disease, for example, facial palsy or meningitis. If the illness is unrelated to infection by *B. burgdorferi*, the C6 or VlsE assay may be negative and the whole-cell EIA positive due to the persistence of antibodies elicited by prior Lyme disease that was successfully treated. C6 titers do not wane as rapidly in patients treated for later manifestations of Lyme disease (Peltomaa et al., 2003), and they may not be useful for evaluating patients with post-treatment Lyme disease syndrome (Fleming et al., 2004).

Full-length VlsE, expressed as a recombinant protein, is the other leading antigen that has been evaluated as an alternative to two-tiered serology in US patients with encouraging results. After the initial description of VlsE as a serodiagnostic antigen (Lawrenz et al., 1999), whole VlsE was identified as the most sensitive and specific of 11 candidate recombinant antigens for evaluation of early Lyme disease by EIA (Magnarelli et al., 2002). Indirect chemiluminescent immunoassays (CLIAs) are commercially available based on recombinant VlsE. In Europe, the Liaison assay produced by DiaSorin contains not only a VlsE cloned from *B. garinii* but also recombinant OspC from *B. afzelii*, bound to magnetic particles for the analysis of IgG and IgM, respectively (Riesbeck and Hammas, 2007). In the United States, the Diasorin assay contains VlsEs from both *B. burgdorferi* sensu stricto and *B. garinii* but does not include OspC. It has been evaluated (Ledue et al., 2008) and judged by the FDA to be substantially equivalent to the predicate Immunetics, Inc. C6 assay and, as noted earlier, has been approved for use as a first-tier assay.

Recent work indicates that C6 and whole VlsE antigens detect different activities in the antibody responses to *Borrelia* infection (Embers et al., 2007). IgG antibodies to C6 peptide were commonly seen in serum samples that lacked detectable IgG reactive with recombinant VlsE, whereas the converse was rarely observed. In contrast, IgM antibodies were more frequently reactive with VlsE than with C6 antigen. The frequency of IgG reactivity alone to the C6 peptide exceeded the combined frequency of either IgM or IgG reactivity with VlsE in this study of a small number ($n = 39$) of well-characterized samples. Diagnostic tests based on VlsE may primarily detect antibodies to conformational epitopes and/or variable regions of the molecule, since the invariant region reproduced in the C6 assay appears to be largely buried within the protein structure, and therefore inaccessible to antibody.

APPROPRIATE USE OF SEROLOGIC TESTS

Principles for the use and interpretation of diagnostic data in clinical medicine are well established and described in numerous texts (e.g., Sackett et al., 1991). The value of serologic test results depends on their diagnostic predictive values, both positive and negative. Although much of this chapter has focused on the diagnostic sensitivities and specificities of various types of serologic assays, it is their predictive values that are most relevant clinically. In this context the positive predictive value is the probability that a patient who has a positive test result truly has Lyme borreliosis (expressed as the number of patients who have Lyme disease out of every 100 patients who have positive test results). Negative predictive value is the probability that a patient who has a negative test result does not have Lyme borreliosis (the number of patients who do not have Lyme disease out of every 100 patients who have negative test results). An assay with high diagnostic sensitivity improves negative predictive value; one with high diagnostic specificity improves positive predictive value.

Serologic testing is recommended only for patients who have appropriate pretest probabilities of Lyme disease in order for the results to have useful predictive values. A position paper published by the American College of Physicians (ACP) concluded that laboratory testing should only be done in patients who have a pretest probability of Lyme disease between 0.20 and 0.80 (Tugwell et al., 1997). The pretest probability is estimated from the findings of a careful history and physical examination, coupled with familiarity with the incidence of Lyme disease in the area of residence or travel. In the United States a practical way of assessing risk by area is to consult the CDC's national Lyme disease incidence map and statistical tables (www.cdc.gov/ncidod/dvbid/lyme/ld_statistics.htm), which are updated regularly. A map of the average incidence of Lyme by county for the years 2002 to 2006 is shown in Figure 10.4. The risk of Lyme disease varies greatly by geographic area. As illustrated, the risk is greatest in the northeast and upper midwest and is vanishingly small in some areas of the country. Physicians should consult their county or state health departments for further guidance on the local incidence of Lyme disease, which can be highly focal.

The ACP panel members pointed out that patients who have only nonspecific signs and symptoms of illness such as headache, fatigue, muscle or joint pains, even when they

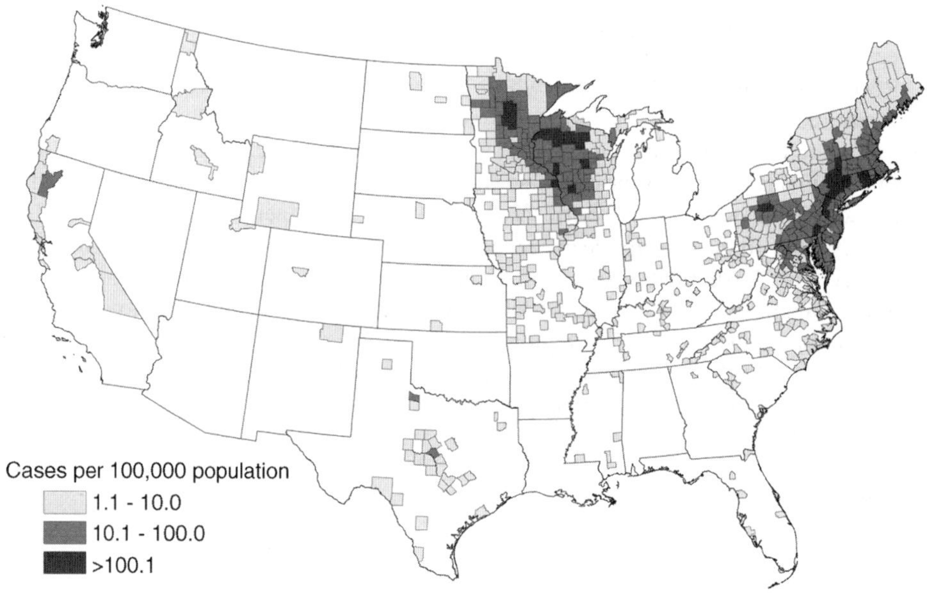

Figure 10.4 Average incidence of Lyme disease by county for 2002 to 2006. Cases met the US national case definition for surveillance and were recorded by state of residence (not state of tick exposure). Population figures were from mid-year 2004 US Census Bureau estimates. Erythema migrans–like rashes sometimes occur after the bites of lonestar ticks (*Amblyomma americanum*) and can be confused with early Lyme disease. Lonestar ticks, which do not transmit Lyme disease bacteria, are common human-biting ticks in the southern and southeastern United States and can be found less commonly in some areas that are endemic for Lyme disease. Source: Centers for Disease Control and Prevention.

reside in a geographic area endemic for Lyme disease, have a pretest probability of Lyme disease of less than 0.20, usually much less. Patients with nonspecific findings and no risk of exposure to infected ticks will have an extremely low pretest probability and certainly should not be tested. This advice may be contrary to what some health care providers received during their medical training. At one time it was commonly said that Lyme disease is one of a group of conditions that can present as almost any syndrome, which we now know is not correct. Routine serologic testing of all patients for whom the diagnosis is unclear at presentation will result in more false-positive results than true positives. A negative test result, if testing is performed despite current guidelines, effectively rules out Lyme disease.

When the pretest probability of Lyme disease is greater than 0.80, laboratory evaluation adds little useful information. An example of this situation is a finding of EM in a patient in an endemic area (Tugwell et al., 1997). Tests for antibodies are not sufficiently sensitive for a negative test result to rule out *B. burgdorferi* infection.

Serologic testing is of significant value when a patient has objective signs (other than EM) compatible with Lyme borreliosis (Table 10.2). IgM test results should be used only within the first month after the onset of initial clinical signs (generally acute neuroborreliosis). Positive IgM serology should not be used to support the diagnosis of late manifestations of *B. burgdorferi* infection. The effect of serologic results on post-test probabilities of Lyme disease in various clinical situations has been calculated and illustrated (Tugwell et al., 1997). This reference can be highly instructive for the nonspecialist. The clinical signs of neuroborreliosis, Lyme carditis, and Lyme arthritis are described elsewhere in this volume and are essential to know to estimate pretest probabilities of Lyme disease.

Specific antibodies to *B. burgdorferi* may be detectable for long periods of time after successful treatment of Lyme borreliosis (Kalish et al., 2001). Their presence in serum samples of patients presenting with other conditions, may result in a diagnostic dilemma. The antibody responses to the C6 synthetic peptide or to recombinant VlsE decline more rapidly than to whole-cell antigens in patients successfully treated for early Lyme disease. Assessment of antibodies to C6 or VlsE may be especially helpful in this situation.

When use of serology is indicated, it is important to select validated laboratory tests. Health care providers are encouraged to select tests that have been established to be clinically useful by publication(s) in the peer-reviewed scientific literature, and/or by approval by regulatory agencies such as the FDA in the United States or by CE marking, the minimum standard for commercial diagnostic test kits in Europe (CDC, 2005). In addition test performance and interpretation should adhere to the recommended guidelines discussed earlier in this chapter.

ACKNOWLEDGMENT

The authors thank Mr. Mark Pilgard and Dr. Susan O'Connell for critically reading the manuscript and Ms. Kiersten Kugeler for preparing Figure 10.4.

REFERENCES

Aguero-Rosenfeld ME, Nowakowski J, Bittker S, Cooper D, Nadelman RB, Wormser GP: Evolution of the serologic response to *Borrelia burgdorferi* in treated patients with culture-confirmed erythema migrans. *J Clin Microbiol* 34:1–9; 1996.

Aguero-Rosenfeld ME, Nowakowski J, McKenna DF, Carbonaro CA, Wormser GP: Serodiagnosis in early Lyme disease. *J Clin Microbiol* 31:3090–3095; 1993.

Aguero-Rosenfeld ME, Roberge J, Carbonaro CA, Nowakowski J, Nadelman RB, Wormser GP: Effects of OspA vaccination on Lyme disease serologic testing. *J Clin Microbiol* 37:3718–3721; 1999.

Aguero-Rosenfeld ME, Wang G, Schwartz I, Wormser GP: Diagnosis of lyme borreliosis. *Clin Microbiol Rev* 18:484–509; 2005.

Akin E, McHugh GL, Flavell RA, Fikrig E, Steere AC: The immunoglobulin (IgG) antibody response to OspA and OspB correlates with severe and prolonged Lyme arthritis and the IgG response to P35 correlates with mild and brief arthritis. *Infect Immun* 67:173–181; 1999.

ASTPHLD: Proceedings of the First National Conference on Lyme Disease Testing. *First National Conference on Lyme Disease Testing*. Dearborn, Michigan: Association of State and Territorial Public Health Laboratory Directors, Washington, DC; 1991.

ASTPHLD: Proceedings of the Second National Conference on Lyme Disease Testing. *Second National Conference on Lyme Disease Testing*. Dearborn, Michigan: Association of State and Territorial Public Health Laboratory Directors, Washington, DC; 1995.

Bacon RM, Biggerstaff BJ, Schriefer ME, Gilmore RD Jr, Philipp MT, Steere AC, Wormser GP, Marques AR, Johnson BJ: Serodiagnosis of Lyme disease by kinetic enzyme-linked immunosorbent assay using recombinant VlsE1 or peptide antigens of *Borrelia burgdorferi* compared with 2-tiered testing using whole-cell lysates. *J Infect Dis* 187:1187–1199; 2003.

Bakken LL, Callister SM, Wand PJ, Schell RF: Interlaboratory comparison of test results for detection of Lyme disease by 516 participants in the Wisconsin State Laboratory of Hygiene/College of American Pathologists Proficiency Testing Program. *J Clin Microbiol* 35:537–543; 1997.

Barbour AG: Isolation and cultivation of Lyme disease spirochetes. *Yale J Biol Med* 57:521–525; 1984.

Brown SL, Hansen SL, Langone JJ: Role of serology in the diagnosis of Lyme disease. *JAMA* 282:62–66; 1999.

Burgdorfer W, Barbour AG, Hayes SF, Benach JL, Grunwaldt E, Davis JP: Lyme disease-a tick-borne spirochetosis? *Science* 216:1317–1319; 1982.

Burkot TR, Schriefer ME, Larsen SA: Cross-reactivity to *Borrelia burgdorferi* proteins in serum samples from residents of a tropical country nonendemic for Lyme disease. *J Infect Dis* 175:466–469; 1997.

Canica MM, Nato F, Du Merle L, Mazie JC, Baranton G, Postic D: Monoclonal antibodies for identification of *Borrelia afzelii* sp. nov. associated with late cutaneous manifestations of Lyme borreliosis. *Scand J Infect Dis* 25:441–448; 1993.

CAP: Tick transmitted disease survey TTD-B; College of American Pathologists, Northfield, Illinois 2007.

CDC: Recommendations for test performance and interpretation from the Second National Conference on Serologic Diagnosis of Lyme Disease. *MMWR Morb Mortal Wkly Rep* 44:590–591; 1995.

CDC: Case definitions for infectious conditions under public health surveillance. Centers for Disease Control and Prevention. *MMWR Recomm Rep* 46:1–55; 1997.

CDC: Notice to readers. Caution regarding testing for Lyme disease. *MMWR Morb Mortal Wkly Rep* 54:125; 2005.

CDC: Lyme disease. United States, 2003–2005. *MMWR Morb Mortal Wkly Rep* 56:573–576; 2007.

Cinco M, Murgia R: Evaluation of the C6 enzyme-linked immunoadsorbent assay for the serodiagnosis of Lyme borreliosis in north-eastern Italy. *New Microbiol* 29:139–141; 2006.

Craven RB, Quan TJ, Bailey RE, Dattwyler R, Ryan RW, Sigal LH, Steere AC, Sullivan B, Johnson BJ, Dennis DT, Gubler DJ: Improved serodiagnostic testing for Lyme disease: results of a multicenter serologic evaluation. *Emerg Infect Dis* 2:136–140; 1996.

Dressler F, Whalen JA, Reinhardt BN, Steere AC: Western blotting in the serodiagnosis of Lyme disease. *J Infect Dis* 167:392–400; 1993.

Eiffert H, Ohlenbusch A, Christen HJ, Thomssen R, Spielman A, Matuschka FR: Nondifferentiation between Lyme disease spirochetes from vector ticks and human cerebrospinal fluid. *J Infect Dis* 171:476–479; 1995.

Eiffert H, Karsten A, Thomssen R, Christen HJ: Characterization of *Borrelia burgdorferi* strains in Lyme arthritis. *Scand J Infect Dis* 30:265–268; 1998.

Embers ME, Jacobs MB, Johnson BJ, Philipp MT: Dominant epitopes of the C6 diagnostic peptide of *Borrelia burgdorferi* are largely inaccessible to antibody on the parent VlsE molecule. *Clin Vaccine Immunol* 14:931–936; 2007.

Engstrom SM, Shoop E, Johnson RC: Immunoblot interpretation criteria for serodiagnosis of early Lyme disease. *J Clin Microbiol* 33:419–427; 1995.

Feder HM Jr, Johnson BJ, O'Connell S, Shapiro ED, Steere AC, Wormser GP, Agger W.A, Artsob H, Auwaerter P, Dumler JS, Bakken JS, Bockenstedt LK, Green J, Dattwyler RJ, Munoz J, Nadelman

RB, Schwartz I, Draper T, McSweegan E, Halperin JJ, Klempner MS, Krause PJ, Mead P, Morshed M, Porwancher R, Radolf JD, Smith RP Jr, Sood S, Weinstein A, Wong SJ, Zemel L: A critical appraisal of "chronic Lyme disease." *N Engl J Med* 357:1422–1430; 2007.

Fingerle V, Schulte-Spechtel UC, Ruzic-Sabljic E, Leonhard S, Hofmann H, Weber K, Pfister K, Strle F, Wilske B: Epidemiological aspects and molecular characterization of *Borrelia burgdorferi* s.l. from southern Germany with special respect to the new species *Borrelia spielmanii* sp. nov. *Int J Med Microbiol* 298:279–290; 2008.

Fleming RV, Marques AR, Klempner MS, Schmid CH, Dally LG, Martin DS, Philipp MT: Pre-treatment and post-treatment assessment of the C(6) test in patients with persistent symptoms and a history of Lyme borreliosis. *Eur J Clin Microbiol Infect Dis* 23:615–618; 2004.

Goettner G, Schulte-Spechtel U, Hillermann R, Liegl G, Wilske B, Fingerle V: Improvement of Lyme borreliosis serodiagnosis by a newly developed recombinant immunoglobulin G (IgG) and IgM line immunoblot assay and addition of VlsE and DbpA homologues. *J Clin Microbiol* 43:3602–3609; 2005.

Gomes-Solecki MJ, Meirelles L, Glass J, Dattwyler RJ: Epitope length, genospecies dependency, and serum panel effect in the IR6 enzyme-linked immunosorbent assay for detection of antibodies to *Borrelia burgdorferi*. *Clin Vaccine Immunol* 14:875–879; 2007.

Haddad FA, Nadelman RB: Lyme disease and the heart. *Front Biosci* 8:s769–s782; 2003.

Halperin JJ, Shapiro ED, Logigian E, Belman AL, Dotevall L, Wormser GP, Krupp L, Gronseth G, Bever CT Jr.: Practice parameter. Treatment of nervous system Lyme disease (an evidence-based review). Report of the Quality Standards Subcommittee of the American Academy of Neurology. *Neurology* 69:91–102; 2007.

Hansen K, Asbrink E: Serodiagnosis of erythema migrans and acrodermatitis chronica atrophicans by the *Borrelia burgdorferi* flagellum enzyme-linked immunosorbent assay. *J Clin Microbiol* 27:545–551; 1989.

Hauser U, Lehnert G, Lobentanzer R, Wilske B: Interpretation criteria for standardized Western blots for three European species of *Borrelia burgdorferi* sensu lato. *J Clin Microbiol* 35:1433–1444; 1997.

Jaulhac B, Heller R, Limbach FX, Hansmann Y, Lipsker D, Monteil H, Sibilia J, Piemont Y: Direct molecular typing of *Borrelia burgdorferi* sensu lato species in synovial samples from patients with lyme arthritis. *J Clin Microbiol* 38:1895–1900; 2000.

Johnson BJ, Robbins KE, Bailey RE, Cao BL, Sviat SL, Craven RB, Mayer LW, Dennis DT: Serodiagnosis of Lyme disease: Accuracy of a two-step approach using a flagella-based ELISA and immunoblotting. *J Infect Dis* 174:346–353; 1996.

Johnson BJB: Lyme serologic assays for antibodies to *Borrelia burgdorferi*. *In* Detrick B, Hamilton RG, Folds JD (eds): *Manual of Molecular and Clinical Laboratory Immunology*. Washington, DC, ASM Press; 2006.

Kaell AT, Redecha PR, Elkon KB, Golightly MG, Schulman PE, Dattwyler RJ, Kaell DL, Inman RD, Christian CL, Volkman DJ: Occurrence of antibodies to *Borrelia burgdorferi* in patients with nonspirochetal subacute bacterial endocarditis. *Ann Intern Med* 119:1079–1083; 1993.

Kalish RA, McHugh G, Granquist J, Shea B, Ruthazer R, Steere AC: Persistence of immunoglobulin M or immunoglobulin G antibody responses to *Borrelia burgdorferi* 10–20 years after active Lyme disease. *Clin Infect Dis* 33:780–785; 2001.

Kannian P, McHugh G, Johnson BJ, Bacon RM, Glickstein LJ, Steere AC: Antibody responses to *Borrelia burgdorferi* in patients with antibiotic-refractory, antibiotic-responsive, or non-antibiotic-treated Lyme arthritis. *Arthritis Rheum* 56:4216–4225; 2007.

Klempner MS, Hu LT, Evans J, Schmid CH, Johnson GM, Trevino RP, Norton D, Levy L, Wall D, McCall J, Kosinski M, Weinstein A: Two controlled trials of antibiotic treatment in patients with persistent symptoms and a history of Lyme disease. *N Engl J Med* 345:85–92; 2001.

Lawrenz MB, Hardham JM, Owens RT, Nowakowski J, Steere AC, Wormser GP, Norris SJ: Human antibody responses to VlsE antigenic variation protein of *Borrelia burgdorferi*. *J Clin Microbiol* 37:3997–4004; 1999.

Ledue TB, Collins MF, Young J, Schriefer ME: Evaluation of the recombinant VlsE-based liaison chemiluminescence immunoassay for detection of *Borrelia burgdorferi* and diagnosis of Lyme disease. *Clin Vaccine Immunol* 15:1796–1804; 2008.

Liang FT, Steere AC, Marques AR, Johnson BJ, Miller JN, Philipp MT: Sensitive and specific serodiagnosis of Lyme disease by enzyme-linked immunosorbent assay with a peptide based on an immunodominant conserved region of *Borrelia burgdorferi* vlsE. *J Clin Microbiol* 37:3990–3996; 1999.

Liang FT, Aberer E, Cinco M, Gern L, Hu CM, Lobet YN, Ruscio M, Voet PE Jr., Weynants VE, Philipp MT: Antigenic conservation of an immunodominant invariable region of the VlsE lipoprotein among European pathogenic genospecies of *Borrelia burgdorferi* SL. *J Infect Dis* 182:1455–1462; 2000.

Magnarelli LA: Quality of Lyme disease tests. *JAMA* 262:3464–3465; 1989.

Magnarelli LA: Current status of laboratory diagnosis for Lyme disease. *Am J Med* 98:10S–12S; discussion 12S–14S; 1995.

Magnarelli LA, Lawrenz M, Norris SJ, Fikrig E: Comparative reactivity of human sera to recombinant VlsE and other *Borrelia burgdorferi* antigens in class-specific enzyme-linked immunosorbent assays for Lyme borreliosis. *J Med Microbiol* 51:649–655; 2002.

Marangoni A, Sparacino M, Mondardini V, Cavrini F, Storni E, Donati M, Cevenini R, Sambri V: Comparative evaluation of two enzyme linked immunosorbent assay methods and three Western blot methods for the diagnosis of culture-confirmed early Lyme borreliosis in Italy. *New Microbiol* 28:37–43; 2005.

Marangoni A, Sambri V, Accardo S, Cavrini F, Mondardini V, Moroni A, Storni E, Cevenini R: A decrease in the immunoglobulin G antibody response against the VlsE protein of *Borrelia burgdorferi* sensu lato correlates with the resolution of clinical signs in antibiotic-treated patients with early Lyme disease. *Clin Vaccine Immunol* 13:525–529; 2006.

Margos G, Vollmer SA, Cornet M, Garnier M, Fingerle V, Wilske B, Bormane A, Vitorino L, Collares-Pereira M, Drancourt M, Kurtenbach K: A new *Borrelia* species defined by multilocus sequence analysis of housekeeping genes. *Appl Environ Microbiol* 75:5410–5416; 2009.

NCCLS: Western blot assay for antibodies to *Borrelia burgdorferi*. Approved Guideline. NCCLS document M34-A 2000, Vol. 20 No. 20. National Committee for Clinical Laboratory Standards; 2000.

Ohlenbusch A, Matuschka FR, Richter D, Christen HJ, Thomssen R, Spielman A, Eiffert H: Etiology of the acrodermatitis chronica atrophicans lesion in Lyme disease. *J Infect Dis* 174:421–423; 1996.

Panelius J, Lahdenne P, Saxen H, Carlsson SA, Heikkila T, Peltomaa M, Lauhio A, Seppala I: Diagnosis of Lyme neuroborreliosis with antibodies to recombinant proteins DbpA, BBK32, and OspC, and VlsE IR6 peptide. *J Neurol* 250:1318–1327; 2003.

Peltomaa M, McHugh G, Steere AC: Persistence of the antibody response to the VlsE sixth invariant region (IR6) peptide of *Borrelia burgdorferi* after successful antibiotic treatment of Lyme disease. *J Infect Dis* 187:1178–1186; 2003.

Peltomaa M, McHugh G, Steere AC: The VlsE (IR6) peptide ELISA in the serodiagnosis of lyme facial paralysis. *Otol Neurotol* 25:838–841; 2004.

Philipp MT, Bowers LC, Fawcett PT, Jacobs MB, Liang FT, Marques AR, Mitchell PD, Purcell JE, Ratterree MS, Straubinger RK: Antibody response to IR6, a conserved immunodominant region of the VlsE lipoprotein, wanes rapidly after antibiotic treatment of *Borrelia burgdorferi* infection in experimental animals and in humans. *J Infect Dis* 184:870–878; 2001.

Philipp MT, Wormser GP, Marques AR, Bittker S, Martin DS, Nowakowski J, Dally LG: A decline in C6 antibody titer occurs in successfully treated patients with culture-confirmed early localized or early disseminated Lyme Borreliosis. *Clin Diagn Lab Immunol* 12:1069–1074; 2005.

Pohl-Koppe A, Wilske B, Weiss M, Schmidt H: *Borrelia* lymphocytoma in childhood. *Pediatr Infect Dis J* 17:423–426; 1998.

Richter D, Postic D, Sertour N, Livey I, Matuschka FR, Baranton G: Delineation of *Borrelia burgdorferi* sensu lato species by multilocus sequence analysis and confirmation of the delineation of *Borrelia spielmanii* sp. nov. *Int J Syst Evol Microbiol* 56:873–881; 2006.

Riesbeck K, Hammas B: Comparison of an automated *Borrelia* indirect chemiluminescent immunoassay (CLIA) with a VlsE/C6 ELISA and Immunoblot. *Eur J Clin Microbiol Infect Dis* 26:517–519; 2007.

Roux F, Boyer E, Jaulhac B, Dernis E, Closs-Prophette F, Puechal X: Lyme meningoradiculitis. Prospective evaluation of biological diagnosis methods. *Eur J Clin Microbiol Infect Dis* 26:685–693; 2007.

Russell H, Sampson JS, Schmid GP, Wilkinson HW, Plikaytis B: Enzyme-linked immunosorbent assay and indirect immunofluorescence assay for Lyme disease. *J Infect Dis* 149:465–470; 1984.

Ruzic-Sabljic E, Strle F, Cimperman J, Maraspin V, Lotric-Furlan S, Pleterski-Rigler D: Characterisation of *Borrelia burgdorferi* sensu lato strains isolated from patients with skin manifestations of Lyme borreliosis residing in Slovenia. *J Med Microbiol* 49:47–53; 2000.

Ruzic-Sabljic E, Lotric-Furlan S, Maraspin V, Cimperman J, Pleterski-Rigler D, Strle F: Analysis of *Borrelia burgdorferi* sensu lato isolated from cerebrospinal fluid. *APMIS* 109:707–713; 2001.

Sackett DL, Haynes RB, Guyatt GH, Tugwell P: The interpretation of diagnostic data. *Clinical Epidemiology: A Basic Science for Clinical Medicine.* Boston, Little, Brown, pp 69–152; 1991.

Schulte-Spechtel U, Lehnert G, Liegl G, Fingerle V, Heimerl C, Johnson BJ, Wilske B: Significant improvement of the recombinant *Borrelia*-specific immunoglobulin G immunoblot test by addition of VlsE and a DbpA homologue derived from *Borrelia garinii* for diagnosis of early neuroborreliosis. *J Clin Microbiol* 41:1299–1303; 2003.

Schulte-Spechtel U, Fingerle V, Goettner G, Rogge S, Wilske B: Molecular analysis of decorin-binding protein A (DbpA) reveals five major groups among European *Borrelia burgdorferi* sensu lato strains with impact for the development of serological assays and indicates lateral gene transfer of the dbpA gene. *Int J Med Microbiol* 296(suppl 40): 250–266; 2006.

Sillanpaa H, Lahdenne P, Sarvas H, Arnez M, Steere A, Peltomaa M, Seppala I: Immune responses to borrelial VlsE IR6 peptide variants. *Int J Med Microbiol* 297:45–52; 2007.

Smismans A, Goossens VJ, Nulens E, Bruggeman CA: Comparison of five different immunoassays for the detection of *Borrelia burgdorferi* IgM and IgG antibodies. *Clin Microbiol Infect* 12:648–655; 2006.

Steere AC, Batsford WP, Weinberg M, Alexander J, Berger HJ, Wolfson S, Malawista SE: Lyme carditis. Cardiac abnormalities of Lyme disease. *Ann Intern Med* 93:8–16; 1980.

Steere AC, Coburn J, Glickstein L: The emergence of Lyme disease. *J Clin Inves*, 113:1093–1101; 2004.

Steere AC, Sikand VK, Meurice F, Parenti DL, Fikrig E, Schoen RT, Nowakowski J., Schmid CH, Laukamp S, Buscarino C, Krause DS: Vaccination against Lyme disease with recombinant *Borrelia burgdorferi* outer-surface lipoprotein A with adjuvant. Lyme Disease Vaccine Study Group. *N Engl J Med* 339:209–215; 1998.

Strle F, Nadelman RB, Cimperman J, Nowakowski J, Picken RN, Schwartz I, Maraspin V, Aguero-Rosenfeld ME, Varde S, Lotric-Furlan S, Wormser GP: Comparison of culture-confirmed erythema migrans caused by *Borrelia burgdorferi* sensu stricto in New York State and by *Borrelia afzelii* in Slovenia. *Ann Intern Med* 130:32–36; 1999.

Tjernberg I, Kruger G, Eliasson I: C6 peptide ELISA test in the serodiagnosis of Lyme borreliosis in Sweden. *Eur J Clin Microbiol Infect Dis* 26:37–42; 2007.

Tugwell P, Dennis DT, Weinstein A, Wells G, Shea B, Nichol G, Hayward R, Lightfoot R, Baker P, Steere AC: Laboratory evaluation in the diagnosis of Lyme disease. *Ann Intern Med* 127:1109–1123; 1997.

Vasiliu V, Herzer P, Rossler D, Lehnert G, Wilske B: Heterogeneity of *Borrelia burgdorferi* sensu lato demonstrated by an ospA-type-specific PCR in synovial fluid from patients with Lyme arthritis. *Med Microbiol Immunol* 187:97–102; 1998.

Wang G, van Dam AP, Schwartz I, Dankert J: Molecular typing of *Borrelia burgdorferi* sensu lato: taxonomic, epidemiological, and clinical implications. *Clin Microbiol Rev* 12:633–653; 1999.

Wilske B, Preac-Mursic V, Gobel UB, Graf B, Jauris S, Soutschek E, Schwab E, Zumstein G: An OspA serotyping system for *Borrelia burgdorferi* based on reactivity with monoclonal antibodies and OspA sequence analysis. *J Clin Microbiol* 31:340–350; 1993.

Wilske B, Busch U, Eiffert H, Fingerle V, Pfister HW, Rossler D, Preac-Mursic V: Diversity of OspA and OspC among cerebrospinal fluid isolates of *Borrelia burgdorferi* sensu lato from patients with neuroborreliosis in Germany. *Med Microbiol Immunol* 184:195–201; 1996a.

Wilske B, Busch U, Fingerle V, Jauris-Heipke S, Preac-Mursic V, Rossler D, Will G: Immunological and molecular variability of OspA and OspC. Implications for *Borrelia* vaccine development. *Infection* 24:208–212; 1996b.

Wilske B, Habermann C, Fingerle V, Hillenbrand B, Jauris-Heipke S, Lehnert G, Pradel I, Rossler D, Schulte-Spechtel U: An improved recombinant IgG immunoblot for serodiagnosis of Lyme borreliosis. *Med Microbiol Immunol* 188:139–144; 1999.

Wilske B, Zöller L, Brade V, Eiffert H, Göbel UB, Stanek G: MIQ 12, Lyme-Borrelios. *In* Mauch H, Lütticken RE (eds): *Qualitätsstandards in der mikrobiologisch-infektiologischen Diagnostik*. Munich, Urban, Fischer; 2000.

Wilske B, Fingerle V, Schulte-Spechtel U: Microbiological and serological diagnosis of Lyme borreliosis. *FEMS Immunol Med Microbiol* 49:13–21; 2007a.

Wilske B, Johnson BJB, Schriefer ME: *Borrelia*. *In* Murray PR, Baron EJ, Jorgensen JH, Landry ML, Pfaller AE (eds): *Manual of Clinical Microbiology*, 9th ed. Washington, DC, ASM Press; 2007b.

Wormser GP, Horowitz HW, Nowakowski J, McKenna D, Dumler JS, Varde S, Schwartz I, Carbonaro C, Aguero-Rosenfeld M: Positive Lyme disease serology in patients with clinical and laboratory evidence of human granulocytic ehrlichiosis. *Am J Clin Pathol* 107:142–147; 1997.

Wormser GP, Carbonaro C, Miller S, Nowakowski J, Nadelman RB, Sivak S, Aguero-Rosenfeld ME: A limitation of 2-stage serological testing for Lyme disease: enzyme immunoassay and immunoblot assay are not independent tests. *Clin Infect Dis* 30:545–548; 2000.

Wormser GP, Dattwyler RJ, Shapiro ED, Halperin JJ, Steere AC, Klempner MS, Krause PJ, Bakken JS, Strle F, Stanek G, Bockenstedt L, Fish D, Dumler JS, Nadelman RB: The clinical assessment, treatment, and prevention of lyme disease, human granulocytic anaplasmosis, and babesiosis: clinical practice guidelines by the Infectious Diseases Society of America. *Clin Infect Dis* 43:1089–1134; 2006.

Zhang JR, Hardham JM, Barbour AG, Norris SJ: Antigenic variation in Lyme disease borreliae by promiscuous recombination of VMP-like sequence cassettes. *Cell* 89:275–285; 1997.

11

PROGNOSIS OF PERSONS WITH LYME BORRELIOSIS

Eugene D. Shapiro and Sunil K. Sood

While most studies indicate that the short-term prognosis of persons treated for Lyme disease (Lyme borreliosis) is excellent, there are conflicting opinions about the long-term outcomes, and this has contributed to the controversy about this illness. Studies that have addressed the issue of long-term prognosis include case reports, case series, and cohort studies, as well as clinical trials of treatment of persons with persistent symptoms. The best data available are from series of antibiotic-treated erythema migrans patients. These include both European and American studies (Feder et al., 2007; Marques, 2008). The presence of post–Lyme disease symptoms of unknown cause one year or more after treatment ranged from 0% to 0.5% in children (Gerber et al., 1996; Arnez et al., 2002) to 23% in adults (Strle et al., 1993). However, the validity of concluding there is a causal association between Lyme disease and the measured outcomes can be questioned.

SHORT-TERM OUTCOMES

There are a considerable number of clinical trials and observational studies of antibiotic treatment of patients who present at various stages of Lyme disease. In most instances, the rates of short-term cure after a single course of conventional treatment with antimicrobials is ≥90% (Nadelman et al., 1992; Luger et al., 1995; Nowakowski et al., 1995; Gerber et al.,

Lyme Borreliosis in Europe and North America: Epidemiology and Clinical Practice, First Edition. Edited by Sunil K. Sood

1996; Luft et al., 1996; Dattwyler et al., 1997; Wormser et al., 2006; Smith et al., 2002; Stanek and Strle, 2003; Halperin, 2008; Marques, 2008; Cerar et al., 2010; Kowalski et al., 2010). Moreover those patients who were not cured in the short-term generally have nonspecific symptoms, such as fatigue or myalgia, rather than objective signs, such as erythema migrans, facial nerve palsy, or synovitis. In most instances those who went on to develop signs of later stage Lyme disease, despite treatment, actually had some evidence of later-stage disease (e.g., neurologic signs) that was present at the time that treatment was begun. A possible exception is Lyme arthritis, in which rates of recurrence or persistence, at least in the short term, may exceed 5% (Wormser et al., 2006). However, arthritis resolves in the ensuing several months in the vast majority of such patients. The significance of reports of nonspecific complaints after treatment is unclear. In most instances even these complaints resolve within weeks to months.

LONG-TERM OUTCOMES

Obviously it is not possible to conduct clinical trials in which, after a baseline assessment of representative subjects, some patients are randomized to develop Lyme disease, followed for a prolonged period, and then outcomes are assessed by blinded investigators. We are left instead primarily with observational studies that assess outcomes of persons with a history of Lyme disease. Another approach is to conduct a randomized clinical trial to assess the effect of antibiotic treatment versus placebo on a group of patients with chronic symptoms suspected to be due to persistent infection with *Borrelia burgdorferi*, the assumption being that if those who receive the antibiotic improve, it is an indication that their symptoms are due to Lyme disease. There are many potential problems with the validity of both types of studies.

First, consider the observational studies (Figure 11.1). These studies are done in a cross-sectional manner (i.e., there is no assessment of the patient's baseline state before the onset of Lyme disease). In most instances it is assumed that abnormalities at follow-up were not present at baseline, an assumption that is not necessarily valid. Second, patients receive a variety of different treatments (or no treatment, in the case of some older studies). Differences in treatment may affect the outcomes. Other factors that may affect the outcomes are comorbid illnesses or injuries, normal aging, and factors such as stress, publicity about Lyme disease, and development of functional somatic syndromes (Barsky and Borus, 1999; Hatcher and Arroll, 2008).

An additional major problem is the high frequency of misdiagnosis, attributable in part to inappropriate use of serologic tests for Lyme disease and/or interpretation of the results

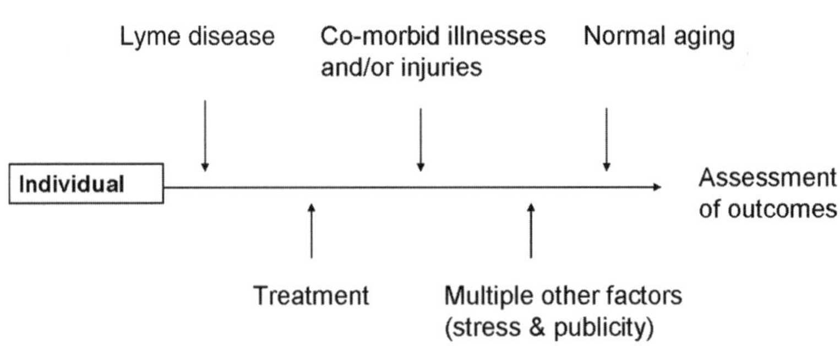

Figure 11.1 Longitudinal study to assess long-term outcomes of persons with Lyme disease.

(Steere et al., 1993; Seltzer and Shapiro, 1996; Tugwell et al., 1997; Reid et al., 1998). Because serologic tests remain positive for many years after infection with *B. burgdorferi*, new abnormalities that are unrelated to a previous infection may be erroneously attributed to Lyme disease (Feder et al., 1992; Hilton et al., 1997; Kalish et al., 2001b).

It is important to understand that the predictive value of antibody tests, even highly accurate ones, is highly dependent on the prevalence of the infection among patients who are tested. Antibody tests for Lyme disease should not be used as screening tests (Seltzer and Shapiro, 1996; Tugwell et al., 1997). Unfortunately, demands for testing are commonly fulfilled because many lay persons, and many physicians, have the erroneous belief that chronic, nonspecific symptoms such as arthralgia or fatigue by themselves may be manifestations of Lyme disease. Lyme disease will be the cause of the nonspecific symptoms in very few such patients, if any, since these complaints are extremely common in the general population (Buchwald et al., 1995; Wessely, 2001; Luo et al., 2005). Because the specificity of even the best antibody tests for Lyme disease rarely exceeds 90% to 95%, some of the test results in patients without specific signs of Lyme disease will be positive. The vast majority of these will be false-positive results. Nevertheless, an erroneous diagnosis of Lyme disease, based on the results of these tests, is often made. When the symptoms persist despite antibiotic treatment, such patients may erroneously be considered treatment failures.

Bias is another factor that may affect the validity of studies of the outcomes of persons with Lyme disease. Bias in studies is of several types: investigator bias, recall bias, reporting bias, selection bias, diagnostic bias, and protopathic bias. Investigator bias may occur if persons who assess the outcomes are not blinded to the subject's Lyme disease status. In reporting and recall bias, persons labeled as having Lyme disease may be more likely to recall as well as to report symptoms than are persons with symptoms who were not labeled. Publicity about Lyme disease and information (and misinformation) on the Internet may enhance this potential bias (Sood, 2002; Cooper and Feder, 2004). Selection bias may occur if cases or controls are not representative of all potential cases or controls in the population. An example is when selection of cases is linked to the outcomes, for example, when investigators advertise for persons with persistent symptoms to enter studies of Lyme disease. There is empirical evidence that this occurs (Shadick et al., 1999). A related type of diagnostic bias may occur if patients with nonspecific symptoms such as fatigue and arthralgia are more likely than controls to be tested, and are diagnosed with Lyme disease based on the results of such tests. A form of protopathic bias may also occur when patients are diagnosed with Lyme disease *because* they have the outcome (e.g., problems with memory or chronic fatigue) putatively linked to the disease. Indeed the definition of "chronic Lyme disease" often seems to be simply that a physician declares that the patient has chronic Lyme disease, with no requirement for evidence of either current or past infection (Feder et al., 2007). In reviewing studies that report on the long-term outcomes of persons with Lyme disease, it is important to keep such potential problems in mind.

Observational Studies of Long-Term Outcomes

United States

Case reports and case series have established two rare adverse outcomes that are associated with Lyme disease. These include an autoimmune recurrent arthritis (linked with certain HLA types) and a peripheral radiculopathy that is much more common in Europe than in the United States (Henriksson et al., 1986; Steere et al., 1990; Gross et al., 1998; Stanek and Strle, 2003). Case series have also indicated that a mild encephalopathy very rarely can occur in patients with Lyme disease (Logigian et al., 1990). It occurs primarily in adults with unequivocal evidence of *B. burgdorferi* infection who were not treated with antibiotics and is at least partially reversible by antibiotic treatment (Logigian et al., 1999).

In an uncontrolled follow-up study of 46 largely untreated children originally diagnosed with Lyme arthritis from 1976 to 1979, before the cause and treatment were established, by year seven after diagnosis only one child still had episodes of arthritis (Szer et al., 1991). Other complications were rare.

There have been several controlled observational studies of the outcomes of adults and of children with Lyme disease (Shadick et al., 1994; Shadick et al., 1999; Seltzer et al., 2000; Kalish et al., 2001a; Shadick et al., 2002; Vazquez et al., 2003; Kowalski et al., 2010). In addition to questioning subjects about their symptoms, most of these studies used validated standardized measures of outcomes, such as the short form-36 (SF-36) from the Medical Outcomes Study, a measure of health-related quality of life (Ware and Sherbourne, 1992). In addition, in some studies, patients underwent a physical examination, and in some, they underwent formal neuropsychological testing. Although there was some variation in the results, overall the outcomes were excellent. Compared with controls, at follow-up the adults diagnosed with Lyme disease more frequently reported problems with pain and with memory. However, objective evidence of a higher proportion of abnormalities among patients with Lyme disease, compared with controls, generally could not be documented either on examination or on standardized tests. This suggests that factors such as recall bias as well as reporting bias may account for at least some of the differences that were found. Health-related quality of life, as measured by the SF-36, usually was not significantly different between patients with past Lyme disease and controls. When differences were found, they improved over time (Shadick et al., 2002). In general, the frequency of complaints at follow-up was lower among children than among adults (Gerber et al., 1998; Wang et al., 1998; Seltzer et al., 2000; Vazquez et al., 2003; Kowalski et al., 2010).

Europe

A single genospecies of *B. burgdorferi* causes Lyme disease in the United States. There is much more heterogeneity in the genospecies that cause Lyme disease in Europe, including *B. garinii* that appears to be more neurotropic. Consequently the proportion of patients with neuroborreliosis is higher in Europe than in the United States. In addition several other clinical manifestations of the disease, such as acrodermatitis atrophica and lymphocytoma, occur almost exclusively in Europe, and Bannwarth's syndrome (myeloradiculitis) is much more common there. There are fewer controlled studies of long-term outcomes of patients in Europe and no clinical trials of treatment for "chronic Lyme disease." However, the data available suggest that the long-term outcomes of European patients with Lyme disease are similar to those of patients in the United States. Some of the studies are characterized by the same problems noted previously for the US studies, such as lack of appropriate control groups. This is a particular problem when patients with only nonspecific complaints, such as fatigue, are counted as treatment failures. Despite these shortcomings the data indicate that the outcomes of European patients with Lyme disease are excellent. This is true for studies of patients with both early Lyme disease, most of whom were followed for up to a year (Strle et al., 1993; Barsic et al., 2000; Arnez et al., 2002; Cerar et al., 2010), and for patients with neuroborreliosis (Oksi et al., 1998; Cimperman et al., 1999; Berglund et al., 2002; Oksi et al., 2007; Ljøstad et al., 2008). While the large majority of the patients with neuroborreliosis were well at follow-up, the small proportion with residual abnormalities either had neurologic deficits that were present before treatment was begun or had only nonspecific complaints. No reports suggested progression of neurologic signs despite conventional antibiotic treatment. Even patients with either meningitis or facial palsy who were treated with orally administered doxycycline had excellent outcomes with the exception of a few patients who had subjective complaints (Halperin et al., 2007; Oksi et al., 2007; Ljøstad et al., 2008). One exception to the generally favorable course of most manifestations of Lyme disease are the outcomes of patients with acrodermatitis atrophicans. This appears to be a chronic condition, the outcome of which depends on the timing of antibiotic treatment (Aberer et al., 1996). If treatment is begun early during the acute inflammatory stage of this condition, it usually resolves. However, if treatment is begun after the lesions have become sclerotic, the skin lesions may not be reversible, although there generally will not be further progression.

CLINICAL TRIALS OF TREATMENT IN PERSONS WITH PERSISTENT SYMPTOMS

In the four published randomized clinical trials of treatment, persons with persistent complaints after treatment for Lyme disease were enrolled and treated with either antibiotics or placebo in a double-blind manner (Klempner et al., 2001; Krupp et al., 2003; Fallon et al., 2008). It should be noted that the patients in these studies had evidence of previous Lyme disease (potential subjects with chronic symptoms but who had no previous evidence of Lyme disease were excluded). The investigators had to increase the number of participating centers or the duration of enrollment, or both, to enroll an adequate number of subjects. In one study more than 3300 patients were screened to enroll only 37 subjects (Fallon et al., 2008). This is a reflection of the relatively few patients who have persistent complaints after being treated for well-documented Lyme disease. Whether their symptoms truly were related to Lyme disease can be questioned. Indeed, in the studies by Klempner, 40% of the subjects were seronegative even though the symptoms attributed to Lyme disease persisted for many months.

The largest studies were conducted by Klempner and colleagues (Klempner et al., 2001). They conducted two controlled trials of antibiotic treatment for adult patients with chronic musculoskeletal pain, neurocognitive symptoms, or both that persisted after antibiotic treatment for Lyme disease. One study included 78 patients who were seropositive for IgG antibodies to *B. burgdorferi* at the time of enrollment. The other study included 51 patients who were seronegative but with a history of erythema migrans. In both studies patients were randomly assigned to receive either ceftriaxone administered intravenously for 30 days followed by doxycycline orally for 60 days, or matching regimens with intravenous and oral placebos. The studies were terminated early by the data and safety monitoring board after a scheduled interim analysis indicated that the probability of finding a difference between the treatment and the placebo groups, even if full enrollment was completed, was vanishingly small. There were no significant differences in the outcomes of patients treated with antibiotics compared with those treated with placebo among either the seropositive or the seronegative patients. Symptoms reported by subjects who did complete treatment were quite labile: about a third of patients improved, a third worsened, and a third were unchanged. However, changes in reported symptoms were not related to whether the patient received antibiotics or placebo.

Krupp et al. randomized 55 patients with severe fatigue to receive either ceftriaxone or an identical-appearing placebo for 28 days (Krupp et al., 2003). Although they reported a 13% greater reduction in scores for severity of fatigue (based on an 11-item questionnaire) in the ceftriaxone-treated group, there was no significant difference for the two other outcomes, improvement in cognitive function and clearance of *B. burgdorferi* outer surface protein A from cerebrospinal fluid, an experimental test of CSF infection. There also was no significant difference between groups in the change in score on the SF-36. In this study there was some evidence that blinding of the groups was compromised. A substantial number of subjects developed serious complications from the treatment. The authors concluded that the small difference in score on the severity of fatigue did not justify the treatment. These findings support earlier recommendations that such patients are best treated symptomatically rather than with prolonged courses of antibiotic therapy, which have been associated with serious adverse side effects. The most recent published study randomized subjects with "Lyme encephalopathy" to receive either ceftriaxone or placebo for 10 weeks (Fallon et al., 2008). The entry criteria included (1) a history of either physician-documented erythema migrans or a CDC-defined objective manifestation of Lyme disease and a positive serologic test result for Lyme disease (confirmed by Western blot); (2) a positive IgG Western blot at the time of entry into the study; (3) previous treatment for Lyme disease with at least 3 weeks of IV ceftriaxone, completed at least 4 months before study entry; (4) subjective memory impairment that, by report, started after the onset of Lyme disease; and (5) objective evidence of memory impairment as documented by the Wechsler Memory Scale–III. The investigators and the accompanying editorial concluded that there was no sustainable benefit from treatment, and that there were substantial risks with prolonged treatment (Fallon et al., 2008, Halperin, 2008).

MANAGEMENT OF PATIENTS WHO HAVE BEEN GIVEN A DIAGNOSIS OF CHRONIC LYME DISEASE

Patients labeled as having "chronic Lyme disease" share many of the clinical and epidemiologic features of patients with other functional somatic syndromes (Barsky and Borus, 1999). Recently a practical classification of these patients has been proposed (Feder et al., 2007). It would be useful for the clinician to categorize the patient in order to best direct treatment. (Table 11.1) Most such patients have no evidence of either current or past infection with *B. burgdorferi*. Some patients will have positive test results from laboratories that either use in-house tests that have not been approved by the Food and Drug Administration or interpret approved tests using criteria that have not been validated. A crucial distinction between the very rare patients with true persistent infection with

TABLE 11.1 Classification of patients who may have been given a diagnosis of "chronic Lyme disease"

Category	Clinical Scenario	Antibiotic Treatment Indicated?
1	Symptoms of unknown cause, with no evidence of *Borrelia burgdorferi* infection	No
2	A well-defined illness unrelated to *B. burgdorferi* infection	No
3	Symptoms of unknown cause, with antibodies against *B. burgdorferi* but no history of objective clinical findings that are consistent with Lyme disease	Single course along with counseling that the diagnosis is uncertain and that benefit from treatment is unlikely
4	Post–Lyme disease syndrome	No

Source: Adapted from Feder et al. (2007).

B. burgdorferi and those in category 4 is that patients with true infection will have objective physical signs, such as synovitis (i.e., a frankly inflamed joint) rather than solely subjective symptoms (e.g. pain in the joint).

It is important to acknowledge that the patients with chronic symptoms truly are experiencing these symptoms even though there may be no objective signs of ongoing inflammation. The causes of these "medically unexplained symptoms" are often complex (Stone et al., 2002; Smith and Dwamena, 2007; Fink and Rosendal, 2008) but are extremely unlikely to be related to inadequate treatment with antibiotics. Clinicians who care for patients with Lyme disease should recognize that these patients are likely to be exposed to inaccurate information about a risk of developing "chronic Lyme disease," either on the Internet or from friends or relatives. Anticipatory guidance given at the time of initial diagnosis may help forestall the development of anxiety that such misinformation may induce. Reassurance that treatment is highly effective is an important part of caring for patients with Lyme disease.

CONCLUSIONS

In summary, the short-term prognosis for persons treated for Lyme disease is excellent. It is difficult to conduct high-quality studies of the long-term outcomes of persons with Lyme disease. However, all of the data that are available, which now are considerable, confirm that the long-term outcomes are excellent too. Advice to clinicians, especially infectious disease specialists, rheumatologists, and neurologists to whom patients diagnosed with "chronic Lyme disease" may be referred, is summarized in Table 11.2. Physicians have a collective responsibility to dispel the increasingly prevalent perception that Lyme disease is a reason for unexplained chronic illnesses (Wormser et al., 2006; Kemperman, 2008).

TABLE 11.2 Advice to clinicians on managing patients to misconceptions about the prognosis of Lyme disease

A. *Provide anticipatory counseling about the following to patients with Lyme disease:*

1. The antibiotic-responsive nature of this infectious disease, its lack of resistance, and lack of persistence
2. The limited number of manifestations of the disease
3. Reliable sources of information (e.g., CDC,[a] American Lyme Disease Foundation,[b] EUCALB[c])
4. It is not rare for mild fatigue, musculoskeletal pain, or perceived difficulties with memory to continue beyond the usual treatment duration of 10 to 28 days
5. Retreatment does not accelerate the rate of resolution of these symptoms
6. Return promptly if joint swelling, recurrent skin rash, weakness of facial or other muscles, severe headache, palpitations, or syncope develop

B. *For a patient referred with a diagnosis with chronic Lyme disease, carefully review the evidence upon which the diagnosis was based, especially for patients who did not have Lyme disease but fall into categories 1 to 3:*

1. Emphasize the nonspecific nature of the symptoms and their frequent occurrence in the general population
2. Review that potential exposure in an endemic area or a remote history of rash or "bug" bite is not sufficient to assume that a skin lesion was erythema migrans
3. Point out the unvalidated methods or unproved criteria used to make a diagnosis based on "positive" results in "Lyme specialty" laboratories

C. *For patients with established symptoms, including those with post–Lyme disease syndrome:*

1. Explain that an improvement in symptoms following antibiotic treatment is not confirmation of the diagnosis. It could be from a placebo effect or possible anti-inflammatory effects of commonly used antibiotics
2. Remind the patient of the serious adverse effects of antibiotics (e.g., life-threatening reactions, cholelithiasis, *C. difficile* infection, selection of resistant bacterial flora.)
3. Explain that worsening of symptoms while taking antibiotics, claimed to be a Jarisch–Herxheimer reaction, is not confirmation of the diagnosis of Lyme disease. This reaction only occurs in early disease, usually in the first 24 hours of treatment.
4. Provide emotional and psychological support in addition to symptomatic management of medically unexplained symptoms. Openly address concerns originating from information gathered on "Lyme" from the public domain. For example, reassure that they will not develop brain damage as they are not chronically infected.
5. Establish a collaborative approach between physician and patient, which is crucial to the goals of palliation of symptoms and rehabilitation. The patient should be encouraged to take an active role in the treatment process.

Source: Adapted from Feder et al. (2007).
[a]http://cdc.gov/ncidod/dvbid/lyme/.
[b]http://www.aldf.com/.
[c]http://meduni09.edis.at/eucalb/cms/index.php?lang=en.

REFERENCES

Aberer E, Breier F, Stanek G, Schmidt B: Success and failure in the treatment of acrodermatitis chronica atrophicans. *Infection* 24:85–87; 1996.

Arnez M, Pleterski-Rigler D, Luznik-Bufon T, Ruzic-Sabljic E, Strle F: Solitary erythema migrans in children. Comparison of treatment with azithromycin and phenoxymethylpenicillin. *Wien Klin Wochenschr* 114:498–504; 2002.

Barsic B, Maretic T, Majerus L, Strugar J: Comparison of azithromycin and doxycycline in the treatment of erythema migrans. *Infection* 28:153–156; 2000.

Barsky AJ, Borus JF: Functional somatic syndromes. *Ann Intern Med* 130:910–921; 1999.

Berglund J, Stjernberg L, Ornstein K, Tykesson-Joelsson K, Walter H: 5-y Follow-up study of patients with neuroborreliosis. *Scand J Infect Dis* 34:421–425; 2002.

Buchwald D, Umali P, Umali J, Kith P, Pearlman T, Komaroff AL: Chronic fatigue and the chronic fatigue syndrome. Prevalence in a Pacific Northwest health care system. *Ann Intern Med* 123:81–88; 1995.

Cerar D, Cerar T, Ruzic-Sabljic E, Wormser GP, Strle F: Subjective symptoms after treatment of early Lyme disease. *Am J Med* 123:79–86; 2010.

Cimperman J, Maraspin V, Lotric-Furlan S, Ruzic-Sabljic E, Strle F: Lyme meningitis. A one-year follow up controlled study. *Wien Klin Wochenschr* 111:961–963; 1999.

Cooper JD, Feder HM Jr.: Inaccurate information about lyme disease on the internet. *Pediatr Infect Dis J* 23:1105–1108; 2004.

Fallon BA, Keilp JG, Corbera KM, Petkova E, Britton CB, Dwyer E, Slavov I, Cheng J, Dobkin J, Nelson DR, Sackeim HA: A randomized, placebo-controlled trial of repeated IV antibiotic therapy for Lyme encephalopathy. *Neurology* 70:992–1003; 2008.

Feder HM Jr., Gerber MA, Luger SW, Ryan RW: Persistence of serum antibodies to *Borrelia burgdorferi* in patients treated for Lyme disease. *Clin Infect Dis* 15:788–793; 1992.

Feder HM Jr., Johnson BJ, O'Connell S, Shapiro ED, Steere AC, Wormser GP, Agger WA, Artsob H, Auwaerter P, Dumler JS, Bakken JS, Bockenstedt LK, Green J, Dattwyler RJ, Munoz J, Nadelman RB, Schwartz I, Draper T, McSweegan E, Halperin JJ, Klempner MS, Krause PJ, Mead P, Morshed M, Porwancher R, Radolf JD, Smith RP Jr., Sood S, Weinstein A, Wong SJ, Zemel L: A critical appraisal of "chronic Lyme disease." *N Engl J Med* 357:1422–1430; 2007.

Gross DM, Forsthuber T, Tary-Lehmann M, Etling C, Ito K, Nagy ZA, Field JA, Steere AC, Huber BT: Identification of LFA-1 as a candidate autoantigen in treatment-resistant Lyme arthritis. *Science* 281:703–706; 1998.

Halperin JJ, Shapiro ED, Logigian E, Belman AL, Dotevall L, Wormser GP, Krupp L, Gronseth G, Bever CT Jr.: Practice parameter: treatment of nervous system Lyme disease (an evidence-based review). Report of the Quality Standards Subcommittee of the American Academy of Neurology. *Neurology* 69:91–102; 2007.

Hatcher S, Arroll B: Assessment and management of medically unexplained symptoms. *BMJ* 336:1124–1128; 2008.

Henriksson A, Link H, Cruz M, Stiernstedt G: Immunoglobulin abnormalities in cerebrospinal fluid and blood over the course of lymphocytic meningoradiculitis (Bannwarth's syndrome). *Ann Neurol* 20:337–345; 1986.

Hilton E, Tramontano A, Devoti J, Sood SK: Temporal study of immunoglobin M seroreactivity to *Borrelia burgdorferi* in patients treated for Lyme borreliosis. *J Clin Microbiol* 35:774–776; 1997.

Kalish RA, Kaplan RF, Taylor E, Jones-Woodward L, Workman K, Steere AC: Evaluation of study patients with Lyme disease. 10–20-Year follow-up. *J Infect Dis* 183:453–60; 2001a.

Kalish RA, McHugh G, Granquist J, Shea B, Ruthazer R, Steere AC: Persistence of immunoglobulin M or immunoglobulin G antibody responses to *Borrelia burgdorferi* 10–20 years after active Lyme disease. *Clin Infect Dis* 33:780–785; 2001b.

Kemperman MM, Bakken JS, Kravitz GR: Dispelling the chronic Lyme disease myth. *Minn Med;* 91: 37–41; 2008.

Klempner MS, Hu LT, Evans J, Schmid CH, Johnson GM, Trevino RP, Norton D, Levy L, Wall D, McCall J, Kosinski M, Weinstein A: Two controlled trials of antibiotic treatment in patients with persistent symptoms and a history of Lyme disease. *N Engl J Med* 345:85–92; 2001.

Kowalski TJ, Tata S, Berth W, Mathiason MA, Agger WA: Antibiotic treatment duration and long-term outcomes of patients with early Lyme disease from a Lyme disease-hyperendemic area. *Clin Infect Dis* 50:512–520; 2010.

Krupp LB, Hyman LG, Grimson R, Coyle PK, Melville P, Ahnn S, Dattwyler R, Chandler B: Study and treatment of post Lyme disease (STOP-LD). A randomized double masked clinical trial. *Neurology* 60:1923–1930; 2003.

Ljøstad U, Skogvoll E, Eikeland R, Midgard R, Skarpaas T, Berg A, Mygland A: Oral doxycycline versus intravenous ceftriaxone for European Lyme neuroborreliosis. A multicentre, non-inferiority, double-blind, randomised trial. *Lancet Neurol* 7:690–695; 2008.

Logigian EL, Kaplan RF, Steere AC: Chronic neurologic manifestations of Lyme disease. *N Engl J Med* 323:1438–1444; 1990.

Logigian EL, Kaplan RF, Steere AC: Successful treatment of Lyme encephalopathy with intravenous ceftriaxone. *J Infect Dis* 180:377–383; 1999.

Luo N, Johnson JA, Shaw JW, Feeny D, Coons SJ: Self-reported health status of the general adult U.S. population as assessed by the EQ-5D and Health Utilities Index. *Med Care* 43:1078–1086; 2005.

Oksi J, Nikoskelainen J, Viljanen MK: Comparison of oral cefixime and intravenous ceftriaxone followed by oral amoxicillin in disseminated Lyme borreliosis. *Eur J Clin Microbiol Infect Dis* 17:715–719; 1998.

Oksi J, Nikoskelainen J, Hiekkanen H, Lauhio A, Peltomaa M, Pitkaranta A, Nyman D, Granlund H, Carlsson SA, Seppala I, Valtonen V, Viljanen M: Duration of antibiotic treatment in disseminated Lyme borreliosis. A double-blind, randomized, placebo-controlled, multicenter clinical study. *Eur J Clin Microbiol Infect Dis* 26:571–581; 2007.

Seltzer EG, Gerber MA, Cartter ML, Freudigman K, Shapiro ED: Long-term outcomes of persons with Lyme disease. *JAMA* 283:609–616; 2000.

Seltzer EG, Shapiro ED: Misdiagnosis of Lyme disease: When not to order serologic tests. *Pediatr Infect Dis J* 15:762–763; 1996.

Shadick NA, Phillips CB, Logigian EL, Steere AC, Kaplan RF, Berardi VP, Duray PH, Larson MG, Wright EA, Ginsburg KS, Katz JN, Liang MH: The long-term clinical outcomes of Lyme disease. A population-based retrospective cohort study. *Ann Intern Med* 121:560–567; 1994.

Shadick NA, Phillips CB, Sangha O, Logigian EL, Kaplan RF, Wright EA, Fossel AH, Fossel K, Berardi V, Lew RA; Liang MH: Musculoskeletal and neurologic outcomes in patients with previously treated Lyme disease. *Ann Intern Med* 131:919–926; 1999.

Shadick NA, Phillips CB, Maher NE, Wright L, Al E: Diminished health-related quality-of-life improves over time in Lyme disease. The 12 yr follow up from the Nantucket Lyme disease cohort study. IX International Conference on Lyme Borreliosis and Other Tick-borne Diseases. Alphareta, GA, Imedex; 2002; Abstract #0-36.

Sood SK: Effective retrieval of Lyme disease information on the Web. *Clin Infect Dis* 35:451–464; 2002.

Stanek G, Strle F: Lyme borreliosis. *Lancet* 362:1639–1647; 2003.

Steere AC, Dwyer E, Winchester R: Association of chronic Lyme arthritis with HLA-DR4 and HLA-DR2 alleles. *N Engl J Med* 323:219–223; 1990.

Strle F, Preac-Mursic V, Cimperman J, Ruzic E, Maraspin V, Jereb M: Azithromycin versus doxycycline for treatment of erythema migrans: clinical and microbiological findings. *Infection* 21:83–88; 1993.

Szer IS, Taylor E, Steere AC: The long-term course of Lyme arthritis in children. *N Engl J Med* 325:159–163; 1991.

Tugwell P, Dennis DT, Weinstein A, Wells G, Shea B, Nichol G, Hayward R, Lightfoot R, Baker P, Steere AC: Laboratory evaluation in the diagnosis of Lyme disease. *Ann Intern Med* 127:1109–1123; 1997.

Vazquez M, Sparrow SS, Shapiro ED: Long-term neuropsychologic and health outcomes of children with facial nerve palsy attributable to Lyme disease. *Pediatrics* 112:e93–e97; 2003.

Ware JE Jr., Sherbourne CD: The MOS 36-item short-form health survey (SF-36). I. Conceptual framework and item selection. *Med Care* 30:473–483; 1992.

Wessely S: Chronic fatigue. Symptom and syndrome. *Ann Intern Med* 134:838–843; 2001.

Wormser GP, Dattwyler RJ, Shapiro ED, Halperin JJ, Steere AC, Klempner MS, Krause PJ, Bakken JS, Strle F, Stanek G, Bockenstedt L, Fish D, Dumler JS, Nadelman RB: The clinical assessment, treatment, and prevention of lyme disease, human granulocytic anaplasmosis, and babesiosis. Clinical practice guidelines by the Infectious Diseases Society of America. *Clin Infect Dis* 43:1089–1134; 2006.

12

PREVENTION OF LYME BORRELIOSIS

Sunil K. Sood

Lyme borreliosis is an emerging infectious disease in both the Old and New worlds. The challenge for prevention of this tick-borne infection is greater than with other vector-borne infections because of the complex life cycle of its tick vectors. This can be exploited to decrease transmission to humans at multiple levels. (Hayes and Piesman, 2003). The opportunities for intervention can be divided into three main areas: prevention of tick exposure and of tick bites, prevention of infection after a tick bite, and immunization. Prevention of tick exposure includes the control of ticks and their reservoirs and hosts in nature, by multipronged efforts at landscape management, acaricide application, biological control of ticks, and control of host animals. Tick control and investigations aimed at decreasing the spirochetal burden in nature are discussed briefly in this chapter. For more information the reader is referred to comprehensive reviews, (Hayes et al., 1999; Hayes and Piesman, 2003; Piesman, 2006; Piesman and Eisen, 2008) the book *Lyme Borreliosis: Biology, Epidemiology and Control* by Jeremy Gray and co-editors, and the comprehensive illustrated *Tick Management Handbook* developed by Kirby Stafford of the Connecticut Agricultural Experiment Station (also available on line on the US CDC home page for Lyme disease: http://cdc.gov/ncidod/dvbid/lyme/and at www.ct.gov/caes) (Gray et al., 2002; Stafford, 2007).

Lyme Borreliosis in Europe and North America: Epidemiology and Clinical Practice, First Edition. Edited by Sunil K. Sood

Many of the measures discussed are also useful for the reduction of risk from other tick-borne diseases and from mosquito bites.

PREVENTING EXPOSURE TO TICKS

Personal Protection

Recommendations for personal protection against tick bites have been emphasized ever since Lyme borreliosis became a recognized public health threat (1981). An obvious piece of advice is to avoid infected areas, but because recreational, occupational, and even residential habits make exposure inevitable for most people in endemic areas, other preventive measures need to be implemented (Hayes and Piesman, 2003). The main measures are use of long-sleeved and light-colored clothing, checking the body for ticks, and use of tick-repellents.

Avoidance

Residents and visitors to public parks and nature preserves in endemic areas are familiar with posted signs warning them not to stray from footpaths, and are usually aware of the need to minimize contact with brush, bushes, and heavily wooded areas. However, ticks can attach during even minimal or passing exposure, and can be present on grassy areas and in leaf litter. An additional protective measure is the wearing of long-sleeved clothing, which most people abhor in warm weather, and light-colored clothing that would enable crawling ticks to be seen more readily. The body of evidence for effectiveness of these measures is small. In fact, as discussed in Chapter 3 (on early Lyme borreliosis), ticks seek warm and sequestered areas of the body regardless of their "entry-point" under clothing. Intuitively, tucking long pants into socks and even taping them will prevent tick attachment, but this measure is likely to be more effective with the additional use of repellents if the socks have a fine weave (Stafford, 2007). Patients frequently inquire about the role of pets. Although pets can bring ticks into the home (Curran and Fish, 1989) the likelihood of eggs being laid or of the ticks surviving indoors is very low given a dry environment (Stafford, 2007). Having a pet at home was not statistically associated with Lyme disease in Connecticut (Vazquez et al., 2008). Nevertheless, there is the possibility that unfed ticks could brush off and attach itself to the owners shortly after the pet comes in.

Repellents

The tick repellent in most common use is DEET (*N,N*-diethyl-*m*-toluamide aka *N,N*-diethyl-3-methylbenzamide). DEET is presumed to act by forming an offensive vapor barrier for biting arthropods and ticks. A variety of topical repellents are available commercially, but DEET is singularly the most effective. There is a wide range of concentrations in the formulations sold, but no consensus on the minimum concentration to achieve adequate protection. The more concentrated the preparation, the longer lasting the protection. Formulations with 10% to 30% DEET are adequate to provide protection in most circumstances. Ten percent DEET can be confidently recommended as safe for use on infants and children. It is prudent to wash the child's skin upon returning indoors, a measure that also helps remove attached ticks. Because a 30% formulation provides about 6 hours of protection, the use of even higher concentrations may be superfluous, and has been phased out in Canada.

Concerns about the potential toxicity from transcutaneous absorption of DEET has resulted in underutilization of this very effective modality (Goodyer and Behrens, 1998). In turn there is increasing reliance on plant-based repellents of unproved effectiveness. There are a few pediatric case reports of seizures temporally associated with application of DEET, but as seizures are a common condition in young children, a cause-and-effect relation is far from established. Only a very small proportion of DEET is absorbed after topical application, and its metabolism and elimination are rapid (Selim et al., 1995). Certain DEET-sunscreen combinations and topical retinoids can enhance the absorption of DEET, and DEET decreases the effectiveness of sunscreen (Montemarano et al., 1997; Ross et al., 2004; Katz et al., 2008). The use of combination DEET-sunscreen preparations is not recommended, and if sunscreen is required, it should be applied before DEET. There is no evidence of harm to the fetus when DEET is used during pregnancy or of transfer through breast milk (Koren et al., 2003).

On balance, the evidence does not support a significant health risk from DEET after topical application, whereas the health risks of arthropod and tick bites are substantial (Goodyer and Behrens, 1998). Most reports of serious adverse events documented at national poison control centers in the United States and the United Kingdom were from inhalation or ocular contact, or from ingestion of large amounts of the chemical (Tenenbein, 1987; Veltri et al., 1994; Goodyer and Behrens, 1998). Practical recommendations for safe use of DEET are accessible at http://wwwn.cdc.gov/travel/yellowBookCh2-InsectsArthropods.aspx, http://aapnews.aappublications.org/cgi/content/full/e200399v1 and http://www.pmra-arla.gc.ca/english/consum/insectrepellents-e.html#3, and summarized in Table 12.1.

Permethrin is a synthetic compound that is an insecticide, acaricide, and repellent. It is poorly absorbed through the skin and human toxicity potential is minimal, but it is not approved for use as a repellent because neurotoxic effects are reported with exposure to high doses. It is highly effective in killing ticks on contact when applied to clothing, shoes, and

TABLE 12.1 Tick repellent advice

DEET the repellent of choice

- Use any formulation of DEET with concentration between 10% and 35% under normal exposure circumstances.
- Use safely on babies as young as 2 months, for whom the lowest concentrations are adequate, avoiding the face, and do not leave on overnight.
- Do not use on open wounds, inflamed or sunburned skin
- Use of preparations that are pre-mixed with sunscreens is not recommended. These preparations have been phased out in Canada. Apply sunscreen before applying DEET.

Permethrin

- Apply on clothes, shoes, and surfaces of equipment and patio surfaces. Permethrin is highly lethal to ticks.

Note: Practical recommendations for safe use of DEET are accessible [Accessed 1/19/2011] at
http://wwwn.cdc.gov/travel/yellowBookCh2-InsectsArthropods.aspx
http://aapnews.aappublications.org/cgi/content/full/e200399v1 and
http://www.pmra-arla.gc.ca/english/consum/insectrepellents-e.html#3.

fomites, the mechanism of action being excitation followed by paralysis of the nervous system (Solberg et al., 2003). It is used on clothing by some professional groups at high risk of tick exposure, such as military personnel, hunters, and forestry workers.

The role of garlic and other plant-based natural products, and the synthetic compounds picaridin (KBR 3023), in repelling *Ixodes* ticks remains tentative (Pretorius et al., 2003; Carroll et al., 2005; Jaenson et al., 2005; Katz et al., 2008). A 10% formulation of dodecanoic acid, a naturally occurring carboxylic acid present in coconut and palm kernel oils, delayed the attachment of *I. ricinus* nymphs by a few hours (Schwantes et al., 2008). Although several repellents are marketed under the Skin-So-Soft™ brand, preparations containing diisopropyl adipate and benzophenone demonstrated poor effectiveness even as an *Aedes aegypti* mosquito repellent, while IR3535 and picaridin are not yet proved as tick repellents (Chou et al., 1997; Fradin and Day, 2002).

Tick Checks

It is good practice to perform a tick check under a bright light at the end of each day of possible exposure. This should preferably be a daily routine for persons living in endemic areas because exposure occurs in a residential environment as well. The use of a washcloth may help dislodge recently attached ticks but will not work with *Ixodes* that are well along in the feeding process; special attention should be paid to armpit, groin, back, and scalp skin. In studies in the United States a short duration of attachment of an *Ixodes* tick minimized the risk of acquiring *B. burgdorferi* infection from the bite (Sood et al., 1997; Nadelman et al., 2001). There is a small risk that ticks on clothing can survive washing, so killing them by subjecting them to heat in a dryer for an hour should be considered (Stafford, 2007).

Need for Educational Interventions

In surveys and epidemiologic studies, adherence to recommendations and effectiveness of preventive measures have been variable. For example only 11% of Nantucket, Massachusetts, residents but 79% of Connecticut endemic area residents routinely used tick repellents (Herrington et al., 1997; Phillips et al., 2001). In a study conducted among commuter ferry passengers on Martha's Vineyard, Massachusetts, various tick avoidance behavior rates were prevalent in about a half to two-thirds of people, and possessing "very good knowledge of Lyme disease" did not predict these practices (Shadick et al., 1997). The need for educational interventions is reinforced by findings from another highly endemic focus on Nantucket Island, Massachusetts, where avoidance, repellents, and protective clothing were the least used preventive measures (Phillips et al., 2001). In fact a subsequent educational program conducted aboard a ferry to Nantucket was successful in increasing the use of preventive precautions as well as in reducing the risk of tick-borne illnesses (Daltroy et al., 2007). A tailored educational intervention program in Baltimore County, Maryland, resulted in increased knowledge, improved attitudes especially with regard to repellent use, as well an increase in self-reported preventive behaviors (Malouin et al., 2003).

Effectiveness of Personal Protection Measures

The effectiveness of personal protective measures was assessed in a matched case-control study (Vazquez et al., 2008). A standardized survey was administered to adolescents and adults who had been identified as having Lyme disease between 2000 and 2003 in an active Connecticut-wide surveillance system. A limitation was the self-reported, and therefore unconfirmed, nature of the answers. Surprisingly, the relationship of conventionally accepted risk factors, including frequent outdoor activities, living in grassy or heavily wooded areas, and even occupational exposure, was not demonstrable in their study. Of all personal and periresidential preventive measures analyzed, only the use of protective clothing outdoors and the use of tick repellents on skin or clothing were calculated to be effective (40% and 20%, respectively). Patients with history of definite or possible Lyme disease reported the use of these measures less often than did matched controls. The authors did not rule out the possibility that fastidious use of measures such as repellents and tick checks will demonstrate better effectiveness in prevention of Lyme borreliosis.

Control of Ticks in Nature

Spraying of Acaricides and Other Periresidential Measures

Residential lawns that border woodland vegetation can harbor ticks that are brought in on small mammals. As a short-term measure the sprayed application of acaricides such as carbaryl, chlorpyrifos, and synthetic pyrethroids at the perimeter has been demonstrated to achieve 68% to 100% reduction in ticks (Stafford, 1991; Curran et al., 1993; Piesman, 2006). Acaricides are underutilized because of the widespread perception as well as genuine risks of human, pet, and environmental toxicity. Fewer than 25% of residents in a survey of hyperendemic communities in four northeastern US states reported ever using them on their property (Piesman, 2006).

Straightforward and inexpensive landscape management principles can be applied to reduce the tick burdens in periresidential environments (Stafford, 2007). These measures include clearing leaf litter, sun exposure to reduce humidity in shaded areas since desiccation kills ticks, and spreading wood chips to create a border between lawns and vegetation. Use of certain natural products with putative biocidal effects, as well as the use of entomopathogenic fungi and nematodes, parasitoid wasps, and a variety of other species as biological control agents, need further evaluation at this time. Of these, the Alaska yellow cedar oil extract nootkatone appears to very effective in control of *I. scapularis* and other ticks that transmit pathogens to humans (Samish et al., 2004; Piesman and Eisen, 2008; Dolan et al., 2009).

Host Control

A measure proved to achieve control of *I. scapularis* populations is the reduction or elimination of white-tailed deer from a given geographic area. In one extreme example, elimination of the deer population on Monhegan Island, Maine, has resulted in absence of the tick from the island for several years (Rand et al., 2004). As may be expected, eradication of deer is not a popular measure in most communities. Deer-fencing has instead become a standard technique in efforts to exclude deer from designated recreation areas.

Host-Targeted Acaricides, Antibiotics, and Vaccines

An active area of investigation is the delivery of acaricides to animal hosts in an attempt to diminish their carriage of ticks (Figure 12.1). Host-targeted acaricides have been most successful when applied to deer. The delivery of topical amitraz and permethrin by means of a "four-poster device" reduced questing nymphal *I. scapularis* in the local area by up to 91%

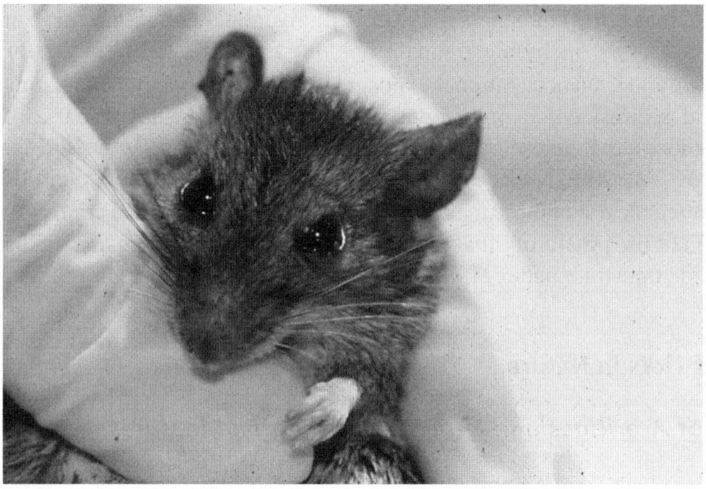

Figure 12.1 *Peromyscus leucopus* with ticks attached (arrow). Source: Kirby Stafford. (*See insert for color representation*).

(Solberg et al., 2003). The device consists of four impregnated paint rollers that the deer must insert its head through in order to access a feeding trough. This approach may be useful in some European deer parks, where deer populations are closely managed within set population limits. Tick control by means of rodent-targeted acaricides has been somewhat less effective. The main borrelial reservoir in the northeastern United States is the white-footed mouse, and permethrin-impregnated cotton balls can be placed in their habitat for them to accumulate as nesting material. Field trials have yielded conflicting results (Piesman, 2006). Current trials are evaluating the acaricide fipronil delivered in bait boxes (Dolan et al., 2004).

A secondary objective is to reduce borrelial infection rates of questing ticks by decreasing bacteremia burdens in the host rodents. This is a loftier goal, but a promising innovative technology uses bait containing *B. burgdorferi*-vaccine or antibiotics for small mammals that sustain transmission in nature (Tsao et al., 2004; Gomes-Solecki et al., 2006; Dolan et al., 2008). The concept derives from the success of oral rabies vaccine in wildlife (Roscoe et al., 1998). Recombinant *E. coli* and vaccinia virus are among the vectors proposed for OspA-based vaccines to be used in this manner (Madurawe et al., 2000; Scheckelhoff et al., 2006). Concerns around the ecological impact of these techniques will need to be addressed before they are implemented on a large scale.

If we are to approach the goal of reducing the occurrence of Lyme borreliosis, a judicious combination of tick control measures should be employed in endemic settings. A major impediment is the inadequacy of systems in place to communicate current research to the public (Piesman and Eisen, 2008).

PREVENTING INFECTION AFTER A TICK BITE

In most cases Lyme borreliosis can be readily diagnosed and easily treated. Still, the apprehension associated with a tick bite, and the uncertainty expressed by many physicians regarding the preferred course of action, makes it valuable to follow an evidence-based approach. Such an approach would allay anxiety, decrease the indiscriminate use of antibiotics, and prevent some cases of *B. burgdorferi* infection.

Tick Removal

Tick removal technique is straightforward. Using an ordinary pair of thin-tipped tweezers or forceps, the tick is grasped;by the mouth end of the tick if discernable—and gently pulled straight up until detached. There is no evidence that remaining embedded mouth parts increase the risk of transmission, or that crushing the tick enhances transmission (Piesman and Dolan, 2002). A technique that involves prying off the tick using a credit card has been proposed, but this should not provide any advantage over the simple removal method. Commercial tick removal devices have not been demonstrated to be superior to tweezers (Piesman and Dolan, 2002). Methods that use petroleum jelly, lidocaine, isopropyl alcohol, volatile substances such as nail polish and gasoline, lighted matches, or heated nails are ineffective, dangerous, and not recommended (Needham, 1985, Stanek and Kahl, 1999).

Tick Identification

In most instances the patient calls the physician because of a suspected tick bite. The first step is to confirm that it is indeed a tick, assuming it has been saved for examination. An important component of education to prevent Lyme borreliosis is to remind people not to discard the suspected tick, but to save it in any dry container (Zip-lock bag, medicine container, etc.), alcohol immersion being unnecessary. Even in an endemic area, almost a third of suspected deer ticks were either other ticks or not a tick at all (Sood et al., 1997). The non-ticks included beetles, lice and their nits, and artifacts including scabs and eraser bits. For this reason the practitioner should attempt to identify the tick. With a little practice it should be possible to distinguish an insect (6-legged) from a nymphal or adult tick (8-legged), differentiate a dog tick and a Lone Star tick from a deer tick, and to identify a nymphal tick because of its small size (Figure 12.2) Speciation of a nymph is difficult in the office setting, but at least in the American northeast, nymphs other than *I. scapularis* rarely attach to humans, with the exception of *I. cookei* in Maine (Hayes and Piesman, 2003; Rand et al., 2007). The availability of tick images on the Internet had made this simple office task much easier (Sood, 2002). The only tools needed are a magnifying glass and pair of tweezers to handle the tick. Alternatively, commercial laboratories perform tick identification, and in endemic counties in the United States it is usually done free of charge at health departments.

At least in eastern North America, as no other species of tick has been shown to transmit *B. burgdorferi*, exclusion of an *Ixodes* tick bite provides immediate reassurance to the patient.

Tick Analysis for Spirochete

The most common request from the patient is to have the tick sent for "testing for Lyme disease." PCR for *B. burgdorferi* DNA is offered in many commercial laboratories, but there is no demonstrable utility of such a test for several reasons. Blood in the tick can inhibit the PCR reaction leading to a false-negative result, and PCR invariably entails the

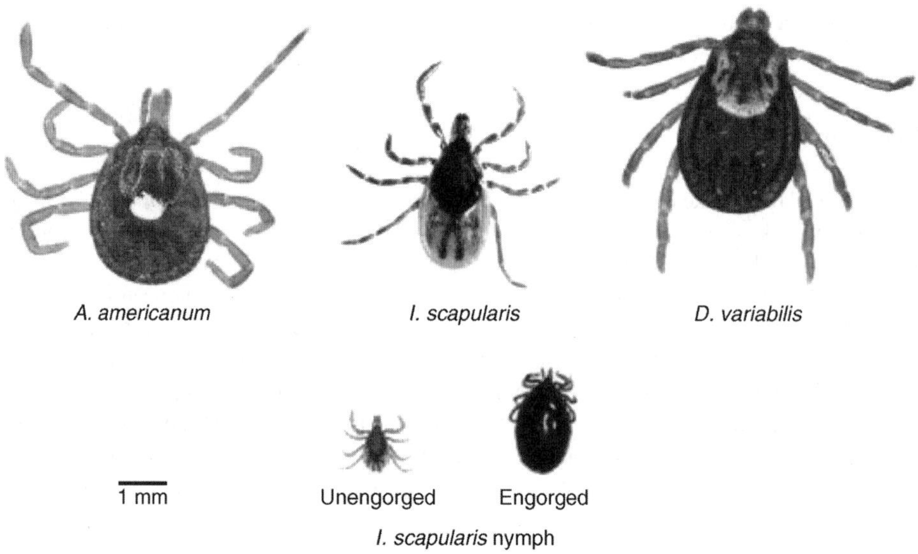

Figure 12.2 Adult female *Amblyomma americanum* (Lone Star Tick), adult Female, and nymphal *Ixodes scapularis* (Deer Ticks), and adult female *Dermacentor variabilis* (Dog Tick). Source: Hayes E and Piesman, J: *N Engl J Med* 348:2424–2430; 2003. Reproduced with permission. (*See insert for color representation*).

risk of false positives. Moreover a variable percentage of *Ixodes* ticks will harbor *B. burgdorferi*, more commonly in an endemic area, but the presence alone does not correlate with transmission.

Assessment of the Risk of Lyme Borreliosis from an *Ixodes* Tick Bite

The incidence of *B. burgdorferi* infection following an *Ixodes* tick bite is low, even in endemic areas, and was 1.2% to 4.4% in US studies (Costello et al., 1989; Salzman et al., 1992; Shapiro et al., 1992; Agre and Schwartz, 1993). In southern Germany, 47 (17%) of 272 *I. ricinus* ticks removed from camp attendees were found to be infected with *B. burgdorferi*, but only 1 of the 47 persons (2.1%) developed symptomatic Lyme disease (Paul et al., 1987). In a larger, two-center prospective study in Germany, an unusually high incidence (16 (26.7%) of 62 persons with PCR-positive ticks) were assessed as having acquired *B. burgdorferi* sensu lato infection (Maiwald et al., 1998). Nine had clinical evidence of Lyme borreliosis, erythema migrans, lymphocytoma, or neuroborreliosis. However, the serologic criteria used for the seven diagnosed by seroconversion were a rise in titer by immunofluorescence assay, new appearance of IgM antibodies, or a twofold rise in IgG antibodies, so some could have represented false positives. Anxiety about consequences of developing Lyme borreliosis, both on the part of the patient or parent and on the part of the physician, leads to an antibiotic commonly being prescribed without further investigation into the circumstances (Murray and Feder, 2001). A decision to treat prophylactically needs to be balanced against the incidence of adverse effects from an antibiotic, which was 30% in an efficacy study (Nadelman et al., 2001). The decision can be made easier if all the variables that influence the risk of infection are taken into consideration. These factors are the geographic location in which the patient acquired the tick, the developmental stage of the tick (which is related to the time of year), and duration of attachment of the tick.

Geographic Location

The risk of *B. burgdorferi* infection following an *Ixodes* tick bite varies with geographic location, even within an endemic area, and even from one year to another, because of the variable rate of *B. burgdorferi* prevalence in ticks. Tick infection rates were 47% to 100% on Shelter Island and Long Island, New York, and 10% to 35% in Connecticut (Anderson, 1988; Burgdorfer, 1989). In contrast, only 1.5% of *I. pacificus* ticks in California were infected. *Borrelia burgdorferi* sensu lato detection rates in Europe have varied widely and by genospecies (see Chapter 2). For example, in Germany, overall 11.1% of *Ixodes ricinus* ticks were infected with *B. burgdorferi*, with *B. garinii* the genospecies in more than 50% of positive ticks (Hildebrandt et al., 2003). Up to 40% of nymphs and 47% of adult ticks on the Swiss Plateau and in an alpine valley were infected (Jouda et al., 2004). Because of the wide range of tick infection rates, geographic location by itself should not be used as a criterion for prophylaxis unless specific local infection rates are available.

Stage of Tick and Time of Year

The risk of acquisition of *B. burgdorferi* infection also varies according to the developmental stage of the tick. Because the nymph feeds in the spring and early summer when people are outdoors, and because it is much smaller than an adult tick and can go unnoticed, most cases of human infection result from the nymphal stage (Nadelman et al., 2001). This reinforces the importance of tick identification.

Duration of Attachment

Duration of attachment is a key factor influencing infection risk. The history is unreliable in determination of an accurate duration of attachment because patients are usually only able to report a broad window of time in which they could have been bitten, for example, a long weekend spent outdoors.

The spirochetes reside and replicate in the midgut of the tick, and there is a delay between the onset of feeding and the appearance of spirochetes in the saliva. In animal studies, the duration of tick attachment correlated closely with the rate of transmission of the spirochete. Laboratory infected *Ixodes* ticks were allowed to feed on the natural host *Peromyscus leucopus* (white-footed mouse) for various lengths of time (Piesman, 1993). With a mean of 15 ticks feeding on each mouse, the transmission rate increased from 7% at 36 hours to 25% at 42 hours and then steeply to 75% at 48 hours. A calculated rate of transmission that assumes that only one tick successfully transmits the infection to a mouse, called the minimal transmission rate (MTR), is probably more relevant with regard to tick-to-human transmission. The MTR was 0.5% at 36 hours, 1.5% at 42 hours, and 5.8% at 48 hours. Additionally ticks that fed on infected rodents for various lengths of time were homogenized and injected into mice. Unfed, 24-hour and 48-hour tick homogenates produced infection rates in mice of 0%, 20%, and 80%, respectively, suggesting that spirochete multiplication occurred during feeding. In experiments where tick removal was performed at serial time points, removal beyond 60 hours was associated with a significant decrease in protection. Thus the occurrence of one or more critical events between about 48 and 60 hours of attachment results in a marked increase in the risk of transmission. Transmission of *B. burgdorferi* sensu stricto by *I. pacificus* nymphs to deer mice began to increase significantly after 72 hours of attachment (Peavey and Lane, 1995). This dynamic may not apply to transmission by *Ixodes spp.* ticks of *B. burgdorferi* genospecies that cause disease in Europe (Crippa et al., 2002; Fingerle et al., 2002). Transmission of *B. afzelii* and *B. burgdorferi* sensu stricto by *Ixodes ricinus* ticks was examined in a mouse infectivity study. The rate of transmission increased with duration of tick attachment, but transmission commenced earlier (at ≤ 48 hours) with *B. afzelii*–infected ticks compared to *B. burgdorferi* sensu stricto infected ticks (Crippa et al., 2002).

In order to establish whether the time-of-feeding dependent rate of transmission applies to deer tick bites in humans, investigators in endemic areas have examined the relationship of duration of attachment to occurrence of Lyme borreliosis. Often a tick that has been attached for several days is visibly engorged. A prospective study of tick bites was conducted in the New York tri-state metropolitan area, which includes several hyperendemic foci of Lyme borreliosis (Sood et al., 1997). Ticks were identified and the duration of attachment (DOA) for *I. scapularis* was determined from the scutal index of engorgement, an objective measure of engorgement that correlates with duration of attachment. *Borrelia burgdorferi* DNA was detectable in 14% of *I. scapularis* ticks. Occurrence of erythema migrans and assay of paired sera by two-step serology revealed that 3.4% of bites resulted in *B. burgdorferi* infection. The incidence of human infection was 20% from ticks attached ≥ 72 hours, which was significantly higher than the 1.1% from ticks attached for < 72 hours (odds ratio, 23.3). This study demonstrated that tick identification and measurement of engorgement could be used to identify a small, high-risk subset of persons, who may benefit from antibiotic prophylaxis. This subset consisted of roughly 1 of every 8 persons for whom the tick's DOA could be determined. The 1 in 5 risk of developing infection in this subset would be viewed as high risk by most practitioners.

Duration of attachment has been accurately determined from the scutal index of engorgement in clinical studies (Sood et al., 1997; Nadelman et al., 2001). It is calculated by dividing the body length, measured from the base of the capitulum to the tip of the abdomen, which increases with time of feeding, by the maximal width of the scutum, an inflexible structure on the dorsal aspect (Figure 12.3). This index has a positive correlation with DOA in an exponential regression model (Falco et al., 1996). The utility of measuring the scutal index was also suggested in a study of *I. ricinus* ticks in an animal model (Meiners et al., 2006). A limitation is the lack of general availability of the technique, which requires use of a stereomicroscope. As a rough substitute, practitioners should be able to recognize fully engorged ticks with some practice (Matuschka and Spielman, 1993; Nadelman and Wormser, 2001) (Figure 12.4). Images of unengorged and engorged *Ixodes* ticks are readily accessible online (Matuschka and Spielman, 1993; Sood, 2002).

Antibiotic Prophylaxis after an *Ixodes* Tick Bite

In a placebo-controlled antibiotic prophylaxis study conducted in the hyperendemic county of Westchester, New York, persons were enrolled if an *I. scapularis* tick was

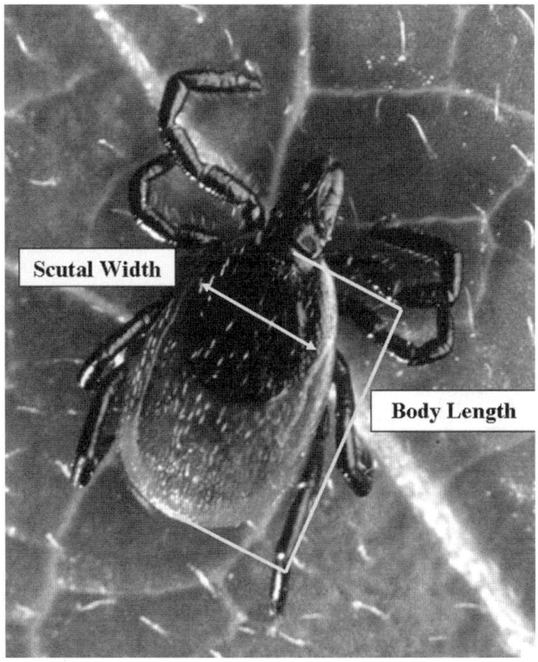

Figure 12.3 Measurements for scutal index with ocular micrometer. For calculation method refer to Falco RC et al., *Am J Epidemiol* 143:187–192; 1996. Source: USDA. Image adapted from http://commons.wikimedia.org/wiki/Image:Adult_deer_tick.jpg/Adult_deer_tick.jpg. (*See insert for color representation*).

brought in within 72 hours of the tick bite (Nadelman et al., 2001). In this study as well, a DOA of 72 hours, as measured objectively by the scutal index method, was found to be the cutoff for significant increase in risk of acquiring *B. burgdorferi* infection (erythema migrans). All infections occurred from the bites of nymphal stage ticks. A single 200-mg dose of doxycycline was 87% efficacious in prevention of Lyme borreliosis, but adverse effects occurred in 30% of doxycycline recipients. In a study in which 3 or 5 days of doxycycline were administered to 261 persons after *I. persulcatus* tick bites in Russia, none developed erythema migrans, and evidence of any symptom considered Lyme borreliosis was 11-fold lower in antibiotic recipients versus 97 untreated controls (Korenberg et al., 1996).

We can see from the epidemiology of tick bites that very few people will qualify for consideration of prophylaxis. Identification of persons at much higher risk of acquiring infection is possible with the help of stage identification (nymph) and assessment of duration of attachment (>72 hours in North American studies, >48 hours based on animal studies and probably >36 hours in the European situation). Therefore antibiotic prophylaxis should be reserved for a bite that is definitively identified as *Ixodes scapularis* attached long enough to transmit infection, ideally as determined by the scutal index method unless the patient is reasonably certain about the DOA (Table 12.2). The efficacy of amoxicillin is unknown, but

(a)

(b)

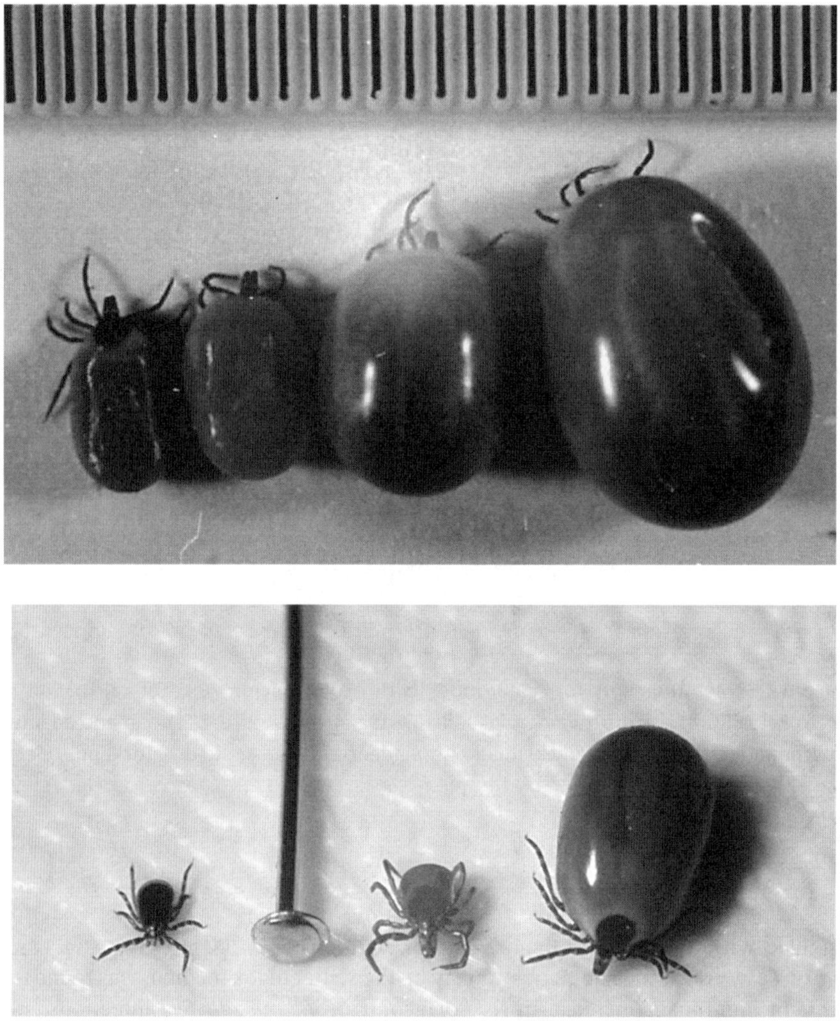

Figure 12.4 (a) Engorgement of *Ixodes* tick. Source: Jeremy Gray, University of Dublin. (b) Flat (unfed) and engorged *Ixodes scapularis* tick. Source: Pfizer. (*See insert for color representation*).

some experts advise a course of amoxicillin (10 days was used in an early study of antibiotic prophylaxis)(Shapiro et al., 1992) in children under 8 years of age (AAP, 2009). In most cases a "wait and watch" approach is completely acceptable given the low risk of Lyme borreliosis following a tick bite, and this is the approach favored in Europe (Stanek and Kahl, 1999).

Asymptomatic seroconversion after a tick bite is a rare event, and the value of acute-and-convalescent paired serum testing for antibodies to *B. burgdorferi* in this setting has not been demonstrated. Therefore the use of serologic testing to aid in management decisions after a tick bite, still commonly considered by physicians in the United States, is not recommended.

TABLE 12.2 Management of an *Ixodes* tick bite

- Removal with simple forceps is the best technique.
- Saving the tick for examination is valuable.
- An adult tick is far less likely to transmit *B. burgdorferi* than a nymph.
- Ticks removed by the next day after attachment are extremely unlikely to transmit *B. burgdorferi*.
- Residual embedded mouth parts do not increase the risk of transmission, but a tick-bite granuloma can develop over time and may require excision.
- Observation of the site of the bite without prophylactic treatment, and monitoring for symptoms of early Lyme borreliosis is the preferred course of action in most situations.
- In North America, antibiotic prophylaxis should be offered:
  - only for an engorged, identified nymphal or female *Ixodes scapularis* (northern deer tick) with attachment more than 48 hours by scutal index method or by accurate history
  - only with single-dose of doxycycline 4 mg/kg to maximum of 200 mg (unless child under 8 years,[a] pregnant woman or other contraindication)

[a]Consider amoxicillin 50 mg/kg divided in 3 doses for 10 days, being mindful of attendant risk of adverse effects.

PREVENTING LYME DISEASE BY IMMUNIZATION

Considering the erratic effectiveness of measures to reduce tick-bite risks, the availability of a vaccine was a valuable addition to our efforts to prevent Lyme disease. The vaccine was developed on a sound biologic basis. Antibodies to several antigens of *B. burgdorferi* are elicited in natural infection, but they do not confer reliable immunity. The antigen in the vaccine was a surface protein of the spirochete, the 31-kilodalton outer surface protein A (OspA), which was shown to prevent infection in mice (Fikrig et al., 1990; Schaible et al., 1990). It was discovered that the antibody to OspA did not kill spirochetes in the vertebrate animal as would be expected for most vaccine-induced antibodies. Anti-OspA in blood ingested by the tick instead inactivated the spirochetes in its gut. This is a novel method to prevent an infectious disease, and is presumed to be the mechanism for vaccine-induced protection against Lyme disease in humans (Thanassi and Schoen, 1999). The vaccine that was marketed between 1999 and 2002 for persons 15 to 70 years old (LYMErix™, GSK) consisted of recombinant OspA lipoprotein (Steere et al., 1998). The vaccine was safe and moderately efficacious (76% after 3 doses), as was a similar OspA vaccine that ultimately was not marketed (Sigal et al., 1998). Safety and immunogenicity was also demonstrated in 2- to 18-year-old children in the United States and Europe (Feder et al., 1999; Beran et al., 2000; Sikand et al., 2001).

Some concern was raised about the long-term safety of OspA vaccines, based on the description of molecular mimicry between an epitope of OspA and that of human-leukocyte function associated antigen 1 (hLFA-1) of human T cells (Gross et al., 1998; Steere et al., 2011). However, neither persons with previous Lyme disease nor normal subjects developed arthritis after vaccination at a higher rate than placebo recipients during 6 years of follow-up. New onset arthritis was reported by $<1\%$ of subjects within 30 days after vaccination and $<3\%$ of subjects after 30 days. These rates probably reflect a background incidence of such symptoms in an adult population. There was no unexpected or unusual pattern of adverse events from reports to the Vaccine Adverse Events Reporting System following administration of the vaccine (Lathrop et al., 2002). There were instead campaigns of misinformation fueled by ready access to Internet sources for answers to medical questions, rather than from authoritative sources (Sood, 2002; Cooper and Feder, 2004; Poland, 2011). Even with the incidence of Lyme disease on the rise, sales for LYMErix declined from about 1.5 million doses in 1999 to a projected 10,000 doses in 2002. Adverse publicity played a major role in the precipitous decline in sales (McSweegan, 2006). It is worth remembering that LYMErix™ was discontinued by the manufacturer for economic reasons, and was not recalled for any safety problems.

This cautionary tale should be heeded lest it threaten the use of other effective vaccines (Abbott, 2006; Anon., 2006; McSweegan, 2007). Whether costs of ongoing and threatened litigation factored into the manufacturer's decision is unknown, but such an economic reality has taken its toll in vaccinology before (Evans, 2006).

Future Lyme Borreliosis Vaccines

Development of a new Lyme disease vaccine is considered a public health priority (Shen et al., 2011; Plotkin et al., 2011). Cost-effectiveness analysis of immunizing against Lyme disease showed that with certain assumptions of high risk, vaccinations will result in net savings (Meltzer et al., 1999). This is because patients commonly undergo an expensive workup, and some are prescribed intravenous treatment. The authors propose that the benefits are likely to be greatest if both local incidence of Lyme disease and the individual's risk for exposure are considered in using the vaccine. In their model a key threshold was an annual incidence of Lyme disease of 0.01 (1%). If it can be assumed that physician-diagnosed cases are up to 90% underreported, several communities in the northeast of the United States and in several European countries have an estimated annual incidence that exceeds a 1% threshold (Coyle et al., 1996; Meek et al., 1996). Given this analysis, development of new vaccines may be economically feasible.

Most of the new candidates are multicomponent or chimeric vaccines that include immunogenic proteins other than, or in addition to OspA: decorin binding protein A (DbpA) fibronectin-binding protein (BBK32), or other outer surface proteins such as OspB or OspC (Hanson et al., 2000; Brown et al., 2005; Schuijt et al., 2011; Livey et al., 2011). DbpA is expressed by *B. burgdorferi* during spirochetemia, and antibodies were protective in mice after needle-challenge but not after tick challenge (Hagman et al., 2000). MedImmune and Sanofi-Aventis intend to develop a combination DbpA–OspA vaccine (NIAID, 2007). A structure-based approach that uses X-ray crystallography to identify protective epitopes can be used to reduce the size of antigens used in a multivalent vaccine (Luft et al., 2002; Livey et al., 2011). Such an approach could facilitate development of a vaccine for worldwide use against Lyme borreliosis caused by species other than *B. burgdorferi* sensu stricto as well. A recombinant OspA chimeric vaccine being developed by Baxter are immunogenic against multiple OspA serotypes, and the vaccine has provided protection against *B. burgdorferi* sensu stricto, *B. afzelii*, and *B. garinii* in a mouse model (Ding et al., 2000; Livey et al., 2011). Another approach exploits the stability of OspC typing-based phylogenetic clusters (Earnhart and Marconi, 2007). OspC has a critical role in infectivity, and antibody to this surface protein is bactericidal (Earnhart et al., 2007). The effort is directed at construction of a chimeric antigen that could protect across many pathogenic genospecies of *B. burgdorferi* sensu lato.

Tick Vaccines

The study of inflammatory and immunomodulatory events at the "tick–host–pathogen interface" have suggested the possibility of tick vaccines to induce broad-spectrum protection against tick-borne infections (Wikel et al., 1997; Schuijt et al., 2011). Among other responses in experimental animals, acquired resistance from tick bites reduces tick viability and ova production, promotes tick detachment, and can partially protect against transmission of pathogens (Wikel, 1996). One current candidate is *Rhipicephalus* tick cement protein 64TRP, which protected mice against *Ixodes ricinus*--transmitted tick-borne encephalitis virus (Labuda et al., 2006).

An understanding of the functions of tick genes by using RNA interference (RNAi) technology may enable genetic manipulation so as to modulate the tick–pathogen interface for the benefit of the accidental human host (de la Fuente et al., 2008).

REFERENCES

AAP: Lyme disease. *In* Pickering LK, Baker CJ, Kimberlin DW, Long SSE (eds): *Red Book: 2009 Report of the Committee on Infectious Diseases*, 28th ed. Elk Grove Village, IL, American Academy of Pediatrics; 2009.

Abbott A: Lyme disease. Uphill struggle. *Nature* 439:524–525; 2006.

Agre F, Schwartz R: The value of early treatment of deer tick bites for the prevention of Lyme disease. *Am J Dis Child* 147:945–947; 1993.

Anderson JF: Mammalian and avian reservoirs for *Borrelia burgdorferi. Ann NY Acad Sci* 539:180–191; 1988.

Anon: Lyme disease vaccine. *Med Lett Drugs Ther* 41:29–30; 1999.

Anon: When a vaccine is safe. *Nature* 439:509; 2006.

Beran J, De Clercq N, Dieussaert I, van Hoecke C: Reactogenicity and immunogenicity of a Lyme disease vaccine in children 2–5 years old. *Clin Infect Dis* 31:1504–1507; 2000.

Brown EL, Kim JH, Reisenbichler ES, Hook M: Multicomponent Lyme vaccine. Three is not a crowd. *Vaccine* 23:3687–3696; 2005.

Burgdorfer W: Vector/host relationships of the Lyme disease spirochete, *Borrelia burgdorferi. Rheum Dis Clin North Am* 15:775–787; 1989.

Carroll JF, Klun JA, Debboun M: Repellency of deet and SS220 applied to skin involves olfactory sensing by two species of ticks. *Med Vet Entomol* 19:101–106; 2005.

CDC: Lyme disease. United States, 1980. *MMWR Morb Mortal Wkly Rep* 30:489–482, 497; 1981.

Chou JT, Rossignol PA, Ayres JW: Evaluation of commercial insect repellents on human skin against *Aedes aegypti* (Diptera: Culicidae). *J Med Entomol* 34:624–630; 1997.

Cooper JD, Feder HM Jr: Inaccurate information about Lyme disease on the internet. *Pediatr Infect Dis J* 23:1105–1108; 2004.

Costello CM, Steere AC, Pinkerton RE, Feder HM Jr: A prospective study of tick bites in an endemic area for Lyme disease. *Conn Med* 53:338–340; 1989.

Coyle BS, Strickland GT, Liang YY, Pena C, McCarter R, Israel E: The public health impact of Lyme disease in Maryland. *J Infect Dis* 173:1260–1262; 1996.

Crippa M, Rais O, Gern L: Investigations on the mode and dynamics of transmission and infectivity of *Borrelia burgdorferi* sensu stricto and *Borrelia afzelii* in *Ixodes ricinus* ticks. *Vector Borne Zoonotic Dis* 2:3–9; 2002.

Curran KL, Fish D: Increased risk of Lyme disease for cat owners. *N Engl J Med* 320:183; 1989.

Curran KL, Fish D, Piesman J: Reduction of nymphal *Ixodes dammini* (Acari: Ixodidae) in a residential suburban landscape by area application of insecticides. *J Med Entomol* 30:107–113; 1993.

Daltroy LH, Phillips C, Lew R, Wright E, Shadick NA, Liang MH: A controlled trial of a novel primary prevention program for Lyme disease and other tick-borne illnesses. *Health Educ Behav* 34:531–542; 2007.

De la Fuente J, Kocan KM, Almazan C, Blouin EF: Targeting the tick-pathogen interface for novel control strategies. *Front Biosci* 13:6947–6956; 2008.

Ding W, Huang X, Yang X, Dunn JJ, Luft BJ, Koide S, Lawson CL: Structural identification of a key protective B-cell epitope in Lyme disease antigen OspA. *J Mol Biol* 302:1153–1164; 2000.

Dolan MC, Maupin GO, Schneider BS, Denatale C, Hamon N, Cole C, Zeidner NS, Stafford KC III: Control of immature *Ixodes scapularis* (Acari: Ixodidae) on rodent reservoirs of *Borrelia burgdorferi* in a residential community of southeastern Connecticut. *J Med Entomol* 41:1043–1054; 2004.

Dolan MC, Zeidner NS, Gabitzsch E, Dietrich G, Borchert JN, Poche RM, Piesman J: A doxycycline hyclate rodent bait formulation for prophylaxis and treatment of tick-transmitted *Borrelia burgdorferi*. *Am J Trop Med Hyg* 78:803–805; 2008.

Dolan MC, Jordan RA, Schulze TL, Schulze CJ, Manning MC, Ruffolo D, Schmidt JP, Piesman J, Karchesy JJ: Ability of two natural products, nootkatone and carvacrol, to suppress *Ixodes scapularis* and *Amblyomma americanum* (Acari: Ixodidae) in a Lyme disease endemic area of New Jersey. *J Econ Entomol* 102:2316–2324; 2009.

Earnhart CG, Marconi RT: An octavalent Lyme disease vaccine induces antibodies that recognize all incorporated OspC type-specific sequences. *Hum Vaccin* 3:281–289; 2007.

Earnhart CG, Buckles EL, Marconi RT: Development of an OspC-based tetravalent, recombinant, chimeric vaccinogen that elicits bactericidal antibody against diverse Lyme disease spirochete strains. *Vaccine* 25:466–480; 2007.

Evans G: Update on vaccine liability in the United States. Presentation at the National Vaccine Program Office Workshop on strengthening the supply of routinely recommended vaccines in the United States, 12 February 2002. *Clin Infect Dis* 42(suppl 3): S130–S137; 2006.

Falco RC, Fish D, Piesman J: Duration of tick bites in a Lyme disease-endemic area. *Am J Epidemiol* 143:187–192; 1996.

Feder HM Jr, Beran J, van Hoecke C, Abraham B, De Clercq N, Buscarino C, Parenti DL: Immunogenicity of a recombinant *Borrelia burgdorferi* outer surface protein A vaccine against Lyme disease in children. *J Pediatr* 135:575–579; 1999.

Fikrig E, Barthold SW, Kantor FS, Flavell RA: Protection of mice against the Lyme disease agent by immunizing with recombinant OspA. *Science* 250:553–556; 1990.

Fingerle V, Rauser S, Hammer B, Kahl O, Heimerl C, Schulte-Spechtel U, Gern L, Wilske B: Dynamics of dissemination and outer surface protein expression of different European *Borrelia burgdorferi* sensu lato strains in artificially infected *Ixodes ricinus* nymphs. *J Clin Microbiol* 40:1456–1463; 2002.

Fradin MS, Day JF: Comparative efficacy of insect repellents against mosquito bites. *N Engl J Med* 347:13–18; 2002.

Gomes-Solecki MJ, Brisson DR, Dattwyler RJ: Oral vaccine that breaks the transmission cycle of the Lyme disease spirochete can be delivered via bait. *Vaccine* 24:4440–4449; 2006.

Goodyer L, Behrens RH: Short report. The safety and toxicity of insect repellents. *Am J Trop Med Hyg* 59:323–324; 1998.

Gray J, Kahl O, Lane RS, Stanek G: *Lyme Borreliosis. Biology, Epidemiology and Control.* New York, CAB International; 2002.

Gross DM, Forsthuber T, Tary-Lehmann M, Etling C, Ito K, Nagy ZA, Field JA, Steere AC, Huber BT: Identification of LFA-1 as a candidate autoantigen in treatment-resistant Lyme arthritis. *Science* 281:703–706; 1998.

Hagman KE, Yang X, Wikel SK, Schoeler GB, Caimano MJ, Radolf JD, Norgard MV: Decorin-binding protein A (DbpA) of *Borrelia burgdorferi* is not protective when immunized mice are challenged via tick infestation and correlates with the lack of DbpA expression by *B. burgdorferi* in ticks. *Infect Immun* 68:4759–4764; 2000.

Hanson MS, Patel NK, Cassatt DR, Ulbrandt ND: Evidence for vaccine synergy between *Borrelia burgdorferi* decorin binding protein A and outer surface protein A in the mouse model of lyme borreliosis. *Infect Immun* 68:6457–6460; 2000.

Hayes EB, Maupin GO, Mount GA, Piesman J: Assessing the prevention effectiveness of local Lyme disease control. *J Public Health Manag Pract* 5:84–92; 1999.

Hayes EB, Piesman J: How can we prevent Lyme disease? *N Engl J Med* 348:2424–2430; 2003.

Herrington JE Jr, Campbell GL, Bailey RE, Cartter ML, Adams M, Frazier EL, Damrow TA, Gensheimer KF: Predisposing factors for individuals' Lyme disease prevention practices: Connecticut, Maine, and Montana. *Am J Public Health* 87:2035–2038; 1997.

Hildebrandt A, Schmidt KH, Wilske B, Dorn W, Straube E, Fingerle V: Prevalence of four species of *Borrelia burgdorferi* sensu lato and coinfection with *Anaplasma phagocytophila* in *Ixodes ricinus* ticks in central Germany. *Eur J Clin Microbiol Infect Dis* 22:364–367; 2003.

Jaenson TG, Palsson K, Borg-Karlson AK: Evaluation of extracts and oils of tick-repellent plants from Sweden. *Med Vet Entomol* 19:345–352; 2005.

Jouda F, Perret JL, Gern L: Density of questing *Ixodes ricinus* nymphs and adults infected by *Borrelia burgdorferi* sensu lato in Switzerland. Spatio-temporal pattern at a regional scale. *Vector Borne Zoonotic Dis* 4:23–32; 2004.

Katz TM, Miller JH, Hebert AA: Insect repellents. Historical perspectives and new developments. *J Am Acad Dermatol* 58:865–871; 2008.

Koren G, Matsui D, Bailey B: DEET-based insect repellents Safety implications for children and pregnant and lactating women. *CMAJ* 169:209–212; 2003.

Korenberg EI, Vorobyeva NN, Moskvitina HG, Gorban L: Prevention of borreliosis in persons bitten by infected ticks. *Infection* 24:187–189; 1996.

Labuda M, Trimnell AR, Lickova M, Kazimirova M, Davies GM, Lissina O, Hails RS, Nuttall PA: An antivector vaccine protects against a lethal vector-borne pathogen. *PLoS Pathog* 2:e27; 2006.

Lathrop SL, Ball R, Haber P, Mootrey GT, Braun MM, Shadomy SV, Ellenberg SS, Chen RT, Hayes EB: Adverse event reports following vaccination for Lyme disease. December 1998–July 2000. *Vaccine* 20:1603–1608; 2002.

Livey I, O'Rourke M, Traweger A, Savidis-Dacho H, Crowe BA, Barrett PN, Yang X, Dunn JJ, Luft BJ: A new approach to a Lyme disease vaccine. *Clin Infect Dis* 52(Suppl 3):s266–270; 2011.

Luft BJ, Dunn JJ, Lawson CL: Approaches toward the directed design of a vaccine against *Borrelia burgdorferi*. *J Infect Dis* 185(suppl 1): S46–S51; 2002.

Madurawe RD, Chase TE, Tsao EI, Bentley WE: A recombinant lipoprotein antigen against Lyme disease expressed in *E. coli*. Fermentor operating strategies for improved yield. *Biotechnol Prog* 16:571–576; 2000.

Maiwald M, Oehme R, March O, Petney TN, Kimmig P, Naser K, Zappe HA, Hassler D, von Knebel Doeberitz M: Transmission risk of *Borrelia burgdorferi* sensu lato from *Ixodes ricinus* ticks to humans in southwest Germany. *Epidemiol Infect* 121:103–108; 1998.

Malouin R, Winch P, Leontsini E, Glass G, Simon D, Hayes EB, Schwartz BS: Longitudinal evaluation of an educational intervention for preventing tick bites in an area with endemic lyme disease in Baltimore County, Maryland. *Am J Epidemiol* 157:1039–1051; 2003.

Matuschka FR, Spielman A: Risk of infection from and treatment of tick bite. *Lancet* 342:529–530; 1993.

McSweegan E: Lyme vaccine demonized by advocacy groups. *Nature* 440:278; 2006.

McSweegan E: The Lyme vaccine. A cautionary tale. *Epidemiol Infect* 135:9–10; 2007.

Meek JI, Roberts CL, Smith EV Jr, Cartter ML: Underreporting of Lyme disease by Connecticut physicians, 1992. *J Public Health Manag Pract* 2:61–65; 1996.

Meiners T, Hammer B, Gobel UB, Kahl O: Determining the tick scutal index allows assessment of tick feeding duration and estimation of infection risk with *Borrelia burgdorferi* sensu lato in a person bitten by an *Ixodes ricinus* nymph. *Int J Med Microbiol* 296(suppl 40): 103–107; 2006.

Meltzer MI, Dennis DT, Orloski KA: The cost effectiveness of vaccinating against Lyme disease. *Emerg Infect Dis* 5:321–328; 1999.

Montemarano AD, Gupta RK, Burge JR, Klein K: Insect repellents and the efficacy of sunscreens. *Lancet* 349:1670–1671; 1997.

Murray T, Feder HM Jr: Management of tick bites and early Lyme disease. A survey of Connecticut physicians. *Pediatrics* 108:1367–1370; 2001.

Nadelman R, Wormser GP: Single-dose doxycycline for the prevention of Lyme disease. *N Engl J Med* 345:1348–1350; 2001.

Nadelman RB, Nowakowski J, Fish D, Falco RC, Freeman K, McKenna D, Welch P, Marcus R, Aguero-Rosenfeld ME, Dennis DT, Wormser GP: Prophylaxis with single-dose doxycycline for the prevention of Lyme disease after an *Ixodes scapularis* tick bite. *N Engl J Med* 345:79–84; 2001.

Needham GR: Evaluation of five popular methods for tick removal. *Pediatrics* 75:997–1002; 1985.

NIAID: *Lyme Disease: Vaccine Production* [Online]; 2007. Available: http://www3.niaid.nih.gov/topics/lymeDisease/research/vaccine.htm [Accessed January 27, 2011].

Paul H, Gerth HJ, Ackermann R: Infectiousness for humans of *Ixodes ricinus* containing *Borrelia burgdorferi*. *Zentralbl Bakteriol Mikrobiol Hyg [A]* 263:473–476; 1987.

Peavey CA, Lane RS: Transmission of *Borrelia burgdorferi* by *Ixodes pacificus* nymphs and reservoir competence of deer mice (*Peromyscus maniculatus*) infected by tick-bite. *J Parasitol* 81:175–178; 1995.

Phillips CB, Liang MH, Sangha O, Wright EA, Fossel AH, Lew RA, Fossel KK, Shadick NA: Lyme disease and preventive behaviors in residents of Nantucket Island, Massachusetts. *Am J Prev Med* 20:219–224; 2001.

Piesman J: Dynamics of *Borrelia burgdorferi* transmission by nymphal *Ixodes dammini* ticks. *J Infect Dis* 167:1082–1085; 1993.

Piesman J: Strategies for reducing the risk of Lyme borreliosis in North America. *Int J Med Microbiol* 296(suppl 40): 17–22; 2006.

Piesman J, Dolan MC: Protection against lyme disease spirochete transmission provided by prompt removal of nymphal *Ixodes scapularis* (Acari: Ixodidae). *J Med Entomol* 39:509–512; 2002.

Piesman J, Eisen L: Prevention of tick-borne diseases. *Annu Rev Entomol* 53:323–543; 2008.

Plotkin SA: Correcting a public health fiasco: The need for a new vaccine against Lyme disease. *Clin Infect Dis* 52(Suppl 3):s271–275; 2011.

Poland GA: Vaccines against Lyme disease: What happened and what lessons can we learn? *Clin Infect Dis* 52(Suppl 3):s253–258; 2011.

Pretorius AM, Jensenius M, Clarke F, Ringertz SH: Repellent efficacy of DEET and KBR 3023 against *Amblyomma hebraeum* (Acari: Ixodidae). *J Med Entomol* 40:245–248; 2003.

Rand PW, Lubelczyk C, Holman MS, Lacombe EH, Smith RP Jr: Abundance of *Ixodes scapularis* (Acari: Ixodidae) after the complete removal of deer from an isolated offshore island, endemic for Lyme disease. *J Med Entomol* 41:779–784; 2004.

Rand PW, Lacombe EH, Dearborn R, Cahill B, Elias S, Lubelczyk CB, Beckett GA, Smith RP Jr: Passive surveillance in Maine, an area emergent for tick-borne diseases. *J Med Entomol* 44:1118–1129; 2007.

Roscoe DE, Holste WC, Sorhage FE, Campbell C, Niezgoda M, Buchannan R, Diehl D, Niu HS, Rupprecht CE: Efficacy of an oral vaccinia-rabies glycoprotein recombinant vaccine in controlling epidemic raccoon rabies in New Jersey. *J Wildl Dis* 34:752–763; 1998.

Ross EA, Savage KA, Utley LJ, Tebbett IR: Insect repellent [correction of repellant] interactions: sunscreens enhance DEET (*N*,*N*-diethyl-*m*-toluamide) absorption. *Drug Metab Dispos* 32:783–785; 2004.

Salzman MB, Rubin LG, Sood SK: Incidence of seroconversion to *Borrelia burgdorferi* by immunoblot after a tcik bite in an endemic area for Lyme disease (abstract). *Am J Dis Child* 146:515; 1992.

Samish M, Ginsberg H, Glazer I: Biological control of ticks. *Parasitology* 129(suppl): S389–S403; 2004.

Schaible UE, Kramer MD, Eichmann K, Modolell M, Museteanu C, Simon MM: Monoclonal antibodies specific for the outer surface protein A (OspA) of *Borrelia burgdorferi* prevent Lyme borreliosis in severe combined immunodeficiency (scid) mice. *Proc Natl Acad Sci USA* 87:3768–3772; 1990.

Scheckelhoff MR, Telford SR, Hu LT: Protective efficacy of an oral vaccine to reduce carriage of *Borrelia burgdorferi* (strain N40) in mouse and tick reservoirs. *Vaccine* 24:1949–1957; 2006.

Schuijt TJ, Hovius JW, van der Poll T, van Dam AP, Fikrig E: Lyme borreliosis vaccination: The facts, the challenge, the future. *Trends Parasitol* 27:40–47; 2011.

Schwantes U, Dautel H, Jung G: Prevention of infectious tick-borne diseases in humans. Comparative studies of the repellency of different dodecanoic acid-formulations against *Ixodes ricinus* ticks (Acari: Ixodidae). *Parasit Vectors* 1:8; 2008.

Selim S, Hartnagel RE Jr, Osimitz TG, Gabriel KL, Schoenig GP: Absorption, metabolism, and excretion of *N*, *N*-diethyl-*m*-toluamide following dermal application to human volunteers. *Fundam Appl Toxicol* 25:95–100; 1995.

Shadick NA, Daltroy LH, Phillips CB, Liang US, Liang MH: Determinants of tick-avoidance behaviors in an endemic area for Lyme disease. *Am J Prev Med* 13:265–270; 1997.

Shapiro ED, Gerber MA, Holabird NB, Berg AT, Feder HM Jr, Bell GL, Rys PN, Persing DH: A controlled trial of antimicrobial prophylaxis for Lyme disease after deer-tick bites. *N Engl J Med* 327:1769–1773; 1992.

Shen AK, Mead PS, Beard CB: The Lyme disease vaccine–a public health perspective. *Clin Infect Dis* 52(Suppl 3):s247–252; 2011.

Sigal LH, Zahradnik JM, Lavin P, Patella SJ, Bryant G, Haselby R, Hilton E, Kunkel M, Adler-Klein D, Doherty T, Evans J, Molloy PJ, Seidner AL, Sabetta JR, Simon HJ, Klempner MS, Mays J, Marks D, Malawista SE: A vaccine consisting of recombinant *Borrelia burgdorferi* outer-surface protein A to prevent Lyme disease. Recombinant Outer-Surface Protein A Lyme Disease Vaccine Study Consortium. *N Engl J Med* 339:216–222; 1998.

Sikand VK, Halsey N, Krause PJ, Sood SK, Geller R, van Hoecke C, Buscarino C, Parenti D: Safety and immunogenicity of a recombinant *Borrelia burgdorferi* outer surface protein A vaccine against Lyme disease in healthy children and adolescents. A randomized controlled trial. *Pediatrics* 108:123–128; 2001.

Solberg VB, Miller JA, Hadfield T, Burge R, Schech JM, Pound JM: Control of *Ixodes scapularis* (Acari: Ixodidae) with topical self-application of permethrin by white-tailed deer inhabiting NASA, Beltsville, Maryland. *J Vector Ecol* 28:117–134; 2003.

Sood SK: Effective retrieval of Lyme disease information on the Web. *Clin Infect Dis* 35:451–464; 2002.

Sood SK, Salzman MB, Johnson BJ, Happ CM, Feig K, Carmody L, Rubin LG, Hilton E, Piesman J: Duration of tick attachment as a predictor of the risk of Lyme disease in an area in which Lyme disease is endemic. *J Infect Dis* 175:996–999; 1997.

Stafford KC III: Effectiveness of carbaryl applications for the control of *Ixodes* dammini (Acari: Ixodidae) nymphs in an endemic residential area. *J Med Entomol* 28:32–36; 1991.

Stafford KC III: *Tick Management Handbook*. New Haven, The Connecticut Agricultural Experiment Station; 2007.

Stanek G, Kahl O: Chemoprophylaxis for Lyme borreliosis? *Zentralbl Bakteriol* 289:655–665; 1999.

Steere AC, Sikand VK, Meurice F, Parenti DL, Fikrig E, Schoen RT, Nowakowski J, Schmid CH, Laukamp S, Buscarino C, Krause DS: Vaccination against Lyme disease with recombinant *Borrelia burgdorferi* outer-surface lipoprotein A with adjuvant. Lyme Disease Vaccine Study Group. *N Engl J Med* 339:209–215; 1998.

Steere AC, Drouin EE, Glickstein LJ: Relationship between immunity to *Borrelia burgdorferi* outer-surface protein A (OspA) and Lyme arthritis. *Clin Infect Dis* 52 (Suppl 3):s259–265; 2011.

Tenenbein M: Severe toxic reactions and death following the ingestion of diethyltoluamide-containing insect repellents. *JAMA* 258:1509–1511; 1987.

Thanassi WT, Schoen RT: Successful vaccination for Lyme disease. A novel mechanism. *Expert Opin Investig Drugs* 8:29–35; 1999.

Tsao JI, Wootton JT, Bunikis J, Luna MG, Fish D, Barbour AG: An ecological approach to preventing human infection. Vaccinating wild mouse reservoirs intervenes in the Lyme disease cycle. *Proc Natl Acad Sci USA* 101:18159–18164; 2004.

Vazquez M, Muehlenbein C, Cartter M, Hayes EB, Ertels S, Shapiro ED: Effectiveness of personal protective measures to prevent Lyme disease. *Emerg Infect Dis* 14:210–216; 2008.

Veltri JC, Osimitz TG, Bradford DC, Page BC: Retrospective analysis of calls to poison control centers resulting from exposure to the insect repellent *N,N*-diethyl-*m*-toluamide (DEET) from 1985–1989. *J Toxicol Clin Toxicol* 32:1–16; 1994.

Wikel SK: Host immunity to ticks. *Annu Rev Entomol* 41:1–22; 1996.

Wikel SK, Ramachandra RN, Bergman DK, Burkot TR, Piesman J: Infestation with pathogen-free nymphs of the tick *Ixodes scapularis* induces host resistance to transmission of *Borrelia burgdorferi* by ticks. *Infect Immun* 65:335–338; 1997.

INDEX

Lyme Borreliosis in Europe and North America: Epidemiology and Clinical Practice, First Edition.
Edited by Sunil K. Sood